Praise for *Your Baby's Brain*

"Give your child the greatest opportunity to reach her fullest potential, both emotionally and intellectually. In [*Your Baby's Brain*], Dr. Gross gives new meaning to every cuddle, every hug, every touch, with explanations of how they effect a baby's brain development. This is must reading for parents and grandparents and settles the old argument of nature vs. nurture with enough neuroscience to explain the gene factor and helpful advice for the nurturing."

—Pat Mitchell, media executive, producer, curator of TEDWomen

"'Every touch, sight, smell, and interaction . . . impacts the wiring of your child's brain.' In the face of such a formidable statement, how very lucky we are to have Gail's beautiful, wise, important book to guide us toward being the best that we can be for our children. Ultimately, [*Your Baby's Brain*] is not only about helping kids grow, it is about building a better world. As always, Gail builds her case and teaches us with rigor, intelligence, and above all, her trademark compassion."

—Mariska Hargitay, Golden Globe and Emmy Award–winning actress

"In [*Your Baby's Brain*], Dr. Gail Gross tells us about the neuroscience of early childhood development, teaching parents not only the stages of brain growth, but also how they can give their children the greatest opportunity to reach their full potential, both emotionally and intellectually. A must-read for all parents."

—Arianna Huffington, founder & CEO
of Thrive Global and founder of *The Huffington Post*

"Though your genes are a blueprint, they're only a two-dimensional look at what will be a three-dimensional child. And now we know that the old argument between the influence of nature versus nurture has been settled, pointing to a 50/50 split of equal impact. Though nature supplies your genes, it is the experiences your child has that determine which genes are expressed and which are suppressed. In a sense, your child's brain develops in reaction to the stimulation it receives, and every cuddle, every hug, every touch, will affect her brain development. As Dr. David Rice stated, 'biology is not destiny.' [*Your Baby's Brain*] is about the neuroscience of early childhood development, teaching parents not only the stages of brain growth, but also how to positively affect them. This will give your child the greatest opportunity to reach her fullest potential, both emotionally and intellectually."

—Goldie Hawn, Academy Awar

"Dr. Gross teaches you how your baby's growing brain is a work in progress, and how you can be part in helping your child attain their fullest potential. The science is there. Make this your manual for giving your child or grandchild the greatest gift you can offer them, the gift of higher intelligence."

—Alberto Villoldo, PhD, bestselling author of *One Spirit Medicine*

"Even the most loving and well-meaning parents can inadvertently make mistakes because they don't understand how a child's brain grows and develops in those formative first years. In this pioneering book, child development and parenting expert Dr. Gail M. Gross explains steps you can take to boost your child's ability to learn and succeed in school and life. This practical approach to nurturing young minds is a must-read for every new parent."

—Lynda Resnick, entrepreneur, businesswoman, and owner of The Wonderful Company

"A 'loving, nurturing, present parent' is the most important element in the development of a child's brain, says Dr. Gail Gross. A must-read for all new parents."

—Marlene Malek, vice chairman of Friends of Cancer Research

"We all want our children to reach their maximum potential. But we are not all aware that we already possess the power to do so. With her signature brilliance and heart, Dr. Gail Gross proves in relatable terms how YOU can shape your child's brain—and future."

—Lyn Davis Lear, MFT, PhD, psychologist, film producer, Sundance Board of Trustee, social and political activist and philanthropist

"Dr. Gail Gross has written another outstanding book, [*Your Baby's Brain*]. When you find out you are having your first child, you experience both happiness and fright. The frightening part is that you have the responsibility of raising this child. You as a parent have that power. You build your child's brain by stimulation—cuddling, reading, singing, etc. Bond and nurture your child; your time with them is powerful. Take control and mold this baby into a healthy, happy child who is ready to take on the world. [*Your Baby's Brain*] will point out the tools you need to do this. Know in your hear that you have these tools."

—C. R. "Bob" Bell, Vice Admiral (retired) United States Navy

"Gail Gross is a genius in taking complex issues and making them easy to understand. Every young couple—as well as grandparents—should read [*Your Baby's Brain*]. It is powerful in teaching us how to be a major influence on our child's brain development."

—Michael B. Yanney, Chairman Emeritus of the Board of Burlington Capital

"We all want the children in our lives to grow into happy, successful adults. In her new book, [*Your Baby's Brain*], Gail offers clinically proven guidance and actionable advice for boosting your child's positive mental and physical trajectory."

—Renee Parsons, businesswoman and philanthropist, founder of the Bob & Renee Parsons Foundation

"Dr. Gail Gross insightfully and persuasively affirms parents' ability to affect the mental, emotional and psychological identify of their children: they become who they are largely through the experiences we share with them. This is a welcome and timely reminder of the gravity and importance of our children's formative years: a must-read for all present and prospective parents.

Rich, stimulating experience and loving, compassionate relationships are the foundation to becoming all you can be. With important new data and incisive wisdom, Dr. Gail Gross is our guide to being a fulfilled parent of a child who is eager to learn and filled with wonder about the world and their place in it.

In these days when we connect to each other through devices and data, Dr. Gail Gross reminds us of the vital importance of emotional bonding, physical connection, and quality time in raising a child that is healthy and happy in body, mind, and spirt. There is much compassionate wisdom in these pages, and I encourage you to experience it."

—Tara Guber, president and founder of Yoga Ed

"[*Your Baby's Brain*] is a how-to guide on best practices for parents to ensure a baby's optimal brain health. An engrossing read."

—Michelle King Robson, founder of EmpowHER, and CEO of Safeface cosmetics and founder of HER Inc.

"Dr. Gail Gross has written a book with a keen observation that escapes many mothers but is an absolute. Bonding cannot be done by proxy; Mom has only one chance . . . the key to early childhood development is being there."

—Ambassador Joseph and Alma Gildenhorn

"In 1980, my husband and I started our family of four children, and began the life-long journey of parenting. For me, an integral part of being a mother was being our children's first teacher. Every day was a day to explore together the world around us. I read the latest, most cutting-edge books on parenting and child development but found nothing to support or explain what I was observing in our children's development. [*Your Baby's Brain*] was exactly the book I was looking for and yearned to read. I can personally attest to the tremendous benefits you will find in your own child's growth and future development—even through their adulthood—by applying the principles and techniques found in Dr. Gail Gross's book. What I was learning by trial-and-error and without understanding why some things worked and others didn't, you will discover in this book. I highly recommend that every parent, teacher, and grandparent read this brilliant work and utilize what you will learn to maximize the potential of the little ones you love and cherish. You will find that you can and will profoundly contribute to their bright future. You will be building your baby's brain!"

—Renée Brinkerhoff, founder and driver, Valkyrie Racing and Valkyrie Gives

"Knowing Dr. Gail Gross as well as I do, knowing how passionate she is about her profession and reaching out to help people, knowing the tremendous amount of love she has in her heart, and not to say the least about her exceptional intelligence, I strongly urge every parent and parent-to-be of a newborn to read every word she has written in [*Your Baby's Brain*]. It can have a very positive impact on your child's future."

—Ronald M. Simon, Founder of RSI Home Products, RSI communities, and The Simon Foundation for Education and Housing

"Dr. Gross has an innate ability to take highly complex subjects, in this case raising our children, and break them down to their most accessible roots. Her writing will both inform and inspire you to take a deeper look into the relationship between parent and child.

What I find particularly remarkable about her writing is how well she blends the science with compassion, a sweet spot that is rare to find in highly personal topics such as this. I wish I had this book when I was raising my kids, but I will be sure to pass it along the day they have kids of their own."

—Sheryl Lowe, jewelry designer, founder & CEO of Sheryl Lowe Jewelry

"Once again, Dr. Gail Gross has provided us with invaluable information that will enhance and improve lives. Every parent should read this scientific, yet approachable book about how our children will thrive when we learn how their brains develop and respond. As in her past writings, Dr. Gross communicates what can be a highly complicated subject, in understandable and loving terms."

—Ann Rubenstein Tisch, founder and president of The Young Women's Network, and founder of seventeen schools around the country

"The importance of early childhood experiences in the development of an individual has been well established. In our busy world, we often look outward towards the latest new gadget or technological advancement to help in our child's growth. Dr. Gross's book is a welcome invitation back into the home, providing parents a practical outline to reengage with their child and foster emotional and social development. [*Your Baby's Brain*] is a great book for the new and seasoned parent alike."

—Dr. Jeff Meyrowitz, MD, pediatrician

"[*Your Baby's Brain*] is bursting with the key insights for parents to ensure they give their child the best start possible in life, and it gives readers a wealth of practical information they can start applying today in the vital quest to optimize their child's future.

Dr. Gail Gross, the author of this authoritative book, is a human behavior expert and family and child development specialist. She serves as a discerning and compassionate guide on the journey to understanding the developing brain by sharing insights from her own commitment to parenting and knowledge gained throughout her career.

With patience and wisdom, Dr. Gross helps parents unlock the importance of genetics, the impact of environment, and the key role of bonding in triggering the blossoming of their child's brain. She encourages parents to 'optimize the window of opportunity' so their children can develop the emotional skills that contribute to social and intellectual growth. And she cheers readers on so they can be perfectly positioned to make the difference in their children's lives that only they can make.

I am honored to call Dr. Gross my friend, and grateful to have her in my life. She understands the intricacy of our human existence and the scientific principles that can generate the results we seek. This book is a magnificent testimony to her devotion and service to others, and a must-read for anyone who has ever wondered if they could be doing more to support their child's developing brain."

—Melani Walton, cofounder of the Rob and Melani Walton Foundation

"We're obsessed with the latest gadgets to make us better. Turns out the most advanced gadget is still the human brain. Dr. Gail Gross just delivered to us the manual."

"[*Your Baby's Brain*] is a beautifully written must-read for parents interested in truly understanding their responsibility and power in shaping their children's developing brains."

"Gail's book has given Extraordinary Clarity of the Miracle of Life. Each page gives the Wisdom and understanding of how early nurturing is essential to life's long growth. I'm in total awe of *this book*. I found it to be so insightful. And on every page, I felt Gail's heart and passion. [*Your Baby's Brain*] takes an in-depth look at the turmoil of our world today. And, it should be a part of our education, as parenting is the most important job we will ever have. I'm honored to be included in this extraordinary journey."

"Dr. Gail Gross is a dynamo! [*Your Baby's Brain*] is a gateway to the deepest understanding of your child's intelligence and well-being. It helps you to teach your children the right things at the right time. Dr. Gross integrates the intellectual, the spiritual, and the psyche into a harmonious whole.

This book will benefit everyone. It lives up to its title and I intend to share it with all of my friends and their children. I could go on and on but I hope everyone will just take my advice and read it!"

"What if all the pre-pre-K schooling, the extra tutors, the special education toys, the latest electronic teaching machines, and best children television programming aren't delivering what parents are promised? Or what they want? Worse, what if all the investment of that time and turns out to be counter-productive? Dr. Gail Gross, in her latest book, argues about a more effective and more productive way for parents to begin their parenting relationship. Her latest effort yields solid research-based recommendations for parents who truly are seeking the best way to bring up their children . . . as well as getting better results than promised by today's trend to earlier and more extensive educational immersion. As a parent of two grown boys, I wish Dr. Gross's book had been available many years ago when we had our first child, but for today's parents just starting out, it offers a welcomed and revealing commentary on some of the best documented child rearing techniques."

—Lloyd M. Bentsen III, president, Bentsen Financial Corp.

YOUR BABY'S BRAIN

HOW TO USE SCIENCE TO RAISE A SMART, SUCCESSFUL CHILD

Dr. Gail Gross

Foreword by *Dean Ornish, M.D.*

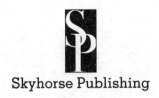

Skyhorse Publishing

Skyhorse Publishing books may be purchased in bulk at special discounts for sales promotion, corporate gifts, fund-raising, or educational purposes. Special editions can also be created to specifications. For details, contact the Special Sales Department, Skyhorse Publishing, 307 West 36th Street, 11th Floor, New York, NY 10018 or info@skyhorsepublishing.com.

Skyhorse® and Skyhorse Publishing® are registered trademarks of Skyhorse Publishing, Inc.®, a Delaware corporation.

Visit our website at www.skyhorsepublishing.com.

10 9 8 7 6 5 4 3 2 1

Library of Congress Cataloging-in-Publication Data is available on file.

Jacket design by Qualcom and Mona Lin
Jacket photographs by iStock

Print ISBN: 978-1-5107-7634-0
Ebook ISBN: 978-1-5107-7872-6

Printed in the United States of America

Previously published as *How to Build Your Baby's Brain* (ISBN: 978-1-5107-3920-8).

To my beloved husband, Jenard Gross, who makes all things possible, including me. You are my sun, my moon, my stars, my heart. You are the love of my life.

Your children are not your children.
They are the sons and daughters of Life's longing for itself.
They come through you but not from you,
And though they are with you yet they belong not to you.

You may give them your love but not your thoughts,
For they have their own thoughts.
You may house their bodies but not their souls,
For their souls dwell in the house of tomorrow,
which you cannot visit, not even in your dreams.

You may strive to be like them,
but seek not to make them like you.
For life goes not backward nor tarries with yesterday.

—Kahlil Gibran

TABLE OF CONTENTS

FOREWORD

This extraordinarily wonderful and important book by Dr. Gail Gross may have a bigger impact on your child's life and development than any other book you've ever read.

As she writes, *you* are the single greatest determinant of your child's personality, intellect, and future. This book will profoundly empower you to nurture, guide, and support your child in the most meaningful ways for both of you.

Many people are surprised to learn that much of this development occurs in the first one hundred days and especially during the first four years of a child's life. And while a child's genes are a factor, what we do as parents plays an even more important role. Genes are only a predisposition, not their fate.

Scientists used to believe that education began at kindergarten. We now know that it actually starts at the moment of birth—and as some studies have shown, even in utero. Children who have the positive parenting experiences that Gail describes in this book during their first four years of life have a significant advantage over children who do not.

As Gail writes, "Your child's brain builds and grows in response to the stimulation it receives, which means *each and every one* of your child's physical and emotional experiences biologically impacts the development of your child's brain. It's a lot of responsibility—and a lot of power."

The basic, primal instincts that all parents have are the ones that our children most need—to love, nurture, and spend time with them. Just as exercise builds strong muscles, spending time with your child builds a strong brain. Any parent can do it—here, Gail shows how.

Talking to your child, reading to them, playing with them, interacting with them in supportive and nurturing ways builds billions of connections between the neurons in their brains every time this occurs. This increases your child's IQ and potential for success throughout their life. Connections between neurons mirror connections between a parent and child.

This occurs primarily before age four—use it or lose it. Children who have parents who don't spend much time interacting with them by then may have a hard time catching up later.

As Gail explains, "This process, called synaptic pruning, makes it possible for your child's brain to develop correctly. Simply put, stimulation enhances connections and pruning discards what is not being used. And though synaptic pruning extends over the course of a lifetime, it is the most active during early childhood."

This pruning process eliminates billions of connections between neurons that would have been preserved if a parent had spent time talking, playing, singing, reading, and hugging their child.

Spending time on television, iPads, and other devices does not have this beneficial effect. It's why many of the people who invented and built these devices don't allow their kids to use them. Screen time is no substitute for real time.

In short, this is a revolutionary book that can empower our children's lives for the better and, as such, transform the world we live in. It should be required reading for every parent.

—Dean Ornish, MD
Founder and president, Preventive Medicine Research Institute
Clinical professor of medicine, University of California, San Francisco
www.ornish.com

INTRODUCTION

IT TAKES A FAMILY, NOT A VILLAGE

You are well aware that your child's future prospects hinge upon her academic performance. You're inundated on all sides by frenzied statistics, scores, and scholastic stress—and it's all starting earlier and earlier. Our curriculum-obsessed culture has convinced you that to raise a successful, high-achieving child, you need to outsource her education to those who are "more qualified" (with those who stand to benefit doing most of the convincing). You may even believe that scientific advances and new technologies in education and learning can make your child smarter, provided you can secure a spot for her in the right program.

However, contrary to what you've been taught, you don't need talking heads or a host of expensive programs and toys. The truth is you're wasting money and time on programs that put the cart before the developmental horse, ultimately keeping your child from where she needs to go. My forty-eight years of experience as an educator and leading expert on child and family development and human behavior make it easy for me to see what empowers certain children to achieve, and what handicaps others. It is the child who comes to school *ready* to learn, read, think critically, and process on a higher level, instead of frantically accumulating information, who enthusiastically embraces her education, finding out where her true gifts, talents, and efficacy lie.

You, and you alone, can ensure that your child have what she needs to do this, but you have a narrow window: the first five years of her life.

The problem is that you think someone else can do it better, so, like many, you scramble to outsource your child's training too soon, gambling away your child's most precious resource: *you*. You are, in fact, more than just a parent: you are your child's true gene therapist. You have the capacity to alter the expression of your child's genes by the environment you create. This means you can influence which aspects of your child's personality and potential are activated or suppressed. It is the experiences of that early environment that instruct and direct your child's genes, enhancing some and turning others off. Your child's genes are the mixing board, and you are the sound engineer. Once you learn how to tap into that, to flip the right switches, you can expand the limits of your child's potential in ways you may not realize. You can lay the emotional and intellectual groundwork that allows your child to seize opportunities for success fearlessly, naturally, and enthusiastically. As Maria Montessori explained, when discussing childhood education: "It is not acquired by listening to words, but in virtue of experiences in which the child acts on his environment."[1] Therefore, education begins in utero.

It is essential, however, to know how and when to activate those experiences. Your parental superpower wields the most strength during very specific and optimal windows of your child's development. This is critical: what happens within these developmental windows can set the course for the rest of your child's life. It's not just *what* you do that matters, but *when,* as research shows the most significant windows are closed by age five. According to Dr. Alexis Carrell, "The period of infancy is undoubtedly the richest. It should be utilized by education in every possible and conceivable way. The waste of this period of life can never be compensated."[2]

Don't panic. Yes, the stakes are high, but this means parenting is much simpler than you dared to imagine. Great parenting comes down to one mission: you have to be prepped and *present* for those windows, so that you can take full advantage of them and help your child develop into a smart, successful, self-sufficient adult.

That starts with providing an emotionally safe, structured environment. It's the springboard for your child's future. The secure child with a strong central core and good self-esteem isn't likely to fall victim to the influence of the "cool kids" or be pressured to please others who don't have his best interests at heart. Rather, he charts his own course, follows what sparks his intellectual curiosity, and adheres to his own values. For example, the confident, well-loved child is self-actualized, focusing on problem-solving while digging for answers, and doesn't fear the stigma of the science fair or chess match. Children who don't succumb to anxiety and peer pressure are strong enough to explore and express what makes them stand out; they follow their own authority.

In this book, I will teach you how to create parental bonds that inoculate your child against the fear of failure and the discipline problems that can inhibit both intellectual and psychological growth. Through an understanding of the stages of your baby's development, you'll learn to create a world that your little alchemist can explore with wonder, confidence, and ease. I know from my own personal studies and research that as your child's most important teacher, it is your job to create an environment that is not only secure, but rich with printed letters and numbers as well as physical objects he can observe and manipulate. These tools can help him develop the cognitive and emotional skills that in turn contribute to linguistic, cognitive, emotional, and social growth. This not only lays the groundwork for literacy, but expands your child's potential exponentially. And it's not just the environment you create; scientific studies show your presence is the biggest stimulator of linguistic, cognitive, emotional, and social development, so much so that the tension from your absence has the capacity to inhibit and even damage the way your child processes and learns information. I know that to provide a secure life for your child, you can't be there all of the time. Don't worry! In this book, I will show you how to compensate for your time apart by maximizing your time together.

However, you can't *just* be there—you have to know what to do, as well. When you're actively involved with your baby's development, you are present, to observe and enhance those qualities that truly make your child unique. You recognize the potential for a piano protégé and you're there to catch the first signs of a learning or hearing disability, which can be successfully corrected or treated if spotted early enough. The key to being your child's true gene therapist lies in your ability to activate the requisite switches at the appropriate time, which will determine your child's success. In so doing, you will effectively reduce your child's stress, identify his individual gifts, and permanently remove potential obstacles to create a self-actualized child.

Most important, you will gain a full understanding of your child's multiple developmental timelines and how to get them to work in tandem. Too often society conditions you to compartmentalize aspects of your child's growth. As an educator, I saw many bright students who fell behind because their emotional immaturity blocked them from engaging effectively with their school material. The windows in your child's development for progressive and expanded growth are best optimized when they are approached with the full picture in mind. After reading this book, you will have a firm grasp of everything it takes to raise a happy, high-achieving, confident, empathic, and successful child.

This book could not come at a more crucial time in our culture. Our children face a more threatening world than many of us remember from our childhoods. Far too many have been "hurried" to grow up too fast—resulting in an epidemic of stress, mental illness, physical ailments, violence, and emotional and mental shutdown. You, as a parent, want what's best for your child because you love her. I believe your job has never been more important—not only for your child's future, but for ours. We need more children who dare to break from the group and chase the questions that intrigue them. We need the next generation to be grounded in the empathy and connection bred from the security you provide. Most of all, we can't survive without a new generation of fearless innovators and leaders. This book will not only teach you how to provide a happy, brilliant, and successful future for your child—it will help you secure your contribution to our collective success.

MY STORY

My mother did not have the "Donna Reed" model of family life. Her parents were wonderful, loving people who showered her with affection in her formative years. Though my mother's mother died when she was barely five years of age, and her father when she was nine, my grandparents had already instilled a strong central core in my mother that allowed her to not only survive, but to thrive. Her inherent ability to love, connect, and bond made her a strong, wonderful mother (albeit sometimes lacking in practical parenting skills).

My mother created a home environment that was rich in learning, creativity, and exploration. She scoffed at the idea of "toys." Instead, we were encouraged to read a book, paint, play with clay, or pursue any creative endeavor my mother considered of "value." Most important, she actively played with us and incorporated our play into her daily life. I loved to play grocery store, shaping vegetables out of clay as she chopped away making our actual dinner. Playtime and discovery were filled with the connection and communication of ideas. I was encouraged to interact, share, and check in with a mother who was never out of reach.

The transition to kindergarten was jarring. I started school early, at four and a half. I was excited to share my reactions to new materials and discoveries but quickly found that my teacher's job was to educate the class on the benefits of good conduct rather than to foster enthusiasm. I soon picked up on the subtleties and nuances of when to speak and when to be silent.

Frankly, I was completely unprepared for Ms. Meade. A long teaching career had left her short on patience. One afternoon, my class crush knocked over a planter as we raced to get in line. Because I was first, Ms. Meade assumed that I was the culprit. Without a fair trial, she lit into me. Unable to betray my kindergarten love, and completely unaccustomed to screaming as a form of discipline, tears filled my eyes. This only elicited further scolding to "stop crying." At the end of school, traumatized, I bolted out of the classroom and ran all the way home, sobbing and wetting my pants. By the time I reached my mother, I was so distraught that she promised me I would not have to go back to school until I was ready. A little lacking in practical parenting skills, my mother kept me home for three weeks. A call from the school, warning I would have to repeat kindergarten if I didn't immediately return, prompted a parent-teacher conference with Ms. Meade. When my mother explained how Ms. Meade's behavior had traumatized me, she was incredulous. "She's four years old! There's no way she remembers that I yelled at her a month ago!"

I not only remembered then, but I still remember as an adult! It changed my entire educational journey. From that moment on, I was anxious about making mistakes and especially cautious around teachers. As an adult, I realized that we consistently underestimate the impact we have on our children and the lasting effect we can have emotionally and structurally. As a psychologist and educator, I know these events are more than significant; they shape the very neurological makeup of our children and can determine the course of their lives.

When it was my turn to be a parent, I not only sought to create the same environment as my mother, but I took it to the next level. I built a print-rich home full of complex language. I actively taught my children stress-management techniques like meditation, creative imagery, and music. Not only did I want my children to be better prepared for the challenges of school, but I was also keenly aware that their generation was facing an intense, anxiety-ridden educational system with a score-driven, high-stakes atmosphere. After raising my children, my pursuit of multiple advanced degrees in psychology and education opened my eyes to a wealth of crucial parenting information that our culture stifles or even contradicts. Now, it is my mission to share this information with parents to ensure that the next generation gets the foundation it deserves and desperately needs.

Your Baby's Brain will teach you how to transfer information from the latest neuroscience research to your everyday experiences with your child. This will allow you to guide your child through every age and stage of his neurological development, so that you and he can take full advantage of both the information and experiences necessary to lead your child toward emotional maturity and academic success.

By correlating your child's neurological stage with his appropriate age, you can help him unfold into the ultimate expansion of his potential. Not only that, this down-to-earth information will guide your child toward emotional maturity so that he can access and use his abilities. All of this can happen as simply as ABC.

A. Bond with baby and support her emotional development.

B. Coordinate the age and neurological stage of baby's development to enhance his learning potential.

C. Teach stress-reduction techniques, creative visualization, and exercises to help your child focus and concentrate.

Steps A and B will designate every important developmental marker in your baby's life. They will teach you how to incorporate your baby's linguistic, cognitive, emotional, and social development. This parallel development transitions into not only mental and physical maturity, but moral maturity, as well. At every step along the way, I will show you how to help your child integrate all three steps.

As you recognize what your child requires to successfully move from one developmental stage to another, you will be able to structure his environment to create a successful passage. Of course, timing is everything. Neuroscience tells us that there are optimal timelines or windows of opportunity when your baby's brain is uniquely receptive to particular kinds of stimulation. Thus, when you amplify the appropriate ideas and tools at the right time, your baby's brain will be in a heightened state, and thus more receptive to age-appropriate knowledge and skill. As a result, the range of your baby's responses is expanded exponentially with the ease of learning, as she absorbs information naturally. Hence, you and your baby can experience the joy and satisfaction of each educational milestone.

Your Baby's Brain offers you exercises and activities that are not only easy to navigate but fun, with the added bonus of enhancing your child's self-esteem and building a stronger central core. Each exercise and activity is coordinated to your child's age and developmental stage, giving you the opportunity to learn more about your child, so that you can structure an environment uniquely designed for him. By paying attention and getting to know your child, you can create specific learning models that will help merge not only your child's linguistic, cognitive, and social development, but moral and spiritual development, as well.

Step C incorporates stress-reduction techniques in early childhood development. In fact, teaching your child how to cope with stress, as well as how to focus and concentrate, is one of the most important tools in the neuroscience toolbox, yet it is often disregarded by other early childhood development books, perhaps because it is discounted and therefore over-looked. Every stage and age of early childhood growth in *Your Baby's Brain* is accompanied by stress-reduction techniques. For example, massage, yoga, creative visualization, meditation, music, qigong, and so forth are all integrated into each stage of your child's development. These techniques, skills, and tools will help not only your child, but you as well, to lower your anxiety and regulate the stress hormone cortisol, allowing you both to access and process information more effectively. It is not true that you use only a small part of your brain. In reality, when exposed to stress-reduction exercises, your brain is used completely, just like an orchestra. Moreover, neuroscience research states that when you are stressed, anxious, frightened, or unable to cope, you overproduce the stress hormone cortisol, which changes brain architecture and impulse control . . . especially in a developing brain.

Your Baby's Brain will show you how to incorporate stress-reduction techniques into everyday life with your baby, teaching her how to manage stress, lower anxiety, focus, and concentrate. Stress-reduction techniques will show your child how to access her own inner resources. This by itself helps her to build a strong central core, which will increase self-esteem and enhance her ability to not only manage her stress, but also to process information effortlessly. However, children who can't reach inward for stress-reduction techniques, and who don't learn how to cope with stress, may find themselves unable to learn or develop successfully. Cortisol can change the brain, and consistent stress can change the brain irrevocably.

A 24/7 news cycle, technology, and the constant overstimulation of information promote a more threatening world than children experienced even ten years ago. Through the permeation of computer games and television, used all too often as a way to help harried parents, you can see how children can be introduced too early to inappropriate and socially advanced material. Dr. David Elkind, in his books *The Hurried Child: Growing Up Too Fast Too Soon* and *Miseducation: Preschoolers at Risk,* explains the dangers of children growing up more quickly than their internal maturation can accommodate. This accelerated exposure to inappropriate and advanced material causes children to feel anxious and out of control. According to Elkind, "early miseducation can cause permanent damage to a child's self-esteem, the loss of a positive attitude a child needs for learning, the blocking of natural gifts and potential talents."[3] In a sense, children who are pressured to perform or taught the wrong things at the wrong time begin to display stress-related behaviors. By the time they reach the end of concrete operations and enter abstract operations, at approximately the fifth-grade level, they quit rather than try, simply shutting down. Furthermore, there is extensive research to support the idea that children between birth and five years of age who receive such pressure demonstrate not only psychological problems later in life, but intellectual and physical problems, as well. Thus, you can see the danger of putting the brain power of the next generation at risk, which would be a loss of human capital and natural resources for us all. On the other hand, when children in early childhood receive conscious parenting and a time-sensitive education, they unfold in a natural and spontaneous manner, actively and successfully exploring and experiencing their immediate environment.

The exercises and activities that follow are fun to do. They are adapted to each stage of your child's development and will help you, as a parent, to get to know your child better. Most important, these playful interactions will help your child integrate emotional and intellectual as well as moral and spiritual maturation.

By the end, you will be fully equipped to give your child the strategies and skills he will need throughout life to cope with whatever the world throws his way . . . and to succeed.

PART ONE

1

TAP INTO YOUR INNER GENE THERAPIST—THE SCIENCE BEHIND YOUR SECRET PARENTAL POWER

Your child's DNA is not destiny; you are at the helm, guiding his course. The truth is that nature and nurture are in a delicate dance akin to Fred and Ginger's famous choreography: if one goes too fast, the other one falls. Science tells us that early childhood experiences actually have the capacity to structure and alter the brain. That means you didn't just supply your child's DNA—you're still shaping it, and it's only by wielding that power that your child will activate his full potential. You are truly a gene therapist, manipulating and guiding your child's genetic makeup, based on the experiences you create for him. The longer you abdicate your power to shape your child's genetic makeup *after* he's born, the more you leave his development to chance. In this chapter, I'll explain the nuances of your secret parental power—and teach you how to harness its full potency.

As a human behavior expert and family and child development specialist with a PhD in psychology and an EdD in education, I am often asked to comment on how parents can awaken their child's potential. My answer always begins the same way: parents have the power. You are not merely a factor; you are the single greatest determinant of your child's personality, intellect, and future. Your power extends way beyond providing a boost in potential or a push to succeed; you, as a parent, are capable of shaping and are, to a great degree, responsible for the very structure of your child's brain. As a parent, you have the ultimate responsibility for the trajectory your child takes in life. The good news is that you have everything you need to give your baby what she needs.

Your child's genes may be a blueprint, but that's still only a two-dimensional potential mock-up of what will be a three-dimensional person. That old argument of nature versus nurture has been settled, and the truth is that both have about equal influence. Nature may supply the genes, but those genes express themselves in reaction to stimulation from their environment—the environment *you* create and control. So, you can see that you are your child's true gene therapist, and your presence and the environment you create actively determine which of your child's genes are expressed. Your baby's brain builds and grows in response to the stimulation it receives, which means that *each and every one*[1] of her physical and emotional experiences affects the biological development of your baby's brain. It's a lot of responsibility—and a lot of power. And regrettably, far too many parents aren't aware of just how much influence they wield.

Your baby is born with approximately 100 billion neurons and over 50 trillion synapses. This may seem like a lot, but it's only a fraction of the neural connections that she will develop—more than 1,000 trillion in the first year alone. Out of your baby's 24,000 genes, 12,000 of them establish these neural connections in the brain, which designate how the central nervous system will be created and function. However, those 12,000 genes aren't nearly enough to activate all those neural connections. Therefore, it is your baby's heightened experiences, both emotional and physical, that specify and determine those connections. Because the brain is highly efficient, it actually dumps unused neurons while strengthening those used consistently. This process, called *synaptic pruning*,[2] allows your child's brain to develop correctly. Stimulation enhances connections, and pruning discards what is not being used. Synaptic pruning extends over your lifetime, but it is the most active during early childhood. Synaptic pruning means that every experience counts. Every touch, sight, smell, and interaction positively or negatively affects the wiring of your child's brain—each experience, whether positive or negative, is a signal that strengthens, weakens, or reinforces synapses. Think of it as two roads diverging in a yellow wood—except your child's brain will always take the road *most* traveled.

As a result, either the environment will alter your baby's brain architecture, or you will do it on purpose by shaping and influencing baby's environment to that end. This is not a construction process that can or should be outsourced—nature has gone to great pains to signal its preference for parental guidance. Biology ensures through bonding that you hold greater power to stimulate brain development—and the turning on and off of genes—than anyone else in your child's life. Remember that flood of unconditional love you experienced the first time you held your baby? That's a survival instinct (and nature's strongest incentive), put in place to ensure that you will want to be present and engaged in this crucial, formative time of your baby's life. The quality of that experience is determined by bonding: quantity and quality time, attention, care, and nurturing that is physiologically and emotionally essential to your child.

Acts of love like cuddling, soothing your child with your voice, responding to her needs, and reading a book may sound simple, but they are the stimulation your baby's developing brain needs and builds upon most effectively. The more you interact with and stimulate your baby, the more you increase his neuroglial cells. That increase in cells also leads to an increase in activity, and it's easy to see how that promotes faster and more complicated patterns of thought. You're building the highways and infrastructure for high-traffic learning later.

The impact of bonding can't be overstated. The absence of secure bonding and nurturing not only deprives your child of the brain stimulation she needs to thrive, but can cause serious neurological harm. As Laurie Larson points out in her pivotal study on maternal touch, babies who are not fondled or touched can die from lack of physical contact. When that secure bonding is present, the impact is huge: we're talking about influencing your child's IQ by 20 to 40 percent.[3] American psychologist Florence

Goodenough, revered for her work in child psychology, suggested that environmental factors, including complicated language, accounted for between 20 and 40 percent of a person's intelligence score, which she took to be a measure of cognitive development.[4] That can be the difference between average and high achieving—just because you showed up and parented.

HARDWIRED TO LEARN

Babies are hardwired to learn. They are tiny scientists discovering their world through familiar experiments. You don't need formal training or a fancy degree to build your child's brain. Your child—every child—is born with what renowned doctor and educator Maria Montessori called "an inner teacher."[5] Montessori believed that children do not need formal education to learn much of the important social, emotional, and intellectual behavior experienced in their early years. They are naturally driven to explore. What children do need, she argued, is an environment rich with the toys and tools that help them master the progression of skills necessary to build confidence and competence, which leads to good self-esteem and, ultimately, academic success. Your child learns by testing herself against her environment. The very act of venturing out beyond her reach and making discoveries about how the world looks, feels, and tastes stimulates your baby's neurons, which in turn adds to the mass of connections in the brain. With each outing into unknown territory, your child moves to a higher level of intellectual and emotional advancement.

But the most important element in your child's world of exploration—the one thing that will ensure that she reach her full potential—is you. If she can look back and see you or call for you and hear you, she experiences emotional stability, solidifying the intellectual, physical, and emotional progress made in each foray. The secure feeling that comes from strong bonding lowers anxiety, leading to a strong central core, the resource necessary for emotional maturity—which is why your child will learn more at her mother's knee than anywhere else. When your child learns to trust you, she learns to trust herself. At no other point in your child's life will your presence be such a viable and invaluable gift.

WITH BONDING, MORE IS MORE

Until three years of age, your baby sees you as a physical appendage and extension of himself. He does not yet understand that the two of you are separate. And just as you'd be terrified if your child were kidnapped or torn from your arms by a stranger, your baby experiences separation anxiety every time you two are apart. That anxiety bathes your child's brain in potent stress hormones, specifically cortisol, which, while it has other critical functions in the human body, when overproduced can have disastrous effects on its development. Psychologist Daniel Goleman explains, "Cortisol stimulates the amygdala, while it impairs the hippocampus, forcing our attention onto the emotions we feel, while restricting our ability to take in new information."[6] He explains that the amygdala overrides the prefrontal cortex when the brain is in "fight-or-flight" mode.[7] Your hippocampus and prefrontal cortex are the regions of your brain responsible for learning, memory, and high-level thinking (executive function). Therefore, if stress is bathing your baby's developing brain in cortisol, it's also blocking the brain's capacity to build the higher-level thinking and reason needed for your child to thrive.

Not convinced? According to a 2001 study by Flinn et. al., published in *Development and Psychopathology* and cited in the journal *Neuroscience Behaviors*, a child's cortisol levels measurably increase the longer a parent is away from him, which can result in long-term dysfunction in the neurobiological system, with negative effects on emotional health, digestion, and even your child's immune system.

That means you have to be there. Your presence isn't merely a bonus or a positive influence; your absence negatively impacts your child. More important, nursery schools, babysitters, and nannies are not equipped to understand the developmental needs of your child and thus can't deliberately or attentively guide the transition from one stage to the next. Timing is everything. In order to unlock your child's gifted potential, her brain's neurons must be stimulated and guided during her optimal windows of growth. When you're not present, you risk leaving that development to chance, and your absence can cause the overproduction of the stress hormones that may literally change the brain's neurological and emotional framework. When cortisol is produced to excess, or persists over a long duration, it washes over the developing brain like battery acid, changing its structure and affecting neurotransmitters.

I'm not saying that you can't have a career, but you must compensate and accommodate to override the stress that your child experiences when waiting to be reunited with you. Our society does not make it easy to be present—as a working mother, I can attest to the very real obstacles, frustrations, and struggles that working parents experience. But I believe that those obstacles raise the stakes and require an even deeper understanding of which of your emotional assets wields the most influence over your child's growth and success. Nothing is more important than your time.

YOUR TIME IS MORE POWERFUL THAN YOUR MONEY

You may believe, like so many, that more money means more opportunity, and that quality time is a necessary casualty in the rat race to buy your child more things, better schools, memberships, and opportunities to succeed. A study conducted by the Programme for International Student Assessment (PISA) in 2009 indicates that this is a cultural myth. According to PISA's findings, your socioeconomic status accounts for only 10 percent of the variance in your child's academic success.[8]

In a research project in England in 1984, Sarah Bayliss and her team set out to determine whether a parent-involvement program was able to close the gap in education between third graders from poor working-class families and their wealthier upper-middle-class counterparts.[9] They found that the pupils from the poor working-class families, whose parents were involved and supported their children, outperformed those pupils from wealthier families, even those who were given private tutoring from professionals. The only variable in this study was that the children from poorer families were emotionally supported by parents who were involved in their daily activities.

Here in the United States, a similar study confirms the same. Dr. Burton White conducted a three-year study called the Missouri Project, which involved three hundred families and demonstrated that when parents are taught about child development—including how to structure discipline without suppressing natural curiosity and the impulse to explore—children thrive. Students whose parents participated in the study reached higher than average levels of aptitude in linguistic and cognitive ability by the age of three.[10] As a result, it was White who argued that education should begin at birth. White's study led to one of the most groundbreaking programs for parents interested in parental involvement in early education. Because the Missouri Project convinced officials that parents were the most powerful force in early education, Missouri funded PAT (Parents as Teachers) to teach parents how to actively be involved in their child's early education. The PAT program is so successful that it now has both national and international affiliates. The longitudinal results of the PAT programs in California and Missouri indicate that those children whose parents are actively involved in their nurturing and education from birth to three years score significantly higher than comparable children on almost all levels, including linguistic, cognitive, social, and academic abilities.[11]

Because of the results obtained in the Missouri Project, White discovered that after the age of three, it becomes much more difficult to try to remediate both linguistic and intellectual deficits; therefore, a commitment to early childhood education is critical. However, educators now believe that the effects of parental involvement in early education are cumulative and still continue far beyond age three. Children likely retain the positive benefits of the active role their parents played in their early education throughout their lives.[12]

The best news of all? Making that impact isn't nearly as time-consuming as you'd think; you can start seeing results in a matter of weeks, not years. Professor of education Lowell Madden, reporting on the remediation of poor readers in elementary school, states that parents who were taught how to interact with their children by reading in their own home over a six-to-eight-week period multiplied their children's comprehension rate by six times the normal rate.[13] Even more stunning, researchers today believe that 85 percent of all children in the United States labeled educable but mentally challenged could have attained average intelligence had they received sufficient stimulation in their families of origin in their developmental years. What that means, for you and your child, is that regardless of *your* income or education level, you can learn how to expand your child's learning ability if you act during pivotal times in her life.

All this research together illuminates—and refutes—the social fiction that your child needs socioeconomic advantages to have a limitless future. It simply isn't true. You just have to be prepped and present to take advantage of critical, optimal windows of opportunity in your child's development.

OPTIMIZE THE WINDOW OF OPPORTUNITY

So you're a parent, you're ready to get started . . . and you're probably panicking because you don't know what to *do*. You don't need to be a formal teacher or have an advanced degree to foster your child's social, emotional, and intellectual growth. What you *can* do, as your child's most important teacher, is create an environment that is not only secure, but rich in learning materials, print, and objects to manipulate and observe. These tools can help your child develop the emotional skills that in turn contribute to social and intellectual growth—and ultimately academic and personal success.

For example, language starts earlier than you may think, as babies start learning rhythm, meter, and sounds listening to your voice from the fourth month on, in the womb. If you want to expand her potential exponentially, you have to learn to speak in complex language and listen actively.

In this book, I'll teach you how to communicate with your child to spur higher-level neurological development. You'll learn the active listening skills that enable you to catch red flags, spot hidden talents, and internalize the important feedback that your child shares with you. In addition, you'll learn why the old adage "children should speak only when spoken to" rips apart the scaffolding you've worked so hard to build for your child.

The connection between language, reading, and the development of your baby's brain cannot be overemphasized. Talk to your baby constantly. Timing is especially critical where language and reading are concerned. Because the brain stem develops before the cerebral cortex, infants gain control of their five senses first, which means they start out being able to distinguish and imitate sounds, even if they can't make sense of them. This receptivity of language begins four months after gestation; renowned speech scientist and psychologist Dr. Patricia Kuhl says that your baby learns the beginning of her native language from listening to your voice in utero. Thus, your child can learn whatever language she hears. After birth, if your child is exposed to many languages consistently during the window between birth and five years of age, she can learn them all (as long as each language is spoken specifically by one person at a time), and she can learn them with greater ease and speed than at any other time in her life. The important window for language acquisition begins to shut down by the age of five, so if a child learns a new language at the onset of adolescence, she may learn to speak it but will do so with a foreign accent. In due course, language acquisition evolves into reading and writing.[14]

Teachers universally agree that reading is one of the most important factors in your child's academic success. The key to boosting your child's literacy lies in reading to her early and often. And I mean early: while a newborn can't comprehend what you're saying, her associative map is expanded just by the sound and rhythm of your voice, the warmth of your body, and the time spent together. Gradually, your child will learn to anticipate what's coming next and begin to mimic your reading. By allowing your child to "read" to you by reciting what she's memorized, without bothering to correct her, you are paving the way for her to start connecting symbols, sounds, and words. You can also create a print-rich environment by labeling objects in large print, as well as pointing out objects around the house and in the neighborhood.

THE IMPORTANT ROLE OF DAD

While almost any man can father a child, there is so much more to the important role of being Dad in a child's life. Let's look at *who* Father is, and why he is so important.

Fathers are central to the emotional well-being of their children; they are capable caretakers and disciplinarians. Studies show that if your child's father is affectionate, supportive, and involved, he can contribute greatly to her cognitive, linguistic, and social development, resulting in academic achievement, a strong inner core, sense of well-being, good self-esteem, and authenticity.[15]

HOW FATHERS INFLUENCE OUR RELATIONSHIPS

Your child's primary relationship with his father can affect all of his relationships from birth to death, including those with friends, lovers, and spouses. Those early patterns of interactions with Father are the very patterns that will be projected outward onto all relationships: not only your child's intrinsic idea of who he is as he relates to others, but also the range of what your child considers acceptable and loving.

Girls will look for men who hold the patterns of good old Dad, for after all, they know how "to do that." Therefore, if Father was kind, loving, and gentle, they will reach for those characteristics in men. Girls will look for in others what they have experienced and become familiar with in childhood. Because they've gotten used to those familial and historic behavioral patterns, they think that they can handle them in relationships.

Boys, on the other hand, will model themselves after their fathers. They will look for their father's approval in everything they do and copy those behaviors that they recognize as both successful and familiar. Thus, if Dad was abusive, controlling, and dominating, those will be the patterns that his sons will imitate and emulate. However, if Father is loving, kind, supportive, and protective, his son will want to be that.

Human beings are social animals, and we learn by modeling behavior. In fact, all primates learn how to survive and function successfully in the world through social imitation. Those early patterns of interaction are all children know, and it is those patterns that affect how they feel about themselves and how they develop. Your child is vulnerable to those early patterns and incorporates those behavioral qualities in his or her repertoire of social interaction.

It is impossible to overestimate the importance of Dad. For example, girls who have good relationships with their fathers tend to do better in math at the eighth-grade level. Well-bonded boys develop securely with a stable and sustained sense of self. Also, children of involved fathers are less likely to get upset when detached from a parent. This is probably because fathers reassure children that they're okay by giving them more freedom and space to explore their surroundings. This ability to stay back and observe children without too much interference encourages individuation. Parenting styles of fathers seem to reassure and challenge emotional growth, while the parenting styles of mothers is more protective. Fathers allow children to venture out two times the distance that Mother would find comfortable. Moreover, when exposed to a new situation, mothers immediately move in, while fathers stay back and let baby work it out. Both styles are important to baby's psychological growth. Consequently, children of involved fathers have high IQs, greater social skills, greater impulse control, and display less violent behavior.[16] Who we are and who we are to be, we are becoming, and now we know that fathers are central to that outcome.

CHANGING FAMILY ROLES

Only 20 percent of American households consist of married couples with children.[17] Filling the gap are family structures of all kinds, with dads stepping up to the plate and taking on myriad roles. When they are engaged, fathers can really make a difference. They may be classically married, single, divorced, widowed, gay, straight, adoptive, stepfather, a stay-at-home dad, or the primary family provider—the only important thing is that he be involved.

The emergence of women into the job market has forever changed how society views the traditional roles of fathers and mothers. Feminism and financial power have shifted classic parenting trends, and today approximately 60 percent of women work.[18] Add to that the shift in marriage, divorce, lowered birth rates, and family structures of all types, and you can see the emergence of a softening and changing of traditional parenting roles. This transition in economics, urbanization, and sexual roles has led to more open, flexible, and undefined functions for fathers.

A recent study by the National Institute of Child Health and Human Development indicates that dads are more engaged in caretaking than ever before. The reasons for this are varied, but they include mothers working more hours and receiving higher salaries; fathers working less; and more psychological consciousness, better coping skills, mental illness intervention, intimacy in marriage, social connection, and better role-modeling for children.

Children who are well bonded with and loved by involved fathers *tend to have fewer behavioral problems* and are *somewhat inoculated against alcohol and drug abuse.* When fathers are less engaged, children are more likely to drop out of school earlier and to exhibit more problems in behavior and substance abuse. Research indicates that fathers are as important as mothers in their respective roles as caregivers, protectors, financial supporters, and, most important, models for social and emotional behavior. In fact, a relatively new familial structure that has emerged in our culture is the stay-at-home dad. This prototype is growing daily, thanks in part to women's strong financial gain, the recent recession, increase in corporate layoffs, and men's emerging strong sense of self.

Even when fathers are physically removed from their families, there are ways for them to nurture healthy relationships with their children. For instance, recognizing the important role fathers play in daughters' lives,

Angela Patton started a program in which young girls went to visit their fathers in prison for a father-daughter dance. It was a successful program that has spread across the country and not only helped daughters find connection, love, and support from their fathers, but also helped fathers feel important in the lives of their daughters.[19]

When fathers are separated from their children after a divorce, *there are many ways they can remain bonded with their children.* Though divorce is traumatizing to boys and girls alike, strong, consistent, and loving parenting from fathers can help make the transition successful.

2

FROM SERIAL KILLER TO SURGEON— HOW TO TURN YOUR CHILD'S SHORTCOMINGS INTO STRENGTHS

There is a thin line between a serial killer and a surgeon—and which side of the line your child falls on rests entirely in your hands. Now that you've accepted your role as gene therapist, it is up to you to provide the environment and experiences that will transform your child's weaknesses into her greatest strengths. From ADHD to aggression, social detachment to shyness, this chapter will show you how to identify characteristics that might sabotage your child down the line and how to mold those traits into assets.

BE HERE NOW—AVOID PROBLEMS LATER

There is one universal truth that resonates throughout the constellation of early child development: *your child needs your attention.* If you are watching, and listening, you will not only recognize when your child is ready to learn, but you'll also be better able to spot problems as they arise and address them readily. After researching children with reading problems, the National Institute of Health's Child Development and Behavioral Branch found that a twelve-year-old child needs four to five times as much "intervention time" as a five-year-old with similar reading problems. Early intervention is the key to successful remediation across the board.[1]

For example, if your child has a hearing problem that goes unrecognized or untreated in the first few years of life, he is tracking sound, rhythm, grammar, phonemes, and language usage incorrectly. Perhaps sounds are muffled or he's missing the rhythm and intonation of your particular language. While your child's hearing may be corrected later, he will still retain the incorrect rhythm, meter, or intonation in his speech—similar to a foreign accent—because of those incorrect patterns, tracked in his brain, while his hearing was compromised. However, if you're present and able to recognize that there is a problem, a speech pathologist may be able to remediate the speech disorder before that critical window for language acquisition closes.

BEYOND TEST SCORES: SHAPING TALENT AND TEMPERAMENT

The beauty of your parental power as a true gene therapist is that it extends well beyond the realm of intellectual advancement. You're shaping the expression of genes that contribute to talent, giftedness potential, and your child's overall personality. Any teacher will tell you that these components are just as important as intellectual capacity when it comes to academic success.

Regardless of the social cliché "you have to be born a genius," research tells us that the influence of parents in pointing their child in the right direction is statistically significant and can make all the difference in the world. We think of talent as something you're born with, yet giftedness does not always display itself at birth. The late Michael Howe, cognitive scientist and professor at the University of Exeter in England, studied select historical champions and superstars in art, music, tennis, and swimming. His study asserts that high achievers in different fields don't necessarily display their innate talents and gifts when young, not until they are encouraged and supported in those areas by—you guessed it—their parents. Thus, without the special attention of parents, it unlikely that even brilliant or gifted children would realize the full range of their innate abilities.[2]

Even Mozart—who was an obvious and well-known prodigy in composition, theory, and performance by the age of six—was molded and prodded by his father to take it to the next level.

There are some noted traits that gifted and talented high achievers have in common. But the main factor, proven again and again, is that if you as a parent provide self-confidence, support, and encouragement, you will also have the opportunity to develop your child's gifts. This is central to aptitude and development. Only by knowing and paying attention to your child—and recognizing and acknowledging his passions, talents, and abilities—can you create a home conducive to cultivating positive experiences and exploration. Yet if you don't exercise your parental power properly, your gifted child's talent will not necessarily be recognized.

On the flip side, your role as a true gene therapist also applies to nipping in the bud those personality traits that could hinder your child's success. Take the trait of shyness, for example. It was once believed that a predisposition to shyness was permanent; if you were a shy child, you were a shy child—those were just the cards you were dealt. This is no longer true today. We now know that the expression of genes is not set in stone, but rather must be activated to be expressed. Though your child may have the genetic predisposition for shyness, if that gene is not turned on, or if genes that relate to a more outgoing personality are activated instead, she will not be as shy as she might have been.

In his book *The Relationship Code,* psychologist David Reiss describes a twelve-year study at George Washington University in which researchers examined the effect of parental intervention on the shyness gene of 720 pairs of related adolescents. The study indicates that how you raise your child really does makes a difference. "Biology is not destiny," writes Reiss, who was cited in a *Newsweek* article describing the study. "Many genetic factors, powerful as they may be in psychological development, exert their influence only through the good offices of the family."[3] More proof that you are your child's true gene therapist.

It's important to understand that your response to the first appearance of negative personality traits affects the expression and outcome of those genes—and, ultimately, how your child turns out. If your toddler is difficult, cranky, and acting out in aggressive ways, you will most likely respond to his behavior in a heightened state. A problem child can bring out the worst in her parents. When signs of antisocial behavior surface, it can trigger a negative response, which in turn starts a loop of negative responses to this problem behavior. If you aren't conscious and paying attention, you can get caught in a cycle that only serves to stimulate your child's nascent antisocial characteristics. In other words, if you're not careful, you can end up unintentionally reinforcing the very trait you wish to abolish. That's because your social interactions—and reactions—to your child determine which genes are activated and have everything to do with your child's temperament.

Bottom line: when you fail to exert your influence correctly, you might not only reinforce traits that undermine your child's happiness and success, but you may also keep her from ever reaching her full capacity. Your decision to either take control and create an appropriate environment to address your child's behavior or to continue a cycle of negative reactions and negative reinforcement will determine whether your child sets out on a healthy course or develops a behavior disorder. To determine how to meet your child where he is and create an environment that amplifies or represses his innate traits, you have to be there and know your child. This makes all the difference in the world.

Scientists and educators alike have long understood that the blossoming of a child's aptitudes and gifts are not a foregone conclusion; under certain circumstances, her opportunity to develop and realize her innate talents and abilities can be lost. Just as a butterfly must first grow in a cocoon to be nourished and protected, so must your child be enriched before she is ready to fly. Parental involvement in early childhood, including both education and child development, is essential right from the beginning. If you miss the opportunity to influence those critical moments of development, you may miss your chance.

According to psychologist Dr. Benjamin Bloom, children reach half of their IQ by the age of four.[4] Thus, time is of the essence—there really is no time to lose. You and your child are on a challenging journey together, and only you, her parent, has the power to recognize your child's full endowments and direct them. Not only does important learning take place in those critical early years, but also when the actual structure of your child's brain develops and takes shape. It is that architecture that will influence your child's linguistic, cognitive, social, and emotional abilities, from now through adulthood.

Yet each child is an individual, born with a specific, unique personality recognized immediately by her loving parents. Geneticist Dr. Dean Hamer suggested that "we come in large part ready-made from the factory."[5] But neuroscience today tells us that that's only half the story. Nothing happens in a vacuum. We now know that though we are born with a particular set of genes that define us, even the atmosphere in the birthing room affects the expression of those genes. Right from the moment of conception, the environment of the fetus will suppress or enhance her genes' DNA. Right from the beginning, it is mainly you, Mom and Dad, who create those experiences. For example, if Mom is under stress, cortisol can cross her placenta and impact baby. If Mother's stress is consistent, then her baby is getting too much cortisol regularly and as a result is placed on high alert. This is the baby who seems to have a condition similar to ADD, or ADHD, at birth, when actually she is responding to the experience of a highly stressed mother. So when we speak of the effect of the environment on a child's DNA, that environment is for the most part her parents . . . her home team, her only means of support.

On the other hand, studies indicate that there is a reciprocal relationship that develops between parent and child, and it is that relationship that can determine the interaction between you and your baby. For instance, if baby's initial personality appears to be one of calm and quiet, parents respond in kind. However, if baby is cranky or colicky, anxious, or on high alert, Mom and Dad may react in a stressful or even aggressive manner.

Dr. Robert Plomin, one of the contributors to the now-famous book *The Relationship Code*, states that "parents' behavior reflects genetic differences in their children." He goes on to say that basically "if you've got an antisocial kid, you reflect that back in your parenting."[6] In other words, your child's genetic makeup may make him difficult initially, and your reaction to your frustrations can promote anxious and even abusive parenting, which has the effect of negatively reinforcing your baby's difficult behavior. The opposite is also true: an "easy" child stimulates a generous, empathetic, and compassionate parenting style. The key is to pay attention to your child's early behavior, right from birth, and immediately establish an environment that elicits more appropriate child behavior. We used to call this approach *behavior modification*, but now we know that it is so much more than that. In a sense, you are consciously parenting against type, against what would normally be an appropriate response to difficult child behavior. Instead of getting angry, punishing, or even becoming abusive toward a problematic and possibly antisocial baby, you have the opportunity to step back deliberately, recognize and acknowledge your baby's behavior, and take a more consistent, inclusive, and interactive approach, including active listening and heightened ranges of communication. Giving your baby the space to emote, empathically communicating with her right from the beginning, when all she recognizes as calm is the soothing sound of your voice, invests her in the outcome of her behavior while teaching her empathy for herself and others. I call this the *empathic process*, and it can be used in a limited way during the earliest stages of childhood as a strategy that will serve your baby well throughout her life. Here is how it works:

THE EMPATHIC PROCESS/KNOW THE RULES

Step 1: One parent talks about the rules for discussion and creates a safe and trusting environment that includes mutual respect. As we build a win/win environment, we must remember never to embarrass, demean, or discount children's feelings. Never be critical, for in conflict resolution, the key is to model valuing your child, so that he will value himself and, therefore, others. The parent opens the conversation to discuss problems in a constructive way. The key to this communication is to actively listen without defense. The person who speaks has everyone's full attention. Each family member gets to speak an equal amount of time while reserving an equal block of time in which the family interacts to problem-solve.

Step 2: The children are invested in the conversation and are guided to think of positive ways to resolve conflicts—in essence, a win/win brainstorming session, discussing positive options for problem-solving.

Step 3: Finally, the children are invited to pick some positive behavior that is proactive as a solution to the problem discussed that day during the empathic process.

The Empathic Process allows children, through empathy for one another as well as their parents, to learn conflict resolution and problem-solving, as well as five principals of citizenship for a successful empathic relationship:

1. Mutuality—mutual respect.
2. Inner Value—self-value and, therefore, value for others.
3. Responsibility and reliability.
4. Trust.
5. Commitment—obligations.

Each interactive dialogue should be guided by a parent to develop tools for children to cope with stress and become self-empowered. These include choice/change; override the fear of change; proactive/not reactive; and growth.

Finally, the empathic process invests each participant in the outcome of conflict resolution, including the rules and consequences. When your child is invested in the process, he is more likely to follow the rules.

As we mentioned earlier in this chapter, shyness is another obvious trait that presents itself in infancy. The shy child is fearful of change, anxiously crying when assaulted by new sounds, new people, new voices, and new toys. Your shy child is extracautious, having a short fuse when responding to the unexpected. Approximately 20 percent of all babies present characteristics of shyness.

According to psychologist Dr. Jerome Kagan, the characteristics of shyness exhibit a high genetic factor. The shyness gene, therefore, is inherited and presents itself in children who are overly reactive to the unfamiliar. Therefore, neurochemistry has determined one-half of your baby's personality with the emergence of a low threshold for the unexpected. As early as four months, Kagan states that he can identify "better than chance" whether a child will be shy.[7] Yet genes aren't the whole story, according to psychologist David Reiss.[8] Thus, the other 50 percent of your baby's personality, including her shyness, is influenced by her experiences. It is those experiences that can teach your baby how to self-manage and self-regulate her behavior so that she can become socially functional. Will she ever be Jacqueline Kennedy? No. But can she ultimately be comfortable with herself and others? A resounding *yes*. Your baby can be taught to adapt and adjust to her shyness by the environment you create to help her become more socially comfortable. But first you must gain your baby's trust, so that you can modify her behavior. Remember that trust is based on experience. So if baby can learn to trust that Mom is coming to the rescue, even though she is frustrated by a new person, new toy, or small delay in feeding, then she can learn to suspend her reaction for a little while, delaying gratification. By teaching her in small controlled increments of both frustration and trust, you are creating a new habit for baby that allows her to overcome her shyness through a dependable behavior modification model.

If, on the other hand, you are too lenient and mollycoddle your shy child, he might in all probability stay shy. However, if you invite other toddlers over for a designated time period, perhaps five minutes, guaranteeing that the visitors will be gone in that short time, and you keep your word, then you are building your baby's trust and security, while creating a new, positive behavior. It is easy to see that your genes are not the whole story, that it is the environment that amplifies or suppresses those genes. Therefore, what determines which genes direct which behavior is dependent upon the positive and negative reinforcement of each of your baby's experiences within his own environment. At birth, baby displays personality characteristics that either seduce or repel his parents, depending on Mom's and Dad's temperaments. Therefore, the link between nature and nurture is ironically bridged by the addition of parental responses. If baby displays behavior that induces warm and gentle feelings from Mom and Dad, they will respond in kind. If baby is cold and aloof or temperamental and irritable, then parents are more likely to be punishing. This creates a loop in which baby's genes are either positively or negatively reinforced. But if you are a conscious parent and are aware of your baby's inborn temperament, then you can relate to baby in a way that either enhances or tamps down his specific personality characteristics.

Another example of how parents can modify gene expression is in relation to verbal IQ. If baby is talkative, Mom and Dad will most likely talk back, building an associate mass inside baby's developing brain. Then, that chatty toddler can elicit quality reading time from both his parents that will enrich and improve his cognitive, linguistic, and social abilities. This of course leads to confidence and self-esteem, as baby is also responding to the pleasure principle as Mom and Dad delight in his performance. This positive reinforcement leads to competence, as he can now extend out beyond his comfort zone to express himself better, thus having the potential to become an early reader.

The behaviors that build a bridge to influence baby's personality include:

1. Parental response to social or antisocial baby
2. Consistent behavior modification using same approach consistently to alter or change inherited characteristics
3. Nurturing those characteristics that are desirable while demonstrating empathy and compassion consistently for baby's nascent and antisocial behavior
4. Following the empathic process (page 21)
5. Being a trustworthy parent, remembering that trust is based on experience

6. Being a reliable parent so that baby can count on what you say and learn to not only trust you, but to trust himself and the outer world, as well

7. Paying attention, acknowledging, and identifying baby's gifts and deficits so that you can deliberately affect them at the beginning when the plastic brain is still developing

8. Finally, appropriate parenting by meeting your child where he is temperamentally and intervening by orchestrating an applicable learning model

It is in the lab that we see the reflection of how the nature/nurture paradigm manifests. Since monkeys are so metabolically similar to humans, they are often the subject of such research. Looking at how their personalities develop, scientists first studied the relationship between a mother monkey and her baby. Dr. Stephen Suomi determined that 20 percent of the monkeys he observed displayed the same metabolic changes, such as rapid heartbeat, that are present in shy children. Furthermore, 5–10 percent of the baby monkeys demonstrated characteristics that were overly impulsive, causing them to antagonize and challenge older males, as well as to participate in dangerous and risky behavior. Dr. Suomi's study indicated that there was a difference between the metabolism of the shy monkey and that of the overly impulsive monkey. In the brain of the impulsive monkey, there was a lower level of serotonin than normal. Serotonin supports impulse control while suppressing impulsive behavior in all primates. With a low metabolic input of serotonin, both the monkey and the human act out by exhibiting low impulse control, as well as risky activities beyond their capacity to perform. Other characteristics of low serotonin include emotional outbursts and confrontation. This difference in the serotonin-transporter is the culprit, as it determines how much serotonin is distributed to the cells. Monkeys who received a larger serotonin-transporter gene experience a more tranquil and composed demeanor, which allows them to think more clearly and critically. Moreover, states Dr. Suomi, those monkeys who inherited a shorter serotonin-transporter gene have an "impaired serotonin metabolism, leading to aggressive behavior, and a tendency to over consume alcohol."[9]

Yet neither man nor monkey is captive to his inherit genetic makeup. In both cases, baby's social development is largely determined by Mom. For when a nurturing mom replaces a typical mom in the lab, her nurturing changes the outcome of either a high-strung or a stressful baby monkey. Actually, the adoptive mom, who offers more nurturing, alters the stress level of baby, by going out of her way to sidestep anxiety-producing experiences. This behavior approach teaches baby to solicit help in navigating stressful waters, and he often outgrows his anxious sense of self. What is happening here is that the nurturing mom is in effect changing her adoptive baby monkey's biology. It is through her calming techniques that she elevates the serotonin in the metabolism of her adoptive baby, bringing it up to a more average level. Suomi suggests, "Virtually all of the outcomes can be altered substantially by early experiences. Biology just provides a different set of probabilities."[10]

It is within this range of probabilities that environment expresses its most important impact. Though we are born with an inherited and potential persona, it is the effect of our early experiences that molds and shapes those particular genes, deciding which ones are stimulated and which are suppressed. And those early experiences rely profoundly on Mom. There seems to be a 50/50 split between parental responsibility in the nature/ nurture paradigm. In another study, rat pups were observed as their mothers licked and groomed them. The rats whose moms were especially attentive developed brains with genes that appeared to be kicked up a notch, and as a result, these rat pups developed less stress hormone. Therefore, they were in a sense inoculated against stress. According to Dr. Michael Meany, the rats whose mothers nurtured them were less likely to fear new and unusual experiences and were more willing to experiment with trial and error within their surroundings. The rat pups whose moms were less attentive had brain genes that were suppressed and therefore developed more anxiety and stress.

The only variable in this study was the attention Mom paid to her pup through licking and grooming. Dr. Stephen Suomi suggests that "there's complete interaction between genes and rearing condition."[11] So though the nature/nurture relationship creates the structure for how baby adjusts to life experiences, the outcome of his reactions is not completely preordained.

THE SENSITIVE CHILD

When looking at personality characteristics, it is important to remember that your response is paramount in interventions and remediations. For instance, a highly sensitive child is more tuned into the environment around him, picking up the nuances. He senses and often feels when others threaten him, discount him, or don't like him. Dr. Stanley Greenspan suggests that this child should be the subject of extra nurturing to keep him from feeling fearful.[12] Treating this child kindly, and with empathy and determination, helps him approach tests and trials with more confidence. These personality changes can be seen at as early as two years of age if you are consistent and firm in the way you guide baby through stressful situations.

THE HYPERACTIVE CHILD[13]

The hyperactive child is like a perpetual hurricane, always creating storms wherever she goes. It is this baby who is most vulnerable for developmental delays, as her overactive behavior and lack of impulse control can create negative feedback from her parents. Caught in the loop of negative reinforcement, this child can devolve into aggression. As a parent, you can confront this hyperactivity by structuring an environment that is contained and organized with few distractions. This allows baby to self-manage stress and develop control. Teaching baby the rules of what is and is not appropriate through role-playing and particularly self-regulating games can help baby adapt more successfully to her environment.

THE INTROVERTED CHILD[14]

The introverted child appears withdrawn and detached, needing downtime to restore his energy, finding calm and poise in his own company. He's that easy child who experiences discomfort and anxiety when exposed to too much outside stimulation. He is also the child who is extremely creative, since time alone gives him the opportunity to use his imagination. However, he also runs the risk of becoming too self-oriented, lacking in acceptable social skills. With this child, it is important to focus on balance, recognizing that he needs downtime to restore, but also firmly encouraging specific increments of time for social interaction.

THE DISTRACTED CHILD[15]

The distracted child often seems to be lost in a world of his own, daydreaming rather than paying attention to time, directions, and sequencing. He appears to be out of time and out of step with the task at hand. Intervention with the distracted child should include games that reward attention to time and space within specific increments. By teaching your toddler the rules and directions of a game that includes sequencing, he will soon transfer that ability, increasing his connection to time.

THE DIFFICULT CHILD[16]

From the time your baby is born, he is reaching for freedom, independence, and self-control. As a result, the wise parent creates opportunities for baby to experience a sense of control. For example, choosing one pair of socks to put on in the morning from a group of three. By allowing baby to assert his independence, you are suspending the need for him to become controlling—a personality profile that will create later problems within his peer group.

DISCIPLINE

We can all remember the experiments of B. F. Skinner, when he told us that behavior modification (positive and negative reinforcement) was the key to discipline. Though there have been many different philosophies along the way, the one thing that has remained stable is that children do react to positive and negative reinforcement. The elements missing from Skinner's experiment, in which he placed his child in a box to contain her environment while studying her responses to different variables, are love and empathy. When added to consistent positive and negative reinforcement, love and empathy are the necessary elements that complete the process of behavior modification. By positively reinforcing the desired behavior and negatively reinforcing the undesired behavior through rules and consequences, your baby will learn to adapt and adjust her behavior and therefore self-regulate.[17]

From the time your baby is four months old, you become keenly aware of his personality. Is he social? Is he calm? Is he anxious? Is he aggressive? These are all things that you begin to see right at the start. By two years of age, aptly called the Terrible Twos, baby asserts himself with his favorite new word: *no!* Baby is fighting you for control, but there's a method to his madness: he is actually making a cognitive leap. Your two-year-old toddler finds his way into anything that's not out of his reach—cleaning products, medicines, dishes, food—and he delights in experimenting with everything. It is at this point that Mom comes up with the common phrase "no touch," and baby looks directly at his mom and touches anyway. The challenge here is more about your baby testing your response to his behavior. This is how he learns not only about the things around him, but the reactions of the people around him. This is what Albert Bandura called *social learning*. Your two-year-old is at an important cognitive marker and is finding his own sense of self. "No" can easily become a game at this stage, so it's important for you to offer creative choices so that your baby can feel independent while you stay in control.[18]

Hitting is another favorite two-year-old activity, one that often gets out of hand. Not only is it physical, but it also can be a game or a challenge. As with everything else, early intervention is important here. Until your child is a toddler, discipline will be neither understood nor effective. However, after nine months, babies start to recognize what is and is not acceptable. At about eighteen months of age, baby is getting ready emotionally to be able to respond to discipline. But until then, the nervous system is not developed, and discipline is not only ineffective but inappropriate. Discipline is all about being age-appropriate, consistent, and geared to your child's specific developmental period. Your two-year-old takes great pleasure in affecting things, including hitting, throwing, and being physically active. It would be asking too much to expect a toddler to sit for long periods of time or to play with other children. A two-year-old is uncomfortable with other children anyway—and when presented with others, they parallel play rather than socially interact.[19]

WHAT TODDLER TANTRUMS MEAN[20]

Toddlers can sometimes seem like aliens to their parents. One minute your toddler is playing happily with blocks with a big smile on her face, and the next she's throwing those blocks and screaming at the top of her lungs. What causes toddler emotions to go from 0 to 60? While the answer depends on your individual child and circumstances of the moment, her development at different stages also has a lot to do with those tantrums.

TODDLER TANTRUMS: AGE TWO[21]

Your two-year-old is actually experiencing a sense of independence, and you will notice that your toddler wants to do things by himself. For example, he may not want to wear the clothes you choose, or he might resist bedtime, dinnertime, or some particular toy. Your two-year-old will express his temper tantrums in myriad ways: hitting, biting, fighting, crying, kicking. The central theme connecting the temper tantrums is your toddler's desire to "do it by himself," to get his way and resist control.

TODDLER TANTRUMS: AGE THREE[22]

Your three-year-old is most likely less emotional, and her tantrums will reflect that by occurring less often and with less intensity. On the other hand, because temper tantrums typically work and give the child what she desires, it can become a reinforced tactic. The temper tantrum plays out in a similar dynamic at this age; arguing, kicking, screaming, hitting.

TODDLER TANTRUMS: AGE FOUR[23]

By now, your four-year-old has better language and motor skills, so he *is* more independent. Your four-year-old's language capacity now allows him to tell you how he feels, what is on his mind, and why he's angry. This allows your four-year-old to collaborate with you by solving his issues, and, when necessary, even compromising. Temper tantrums become more verbal. For example, your four-year-old may say, "I hate you." Don't take it to heart. He is limited in his ability to express himself and doesn't developmentally understand the word *hate*. His better motor and physical skills allow him to throw things as well as hit others. Furthermore, your four-year-old now possesses better motor skills to either run away from you or hide.

As frustrating as toddler tantrums can be, it is important to remember that your toddler is undergoing important developmental milestones during ages two to four. When tantrums happen, they are often age-appropriate and not deliberately meant to embarrass or harm you. However, it is also important to try your best to prevent toddler tantrums before they start, and then when they do occur, to handle them in ways that can help teach your child appropriate behavior. For example, you're in the middle of the grocery store, and suddenly your toddler starts to have a meltdown. What do you do?

First: with toddlers, it is important to not abandon them when punishing them, so even though you may use timeout as a technique, have a short duration for timeout and don't isolate your toddler from your sight. Understand that during a tantrum, your child is no longer in control. So whenever possible, make eye contact, even if it means getting down physically to his eye level. This will help shift the excitability and energy of the situation and begin to calm things down.

TIPS FOR TAMING TODDLER TANTRUMS: AGE TWO

If a two-year-old eventually gets his way, he'll most likely stop his temper tantrum. But like anything emotional, when feelings continue to escalate, it is harder to defuse. The best course of action is to change your two-year-old's environment: pick him up and take him somewhere else. It breaks the cycle, relieves the tension, and distracts him from the object of his attention.

TIPS FOR TAMING TODDLER TANTRUMS: AGE THREE

At age three, if you take control and do not reward negative behavior, temper tantrums will occur less often and with less conflict. Furthermore, if you give small amounts of control to your toddler—for example, allowing her to select clothing or food from options you have preapproved—your three-year-old will feel a sense of independence that will satisfy her developmental stage and her need to push out in a way that fosters a secure sense of herself. As at age two, distraction still goes a long way in stopping your three-year-old's temper tantrum while you're in the middle of it.

TIPS FOR TAMING TODDLER TANTRUMS: AGE FOUR

Because your four-year-old has better motor and physical skills, he may attempt to strike out during tantrums. It is very important to never allow your four-year-old to hit or punch you. It is never too soon to teach respect, and this lesson is the first time that your child will comprehend a true boundary—one of the most important lessons of his life. Furthermore, your four-year-old has better motor skills to either run away from you or hide, so remember to stay calm, stay cool, and stay in control.

At the end of the day, nothing serves a challenging situation, such as dealing with toddler tantrums, like a good sense of humor and parenting perspective. Don't take these tantrums too seriously and certainly do not take toddler tantrums personally. They're all part of growing up, helping your toddler learn how to handle both new emotions and newfound independence. In the middle of it all, it's important to remember that *this too shall pass*.

PREVENTING TODDLER TANTRUMS

To prevent temper tantrums before they begin:

1. Reward positive behavior and do not reward negative behavior.
2. Choose your battles wisely. If you come down hard on your child and overcontrol him for everything, he may ultimately break out over something small and lose control.
3. Parents are entitled to parent. That means that when you want your child to perform a particular action for you, state it as a declarative sentence, not as a question. For example, don't say: "Do you want to go to sleep?" Say instead: "It's bedtime."
4. If a temper tantrum is about to start, shift the field through distraction and by changing the environment. If it's a young child, just pick him up and take him somewhere else.
5. Sleep is important to our emotions. A tired, cranky child is more likely to have a temper tantrum than a well-rested child.
6. Structure and routine are great ways to defuse temper tantrums, because your child feels secure when he is in a contained environment and knows what's expected of him.
7. Add some humor; don't overreact or take things to heart.
8. Prepare your child for change. Your child is no different from anyone else, and he is especially vulnerable to transitions because of his immaturity. Thus, if there is something he has to end or begin, give him a little notice, and a little time, before you either remove him or insert him into a new activity.
9. Keep your promises and don't make promises you can't keep. Your child thinks concretely, and therefore more emotionally, so if you break your word, you can break his heart.

10. And finally, remember to give your child freedom within limits. Structure the choices that you can live with by presenting your child with those choices and then letting him choose one.

Let's say you have consciously done all you could from the above list to prevent a tantrum, and your child still breaks down. It happens. Know that we moms and dads have most likely all been in your shoes at one time or another.

This doesn't mean that you should ignore your child's acting out, but make the discipline fit the crime. Knowing where your child is developmentally will help you know what kind of discipline is effective for his age and stage. Yet there are times when your toddler is too distraught to focus and give you his attention. In those cases, it is best to change his environment. Take him away from what is upsetting him, to another room or even outside. This will help distract him and give him a chance to recover emotionally. Then, you can reestablish the things that really are important, such as no hitting, no touch when danger is around, and the things that are worth fighting for, like bedtime.

What you're teaching your child, from his earliest stage of development, is how to self-manage his feelings. In effect, nature conspires to help you protect and ensure his survival by making him responsive to both extrinsic and intrinsic encouragement and rewards. As a result, believe it or not, your baby wants rules and regulations. This is how structure leads to security. In a very real way, a loving, firm approach can lead to a discipline model that helps even a difficult child relate to positive reinforcement and freedom within limits.

Children are social learners, and they learn by imitation, so if at all possible, capture your child doing something positive and reinforce it immediately with a hug, a cuddle, a smile, or a positive word or phrase. Soon your baby will reach for those warm fuzzies coming from you and will try hard to elicit them. Most importantly, be what you want to see, remembering that your child, as a social learner, will imitate your behavior. If, like me, you walk when you are on the telephone, your baby, like mine, will do the same. It will make you laugh, it will make you cry, but most important, it should make you realize how important you really are. Those little eyes are following you everywhere.

Because baby will emulate your behavior, you can see how damaging the concept of spanking is. In fact, studies indicate that children who are spanked consistently become more combative.[24] Not only does spanking have only a temporary impact, but it's also embarrassing and profoundly humiliating, as it both stings the body and wounds the soul. Moreover, toddlers generally forget the reason they were spanked in the first place, and the purpose of the discipline is often missed. Your toddler is mostly preoccupied with testing himself against his environment while pushing his behavior limits without a developed moral code. His work includes a full exploration of his local surroundings, where everything is new and interesting. You may find yourself at this point trying to discover for yourself what behavior you're looking for, while determining the best way to implement it. It is easy to see how parents find themselves in a tug-of-war with baby. This is a recipe for stress, not only for you, but also for your toddler. And because parents are under so much stress already, often holding down two jobs, they can easily slip into what may seem like a quick fix and use spanking as a discipline tool. Yet even when caught in the moment, parents have to maintain control by overriding their impulse to spank while finding more positive means of correcting their children's behavior. Often, parents believe that children act out or misbehave on purpose, when in reality, they may simply be trying to get the attention of a parent who has been gone all day.

The discipline choices you make today will in large part determine whether your toddler grows up to be happy and well-adjusted or a difficult, unhappy young adult. Consistent spanking can create a nonempathetic bully. Too many years in timeout can create a child whose desperate need for attention makes him socially uncomfortable. On the other hand, role- modeling and being what you want to see teaches children, by your example, the dos and don'ts of appropriate social interaction. Most importantly, my empathic process connects parent and child, investing them both in the outcome of their mutual behavior.

Here, children are learning by doing and are participating in the consequences of their own discipline. By sharing a range of possibilities to solve the discipline problem, your child is more likely to adhere to the solution she's helped craft. Along the way, your empathic behavior toward your child is modeling empathy for her, a characteristic that she will not only imitate, but also pass on.

To know your child is to know everything, including the prevailing motive for his behavior. By actively listening to your child, while touching his hand and looking him in the eye, you can connect and hear what's on his mind. By using my empathic process, both you and your child have the opportunity to talk about your feelings without defense, giving a safe space in which anger and fear can easily be expressed, in an atmosphere of empathy and love. As a result, your child becomes invested in the consequences of his own behavior and discipline. This discourages uncontrolled outbursts, as your child learns to become the master of his own ship. This is how you teach your child to become self-actualized and less aggressive.

Now you can let your child be your guide and tell you what ails him. In the end, spanking will not incur either love or respect, but remnants of fear, anger, and humiliation which will echo like traces of hurt through the future of your relationship, even into adulthood. To recognize, acknowledge, and understand your child, to really see him, allows you to set the pace: not only for his future, but for yours.

For younger children (under one year of age), who can't possibly understand the concept of discipline, it is important simply to change the environment when things get out of hand or to gently restrain dangerous behavior such as hitting, kicking, and biting. By holding baby securely while speaking in a soothing tone, moving away from the object of his attention, you quickly stop aggressive behavior. It is best when restraining your child from hitting or kicking to have him face you while you hold him and speak to him in a soothing voice, calmly saying "no" to the bad behavior, while expressing love and empathy by your demeanor.

You can support your toddler by helping her express and develop her independence if you allow her the power of choice. Let your child choose from a predetermined, designated set of three of anything, giving her a structure in which you have the final word. This will give your toddler a sense of control, guiding her toward both an intrinsic and extrinsic reward. See your child in context, appreciating that if she doesn't eat everything you put before her, it may be simply because she's a toddler, unable to sit for long periods of time, either in a high chair or at a table. With children under five, it is important to keep mealtime a happy time, rather than a war zone. It's better for your digestion and hers. So go with the flow, keeping in mind that if she's sleeping well and eliminating each day, she's doing okay.

If your child's temperament is anxious or high-strung, overactive or emotional, unable to sit still for short increments of time or focus, he may have ADD or ADHD. Another behavioral red flag is the baby who isn't demonstrating any deliberate grasping, cooing, or facial expressions by eight months. This is the toddler who at two years of age has difficulty with social interactions and cognition. All of these responses signal problems ahead, as they indicate that baby may be experiencing either cognitive or social delays, or possibly both. All of these problems are really problems and require you to seek professional help for both you and baby.

WHAT YOU SHOULD LOOK FOR[25]

0–1 Month	At zero to one month old, baby should react to outside noises, light, and colors. Baby will respond positively to cooing, rocking, touch, and all bonding behavior. He will also be responsive to your voice, your touch, being held and cuddled, and active looking and listening—in general, one-on-one attention. At this stage of development, there is only one person in baby's life: you. In fact, baby doesn't even see you as separate from himself.

2 Months	Baby's only way to let you know how she feels is to vocalize those wants and needs. If she's in distress, she'll cry, if she's comfortable and her needs are being met or if she's contented and joyful, she'll gurgle and coo. But remember that from the time baby is born, you are her entire world. She has no sense of time and space, so when you're out of sight or sound, the baby experiences anxiety and fear. If you are consistently gone for long periods of time, baby feels abandonment. This elevates the cortisol in her blood and can have a long-term effect on the development of baby's brain. When going out and leaving baby with someone other than your mate, be sure baby is familiar with the caretaker.
3 Months	At this point, baby is much more animated, makes eye contact, and expresses pleasure and pain in the usual ways, either smiling or crying. He will let you know exactly how he feels by communicating with you through different tonal cries for Mother, Father, and familial caretakers. It is at this stage baby is starting to differentiate the various people in his social sphere and may even begin to discriminate between those that he likes and doesn't.
4 Months	Now baby's personality begins to shine. She gurgles and smiles when engaging in creative play and may become fussy if that playtime is disturbed. She is still receptive to whatever activity is offered to her; for example, games such as peekaboo or a new cuddly stuffed animal. Here, we see baby's interest in all things on full display as she examines any toy put before her. This is also the beginning of baby exerting her first desire for freedom. Now she may cry to be picked up or wiggle away when someone holds her. At four months, baby has become a little social animal, wanting to participate and be in a relationship. This is when babies start acting out for attention.
5 Months	Baby inserts himself into all possible things. In a sense, he's pushing out beyond his experience by grasping for toys, expressing emotional distress, and starting to learn the give-and-take of social bantering. Emotionally, baby has become aware of how to mediate some of his stress load as the developing brain matures.
6 Months	It is at this stage that baby may negatively react to nonfamily members. He does, on the other hand, like little people closer to his size and age. Now baby is learning how to interact with others. As a result, this is the first opportunity you have as a parent to begin to impress your will on baby's behavior. For example, if baby touches something dangerous or fragile, you can say to him, "No touch," and carefully remove baby from the disqualified object. Furthermore, removing baby from the scene of the crime by changing his environment will also connect baby to the consequence of his behavior. The key here is to be consistent.

7 Months	From the time baby is born, he is seeking freedom. Now he is beginning to learn how to impose his will on others. As baby resists direction by establishing his own authority, it is important to give him the safe space to begin his independence. At this point, baby's feelings are front and center as he makes faces and evokes humor deliberately. Also, baby now recognizes that Mom and Dad and other family members can be bent to his will as he motions to be picked up, carried, hugged, and cuddled. The first pucker of a kiss makes itself seen at this age.
8 Months	Baby is beginning to see the difference between himself and others. He can distinguish between the reflection of his face in a mirror and may even interact with it. Further, your baby is now aware of his attachment to you and doesn't see you as separate, but rather as an appendage. Therefore, he become possessive of you as he simultaneously asserts more independence. In a sense, he reaches out to explore his surroundings while looking back to make sure that you are there and that he's okay. This is the first time that baby actively secures himself to you when strangers appear.
9 Months	Social learning becomes evident in the nine-month-old. As he performs for approval, he acts out for both fun and applause, looking for a positive reaction from those he loves. Your baby at this juncture is beginning to evaluate others' emotions while copying them. For example, if you laugh, baby will try to emulate your laugh. Games such as peekaboo, "how big is baby?" and "where is the light?" become a source of pleasure as he participates while soliciting your positive response.
10 Months	By ten months of age, baby displays a variety of feelings, and as possessiveness raises its ugly head, so does jealousy. Further, the focus of this anxiety is often the one challenge for his mother: a sibling. Your baby may cry or even assault the brother or sister that comes between him and his mother. For now, your baby is socially aware and keenly tuned in to positive and negative reactions.
11 Months	Your baby can now transfer some of his attachment to you onto an inanimate object, such as a favorite toy. Moreover, you may find that your child is exerting himself and finding his place in the family while learning socially, emulating new and interesting noises and motions.
12 Months	At twelve months, your baby expresses his dissatisfaction with your leaving home without him. Because he has no sense of time, he feels frightened and abandoned when you leave. Part of preparing baby for your first outing is to familiarize him with the caretaker who will be watching him while you're gone. Then, practice and rehearse leaving baby for small increments of time, perhaps only ten to fifteen minutes at first, so that baby is prepared. Next, talk baby through the first time you really leave him, making sure that his favorite security toy or blanket is present as an attachment substitute for you. Instruct your babysitter to absolutely not let baby cry it out in his room alone while you are gone, but rather comfort him, rock him, soothe him for as long as it takes for him to self-adjust. If your first excursion is a small one, and you build up time away little by little, your baby will learn to self-soothe and look forward to time with his babysitter.

13 Months	Your baby can now participate in social gatherings. He can have fun running and playing, though he is egocentric and therefore will want to be the center of attention. For the first time, you can really see his persona express itself as he participates with others with laughter and full-on exhibitionism.
14 Months	Your baby is more willing to assert himself. Now a beginning walker, he may even exhibit small moments of rage, tossing toys close at hand to demonstrate his frustration. Until the age of two, baby will remain a parallel player, preferring his own company, his own toys. But he still likes to perform in front of friends and family. Once baby starts walking, it is time to make your house a safe space, including moving sharp objects, medicines, cleaning products, and so forth out of baby's reach.
15 Months	Now baby is able to demonstrate his emotions using specific and definite actions. There is a desire and a point to his behavior. Your child has an objective in mind when he announces his feelings. Baby is cognizant of his sphere of influence and recognizes when those in his community of support are absent. If he shares a toy for a moment, he will almost immediately think better of the idea and retract the overture.
16 Months	Your child is reaching for independence. He is maturing cognitively, socially, emotionally, and physically. He is now developing self-awareness and beginning to rely on his own judgment. For the first time, the word *no* becomes your baby's favorite word, and when upset he may even strike out in frustration. This is the beginning of your child's journey toward autonomy. For the first time, he is testing himself against his environment to gain a sense of control as well as capacity.
17 Months	By seventeen months old, your baby shows a clear understanding of direction, his vocabulary has increased, and he's familiar with your expressions of both approval and disapproval. He is also beginning to recognize appropriate limits. If complimented, he'll smile; if reprimanded, he'll whimper. Baby is also now aware of strangers and may display reticence when he finds himself in an unfamiliar environment. Here, it is important to prepare baby for any unusual circumstance, and to be aware that baby has now displayed a negativism that helps him express his own will against authority.
18 Months	Your child will now begin to escalate his use of the word *no* into the all-too-familiar temper tantrum. As baby becomes socialized, he feels the need to exercise his own desires while experiencing new and intriguing skills. Because your baby is still unsure of appropriate conduct, with minimal comprehension of right and wrong, he engages in unpredictable behavior. Though your toddler still has no interest in sharing, he does need the social experience of relating to others and may exhibit intimacy by cuddling up to Mom or Dad, Grandma or Grandpa.

19 Months	Your toddler explorer now begins to reach beyond his limits as he displays interest not only in playing inside, but exploring outside, as well. You become his safe harbor as he embarks each day on a journey of discovery, looking back for your support. Though he enjoys social interaction, he is still not comfortable playing with other children. Further, your toddler's level of self-awareness makes him susceptible to both positive and negative reinforcement as his willingness to perform for approval gains importance. Therefore, focus on the conduct that involves safety, such as don't go near the street, no touch, no biting, no fighting, etc.
20 Months	Your toddler is still engaging in parallel play. In fact, his anxiety escalates when exposed to other children. Free play is most important at this stage, as baby creatively mimics the world about him. On the other hand, baby's escalating knowledge makes him more vulnerable to fear of the unknown: a rainstorm, a new pet, strangers, and the proverbial fear of the dark. Installing a night light and comforting and soothing baby are simple ways to alleviate the stress of fear and anxiety.
21 Months	Baby's personality is beginning to be on full display as he shows empathy and compassion. He is sensitive to the emotions of those around him, as he begins to self-regulate and delay gratification. Moreover, baby is becoming self-conscious and experiences feelings of guilt, shame, doubt, and empathy. Baby is developing a conscience and is now capable of showing his love through hugs and kisses. While interacting with others, baby still resists sharing, though he may return things that don't belong to him. This is not the time to make baby share; it will only create anxiety and stress. Follow baby's lead and allow him to self-regulate and become autonomous.
22 Months	Though your toddler is coming to the end of parallel play, he will still only back up to the baby he's involved with. He is learning through peer socialization to get along with other children, and if he violates the rules and grabs a toy, he might find himself the recipient of aggressive behavior. He is now developing inhibitory control and may try to do the right thing for an intrinsic reward. This is all part of self-regulation and is connected in a very real way to baby's temperament. Your child is now willing to comply and collaborate with other children. This period of self-regulation foreshadows the confidence of self-reliance that is just around the corner. Therefore, this is the right time to begin to help baby adjust to small increments of time away from Mom and Dad.
23 Months	Your baby is exhibiting a committed compliance, which is the beginning stage of conscience development. Here, your baby starts to internalize your values and rules. Until this point, compliance has been more situational, but now your baby demonstrates specific patterns of behavior and internalization of societal conduct. Your toddler is willing to cooperate when well bonded and securely attached to Mom and Dad. Guidance should be gentle rather than forceful. He is sensitive to unfamiliar situations and may express the fear of rejection. Though he likes alone time, he is also profoundly attracted to his siblings, mimicking their behavior and toddling after them. This is a great opportunity for Mom to support siblings by organizing a specific time for your toddler to interact with them, giving sibs a much-needed break.

GAIL GROSS

24 Months	Welcome to the Terrible Twos, when baby can easily become frustrated. In an effort to become self-actualized, your toddler exerts his will as he strives for independence. Here, Mom and Dad can help baby gain self-control, confidence, and competence by offering him opportunities to choose for himself. Know your child, his temperament and personality, so that you can create an environment that is safe, flexible, and positive. At this stage, baby is articulate and therefore can tell you what he wants and how he feels. If baby has been well bonded, he is beginning to trust himself as he trusts his parents. He will interact with others and primarily learns through imitation. Possessiveness rears its ugly head at this point, and you may see signs of jealousy if a new brother or sister is introduced into the family unit. Such an event, handled with TLC, can help baby accept his new sib. On the other hand, if baby is left alone with his feelings of jealousy and insecurity, he may regress back to an earlier stage of childhood.
25–29 Months	The two-to-three-year-old is narcissistic in his behavior: his life revolves around himself, and his main desire is to have his immediate needs met. His worldview is that everyone is like him. Temper tantrums are most active at this stage, as your toddler tries to manipulate and boss those around him. Your child is refining his skills of interaction and therefore trying out what does and does not work to his benefit. He can tell you when he's happy or sad and will show you if he is fearful or anxious. He is possessively attached to his parents and siblings and may resent the incursion of others. He does, on the other hand, like being around other children and is forming the idea of friendship. Remind your child of the rules when challenged, use timeout when necessary, always be consistent, and never allow yourself to be on the same level as your child. Keep calm, keep cool, and repeat your request gently.
30–36 Months	Your little acorn is beginning to sprout. He is starting to understand the difference between right and wrong and is learning to concentrate. He finds his place in the family unit and is well on his way to demonstrating empathy as well as shame and guilt. The need to be the center of attention has grown, and he resents sharing that attention with sibs. He's caught in the play of star power and doesn't want to give up the spotlight. He is in a stage of early socialization, readying himself for preschool. Of course, this first excursion away from Mom and Dad can create stress and fear, related to attachment anxiety. So it is important to support your toddler through this most important transition. Ultimately, your toddler will adjust to a new environment with new rules as he finds himself away from home several hours a day. It is important now to advocate for your child, be there when he needs you, and guide him through these earliest stages of separation. This is the time to teach your toddler the conduct necessary for childcare so that he can practice and rehearse and be prepared. The most important thing is to find the correct childcare for your particular child.

AGGRESSION

PREDISPOSED TO AGGRESSION[26]

It may surprise you to know that children are predisposed to aggression. As soon as your child gains motor control, he uses his hands and feet to both hit and kick others. The frequency for childhood aggression is escalated at about two years of age and increases until about four, when, through Mother's socializing as well as peer-group socialization, children learn the rule: that it is inappropriate to hit others.

Also, there are sexual differences in aggressive behavior—it appears that girls learn more quickly to sublimate their more violent tendencies through indirect aggression. For example, I'm sure you can all remember the clip of *Mean Girls* that makes one child or another an outcast, telling the others not to play with him or her. This passive-aggressive behavior can even be seen in toddlers. According to Freud, aggression is built into the psyche for survival but must be tamed in order to live in community.

GENETICS AND ENVIRONMENT

Studies of twins inform us that aggression is both genetic and environmental; in fact, it is about a 50/50 split. However, there are certain subsets of children who rarely use aggressive behavior, as well as about 4 percent who are genetically predisposed toward aggression. It is this subset of children who carry aggression into adolescence. Neuroscience tells us that these more genetically aggressive children appear to have low serotonin synthesis. This synthesis deficit promotes problems at home and in school, such as poor social interactions, potential criminality, the use of drugs and alcohol, poor work habits, and antisocial behavior in general.[27]

However, there are things that we can do for these children to lower the cycle of aggression and violence, including:

1. Parental involvement
2. Behavior modification
3. Treating impulse control

4. Social intervention and inclusion
5. Psychotherapy
6. Medication when needed

TEACHING CHILDREN TO COPE WITH AGGRESSION[28]

All of these protocols have the opportunity to change the chronically aggressive child. Most importantly, children can be taught how to cope with aggression by restoring agency and control, a sense of meaning, coping mechanisms, and changes in response time through an environment that supports emotional resiliency. If we don't teach chronically aggressive children empathy, altruism, and impulse control, then violence can become transgenerational. We know, through the science of epigenetics, that altruism and empathy can be taught and passed on to future generations. This requires a child to feel included, supported, and connected to others through a positive environment, role-modeling, and other remediations. You must be what you want to see. Early intervention is the most successful approach. Therefore, parents are called upon to recognize the signals of aggression early, so that they can seek professional psychological help when needed. Early intervention is the key to success.

THE AGGRESSIVE CHILD'S BRAIN[29]

The heightened neurotransmitters that facilitate violence can often be seen in an aggressive child's brain. There may also be problems in the prefrontal cortex and amygdala. In a sense, the primitive brain, which is in all of us, is most frequently activated in the aggressive child and overreacts to perceived offenses. Problems with social signals inhibit an aggressive child and create a state of low impulse control. Therefore, the aggressive child is slow to apply the brakes when necessary and as a result is more likely to crash emotionally, without the inhibitors available from healthy social signals.

SOCIETY AND VIOLENCE[30]

Violence can be contagious, so the question is: how do we keep aggressive and borderline children from inciting violence or joining violent groups? Our own culture romanticizes violence in movies, video games, and certain violent cartoons, which can all overstimulate and excite children who may already have a proclivity toward aggression. The steady diet of violence that children receive daily causes the overproduction of the stress hormone cortisol, which can alter brain patterns and inhibit impulse control. Once brain circuitry is changed, it is very difficult to restore and remediate. As in everything else, there are critical windows of opportunity when the brain is developing and every circuitry system can be affected.

PARENTAL INVOLVEMENT[31]

The one thing you can do as a parent is adopt a comprehensive approach toward the treatment of aggression in your child. Remembering that biology is not destiny, parents can be taught to parent consciously. You can learn to recognize the signs of excessive aggression, creating an environment in early childhood that helps teach your child to self-manage, while constraining the amplifications of his violent tendencies. Bonding is the magic elixir essential to creating a secure environment for your child that enhances, as well as suppresses, certain genes.

UNDERSTANDING YOUR CHILD'S ANGER

As a parent, you know that sometimes your children seem to get angry out of the blue, without warning or reasonable explanation. To understand how to help children work through anger, it first helps to understand where this emotion comes from and how children process anger differently from adults.

Anger is a protective response against physical and emotional injury. Children, in particular, are vulnerable to their feelings until they develop coping skills that help them manage their emotions. Until then, *anger is an instinctive defense for children to use against physical and emotional pain.*

The fight-or-flight response is located in the emotional and more primitive part of the brain. When triggered by a real or perceived threat, we humans are programmed to either attack or run away. In reality, there are times when we must defend ourselves and attack in order to survive. However, young children, who are swimming in a world of emotion, have not yet learned how to distinguish between a real threat and an angry emotion.

ANGER IN VERY YOUNG CHILDREN

Very young children are particularly vulnerable, because they do not have the experience to cope with their feelings and manage their stress. Some very young children repress their feelings, or express their fear and anxiety in the only way they know how, which is usually by getting angry. By the time your child reaches school age, they should be able to both recognize anger and find reasonable ways in which to react to their anger.

ANGER IN SCHOOL-AGED CHILDREN

By the time they reach the fourth and fifth grade, when children start thinking critically and abstractly, some may develop regressive behavior, such as poor impulse control, which can include striking others and temper tantrums. They also may develop headaches and stomachaches, wet the bed, and have sleeping problems.

Because they start moving into abstract operations at this age, children frequently have problems concentrating, focusing, and solving math problems. Finally, their immature behavior often finds these children alienated from their friends.

It is your job as parents to teach your children how to cope with their emotions and to skillfully use the appropriate responses. Now that you understand a bit where this anger stems from and how children at different ages may process these complex emotions, you can start to help your children cope with their anger.

HELPING YOUR CHILD COPE WITH ANGER

Do you find your child lashing out? Are you having trouble communicating with your child during moments of extreme frustration or aggression?

While children are growing and still learning how to cope with anger, they tend to instinctively use anger as a defense against physical and emotional pain. As a parent, there are many ways you can help your child through these emotional moments:

1. **DO recognize and acknowledge your child's feelings.** If you validate your child's feelings, then your child doesn't need to defend those feelings and is less likely to respond in anger. Acknowledging feelings causes your child's anger to soften and leaves a safe space in which she can learn empathy and coping skills. On the other hand, if you discount your child's feelings and experiences, then her anger will intensify as she fights to establish and validate her own sense of self.

2. **DO practice empathy.** By listening to your child's feelings without interruption or defense, you create space for her anger to dissipate, as she no longer needs to use up her energy defending the fairness of her position. By empathizing with your child's feelings, you are helping her regulate the cortisol— the fight-or-flight chemical—that increases from emotional stress. The consistency of your open receptiveness to your child's anger teaches her to react less emotionally and more critically. Ultimately, this is how nature and nurture come into balance, as a child's behavior affects body chemistry and therefore emotional control.

3. **DO teach your child problem-solving skills.** Neurological tracking occurs when your child creatively problem-solves. The more your child practices and rehearses problem-solving rather than emotional reacting, the more his neurological pathways assist him in controlling his impulses. Parents can teach their

children how to recognize, acknowledge, and appropriately cope with their feelings by asking questions that prompt children to think up their own solutions, such as "What do you think would happen if you did Choice A instead of Choice B?" or "What sort of options do you think are available to you and what do you need to do to find a resolution?"

4. **DO establish clear standards for acceptable and unacceptable behavior.** This means that though we want to validate what our child is feeling, allowing those emotions does not mean accepting bad behavior. There are common rules of engagement, which include no hitting, throwing, breaking objects, or disrespect. By involving your child in establishing the consequences for his behavior, you will find that your child is more likely to respect the rules. By limiting your child's aggressive behavior, you are in a sense establishing a safety container for his feelings.

5. **DO teach your child relaxation methods.** By teaching children progressive relaxation, breathing techniques, and other self-managing tools for stress, they can calm themselves when confronted with anger. These techniques not only change the neural pathways, but also affect impulse control. As with every habit, the more you do it, the better you become at it. For example, if a child learns to breathe in before giving in to the impulsive act of hitting, it gives that child a sense of control and lessens the need to establish control by acting out.

6. **DO try a "time in" instead of a "timeout."** As the parent, you are your child's main guide in life, and as his guide, he relies on you to be there with him through his emotional experience, whatever that may be. Therefore, use timeout sparingly and without isolation. Instead, try a "time in"—sit with your child and use the methods in this book; work on breathing with him,

ask him questions about his feelings. The important thing is to be fully present with him to help him through his emotions. Remember, you are teaching your child social cues and skills to be in relationship with others, rather than going it alone. When children are isolated, they often ruminate and feel guilty for their behavior. This only serves to create concrete reasons for low self-esteem, which often cycle back to creating bad behavior.

7. **DON'T attempt to orchestrate your child's feelings.** It is important to value what your child is experiencing. For example, if your child is hurt or crying, never say to him: "Stop crying." Rather, validate your child's experience, saying, "I know that hurts; that would make me cry also." This makes an ally out of you, rather than a target for free-floating anxiety and anger.

   As an ally, your child learns to trust you, realizing you are there for him—no matter what, right or wrong—and that he can count on that. If your child can trust you, he can learn to trust himself and the outer world. If, for example, your child tells you that he hates you, or wants you to leave him alone, it is important to assure him that you will be nearby and that you will always be there for him no matter what.

8. **DON'T go down to your child's level of behavior.** Consciously and deliberately step into your role as the adult and remain there for the entire stressful episode. Little children can really work themselves up emotionally, especially while defending their position. Your job as a parent is to stay composed. Your state of calm allows your child to feel safe in the midst of chaos. A parent is always a child's touchstone, the one they look toward for security and safety. Children become afraid when their parents display anger. By staying in your adult role, you are teaching your child that it is okay to feel angry,

and that when the feeling passes, you are still there, holding a secure space for him.

9. **DO teach your child to recognize anger cues.** If your child can self-monitor, she can self-manage. By recognizing the feelings that accompany anger, your child can recognize the onset of her emotions. This gives her time in which to self-manage before she is caught in the web of feelings. If you see that your child is overtired or cranky, you have the opportunity as a parent to teach her to recognize her oncoming emotions by resting with your child, reading to your child, or spending some cozy time together.

10. **DO teach your child how to bring his feelings to consciousness.** By recognizing the emotions that drive his behavior, your child can learn to skillfully manage that behavior. Writing, drawing, and painting are wonderful ways to express the issues that are bothering your child, especially if he has trouble verbalizing his emotions. When my children were little and reached the point of no return in their emotional intensity, I bought a Shmoo, a balloon that, once punched, pops back up. I gave my children permission to use the pillows on their bed or the Shmoo to release some of their pent-up feelings and emotions. Once those feelings are out in the open, you can collaborate with your child to find ways of coping with these feelings empathically.

11. **Invest your child in the process of managing his anger.** Ask your child to give you some tips on how he could positively manage his emotions. Make a list of five actions he can take—such as breathing deeply for one minute or drawing a picture—and leave the list somewhere your child can see it, such as on his bedroom door or on your refrigerator door.

12. **DO bond with your child.** A well-bonded child can learn to cope and manage his emotions, to problem-solve, to process

information, and to stick with a problem until it is resolved. He is also more adventuresome and will creatively explore different options as solutions to problems. The well-bonded child feels like he can depend on his parents.

In the end, remember that you, as the parent, make all the difference. By following these tips, you can help strengthen your relationship with your child and give him the tools he needs to cope with his anger. If you notice that your child has relationship problems, is a bully, or tries to hurt himself, others, or animals, do consider seeking professional help for both you and your child.

ACCESS TO VIOLENCE ALTERS BABY'S DEVELOPING BRAIN

Children are immersed in technology, and violent programming is altering their brains. Studies show that violence on television—whether it's in a cartoon, children's program, movie, or game—has an adverse effect on your child and the way she thinks and acts. For the most part, children learn from both experience and social learning, or role-modeling. Therefore, when children, especially young children, see violence in media, they have a difficult time differentiating between what is real and what is make-believe, and they tend to emulate or copy what they see. Furthermore, there is a chemical change in the brain similar to that which is seen in posttraumatic stress disorder; if enough violence is viewed, the developing brain reacts as if the viewer has actually been abused.

Dr. Craig A. Anderson, in a study on media violence exposure in youth, found that even short-term viewing of violence can increase physical and verbal aggression, aggressive thought, and aggressive emotion. In fact, according to Anderson, frequent exposure to media violence in childhood can lead to aggressive behavior later in life, including physical and spousal abuse.[32] This research on violent viewing and its effects on children has revealed that chemicals such as cortisol can change the structure of the brain, including impulse control—indicating that children's brains are imagining and storing the violence viewed. In a sense, the mind is rehearsing and imitating the aggressive behavior seen. As a result, aggressive behavior and aggressive responses become an acceptable option later on when children are confronted with conflict.

Dr. John P. Murray calls this brain behavior "encoding aggressive scripts" and states that the posterior cingulate, a part of the brain that holds emotional trauma, stores these neuroimages and retrieves them in a manner similar to the flashback of traumatic memory, present in posttraumatic stress disorder.[33] Excessive viewing of violent Internet and video games also affects brain function in a similar manner.

Research by Dr. Vincent Mathews at Indiana University demonstrates brain changes directly related to viewing only two hours of violent material daily.[34] The brain changes that Mathews's group saw were similar to those seen in teenagers with destructive sociopathic disorders. According to Dr. Murray, "Viewing behavior in media triggers certain areas of the brain that are associated with arousal/attention, detection of threat, episodic memory encoding and retrieval, and motor programming." Murray's study mapped the amygdala and related brain structures, using functional Magnetic Resonance Imaging or MRI to ascertain the neurological changes that resulted from watching violence on television. He concluded that a relationship existed between the chemistry of the brain and viewing violent material, which affected both cognitive and motor behavior.[35]

Dr. Anderson states that "research on violent television, films, video games, and music revealed unequivocal evidence that media violence increases the likelihood of aggressive and violent behavior in both immediate and long-term context."[36] Other studies also cite a finished study by Kaj Bjorkqvist in which he concluded that "even a single exposure increases aggression in the immediate situation."[37] Longitudinal studies show that children who play a lot of violent video games through childhood are more physically aggressive throughout their lives. This is especially true if the violence is one-sided, as in the case of sadistic violence. Add to this the fact that children who watch violence on television have brains that are still developing, and you can see how really dangerous TV, video games, and Internet viewing can be.

We are all familiar with the psychological study in which children who were surrounded by toys, including a plastic bat, watched a cartoon that included hitting. As soon as the cartoon ended, the children reached for the bat and used it in an aggressive manner, hitting the other toys in the room. We know that children are psychologically affected by what they see because they are primates, and therefore social learners. Children who are psychologically more aggressive tend to display less empathy, even as toddlers. We see this characteristic in bullies who are more likely to use aggressive strategies to solve their problems rather than to search for more peaceful conflict resolutions. Bullies, children with low empathy, tend to be more reactive than proactive, relying more on knee-jerk reactions to resolve frustration, and appear to be more fearful of social relationships. This makes them bite before they can be bitten. This perception of danger, when coupled with the lack of empathy, can lead to sadistic behavior. Moreover, children seeing too much violence on TV are more likely to be argumentative, as they have dispensed with the slow caution of inhibitors. These children act out whether at home or at nursery school and are more likely to become a class bully. They are less patient than their counterparts, and studies show that children who watch too much violence on TV, including violent cartoons, appear to be more unwilling to cooperate and delay gratification and are therefore immature. They also harbor a strong sense of entitlement, which can give them feelings of paranoia if their desires go unmet.

You really are your child's first and most influential teacher. Who and what she becomes is completely up to you—and it starts in the womb.

A WOMB WITH A VIEW

It is a common misconception that your baby grows in the womb in a neutral state of unconsciousness. Today, because of technology, you can now see your baby as he interacts with his inner and outer world.

Mothers have long recognized that their babies are learning and actively responding, both to their environment within the womb and the imposition of social stimulation and input from the world at large. In fact, from four months' gestation onward, your baby is both learning your language and recognizing and responding to your voice, while hearing all your body systems—your heart beating, your blood rushing, and various internal processes such as gas, hiccups, etc. Your baby hears all of this through the muffled echo of your body and vocal cords.

Further, ambient sounds from your social environment also reach your baby through music, singing, conversation, reading, and loud noises. Your baby also reacts to light and shadow reflected from the outside, for example, when your OBGYN examines you and shines a light into your uterus.

Moreover, if you are happy, dancing and laughing, your baby will respond in kind by jumping up and down in the womb, kicking and moving around, especially responding to your rhythm, beat, and joyful attitude.

Additionally, your baby will reach for things that invade his space, such as the amniocentesis needle that perforates the uterus in an effort to extract amniotic fluid from the placenta. Your baby also demonstrates a wide range of emotions, including anger and fear.

If twins are growing together, they interact, expressing joy and love as well as frustration and aggression. For instance, twins will move their placentas together so that they can touch each other through the thin membrane separating them.

Your baby is especially responsive to your voice. At four months in utero, he begins to learn your language. He hears the meter and rhythm of that language through the muffled sound of your voice as it echoes through your womb. By the seventh month, your baby is so attached to your voice that if you speak to him in a calm and soothing way, you can affect his mood.

There have been many studies to corroborate a baby's connection to his mother's voice. In one such study, babies were given pacifiers attached to a voice recorder. When a baby heard his mother's voice, as opposed to any other female voice, he reacted by increasing his sucking on the pacifier.

Ultimately, the baby even adapted his sucking rate to the rhythm of his mother's voice in an effort to manipulate the distinct voice of his mother, as opposed to the voice of any other person.

This work by Dr. William Fifer at Columbia University demonstrates not only your baby's attachment to your voice, but also the capacity of your baby to learn and adapt rapidly.[38]

Babies do not connect to their fathers, siblings, or other voices in the same way. So, although your baby may have heard the voices of his father, siblings, and others through the womb—perhaps by reading bedtime stories and singing lullabies—he still has a unique and special attachment to your voice. Of course, it is your voice specifically that is heard for nine months, as it resonates through your abdomen and vocal cords, bonding with baby, while engulfing him in the dulcet tones of love and connection.

HOW YOUR STRESS CAN AFFECT YOUR BABY DURING PREGNANCY

With our society's shift toward more mindful living, you may be aware of how stress impacts *your* well-being. Yet when you become pregnant, you should also be aware of the effects your stress may have on your baby's development.

When you are stressed, your fight-or-flight system causes you to pump cortisol, the stress hormone meant to save you from danger. Cortisol then bathes your brain, temporarily changing your brain structure, so that you react quickly and instinctively.

When you feel attacked, either physically or emotionally, you can't stop to contemplate or use your executive function. Your body, in its wisdom, helps you act quickly to save your hide. This is the same system that your primitive ancestors used to survive.

The problem is that today, most of your threats are emotional, not physical, but your fight-or-flight system can't recognize the difference. Therefore, cortisol is called upon consistently and ultimately wears down the body, like battery fluid, doing untold damage both physically and emotionally.

Now that you are pregnant, that same stress is also taking its toll on the baby growing inside of you. According to Professor Vivette Glover of the Imperial College in London, stress during pregnancy can increase the risk of early cognitive problems.[39]

For example, cortisol stress hormones can cross the placenta. High levels of cortisol in amniotic fluid affect dopamine production in the developing infant brain. It appears that consistent stress to the mother can cause an overly sensitized baby who has a lower stress threshold after birth.

Moreover, a mother's stress can affect her baby permanently. For example, a receptor for stress hormones can cause a biological change in the fetus, which makes it more vulnerable to stress after birth—this links to hyperactive disorders. A correlation to stress in the womb can also lead to later autoimmune problems.

EFFECT OF STRESS ON LANGUAGE-LEARNING ABILITY IN THE WOMB[40]

Did you know that babies learn in the womb, and also that stress can affect their development?

A study by Dr. Patricia Kuhl of the Institute for Learning and Brain Sciences at the University of Washington in Seattle states that babies not only hear their mother's voice and understand their mother's inflection, but they are also already learning her language in the womb. This is the foundation for language. In fact, just hours after birth, a baby can distinguish between a mother's native tongue and the foreign language of another mother.

Because a mother's voice is magnified and amplified by her body, it can be heard by her baby in utero, along with other sounds. Babies also are already making sense of the sounds they hear. By hearing speech patterns and rhythms in the womb, your baby is learning your primary language. Hence, some researchers believe that a mother can facilitate her child's language development, both in the womb and after birth.

TEACHING SOUND RECOGNITION

Studies now indicate that we can even teach babies before birth. We now know that the fetus is so sensitive that stimulation from the mother affects it directly. Studies using EEG sensors, which search for neural traces of memory in utero, indicate that sound repetition becomes a part of memory. Therefore, if the sound is replicated, that memory is activated. When a fetus is introduced to a repeated sound, his memory of that sound stimulates his recognition. As a result, brainwave patterns of the fetus indicate the trace memory of the recognized sound.

A study by cognitive neuroscientist Eino Partanen and others, of the University of Helsinki, discovered that infants' brains not only learned repeated sounds, but also recognized words and their variations. Partanen's study demonstrated that the neural signals for identifying sound, including vowels, are visible as memory traces in a newborn.[41]

Likewise, ten weeks before birth, a fetus uses many of his senses to learn about his inner world, preparing himself for birth. Ultrasounds show us that a fetus will react to noise by kicking, moving, and even dancing around in the womb, bobbing up and down when mother laughs. Further, a fetus's heart rate may lower upon hearing Mother's voice. Even more amazing is the fact that a fetus may touch his face, suck his thumb, stretch his limbs holding his feet, and have enough coordination to grasp his own umbilical cord with his fingers. Fetuses have even been viewed through ultrasound as licking the uterine wall and pushing off of it with their feet. Furthermore, most prenatal sleep occurs in REM. Fetuses sleep for most of the day and night while dreaming—probably about their own environment. Twin fetuses, after twenty weeks, play with each other and even demonstrate fear and anger.

Dr. Christine Moon, a psychologist at Pacific Lutheran University in Tacoma, Washington, along with Dr. Hugo Lagercrantz, a professor at the Karalinska Institute in Sweden and a member of the Nobel Assembly, coauthored a study, with Dr. Patricia Kuhl, which used a pacifier on newborns to measure (by computer) the frequency of sucking by a newborn when she heard her native language. Each suck related to a produced vowel. The infant paused when unfamiliar vowels were introduced, and each new suck produced the next vowel sound. Two sets of vowels sounds were used. Seventeen foreign language sounds were used in conjunction with seventeen native language sounds.[42]

This study indicated that babies remember elementary sounds from their mother as early as thirty weeks before birth. Further, the neurosensory mechanism for hearing is intact at thirty weeks, allowing phonetic learning to occur in the womb. Moreover, past studies assert that the fetus both responds and remembers musical rhythm.[43] Now we know that the fetus is laying the foundation for language development and is in fact partially learning a language. This study, and others like it, indicates that the brain is very sophisticated in utero and is capable of both listening to and learning language.[44]

3

THE UNSTOPPABLE, WELL-BONDED CHILD—HOW TO SPRINGBOARD SUCCESS THROUGH TRUST

Your bond with your baby is the scaffolding upon which her entire future is built. The well-bonded child does better at everything. Even something as simple as your touch or voice has the ability to stimulate immense growth in your child's neurological development. The stronger your bond, the more secure your baby will feel exploring her world, and the more she explores, the more advanced her brain development becomes.

That foundation of trust starts before your baby is even born. It's not just about strengthening the positive attachment between mother and child; your entire family dynamic lays the groundwork for your child's sense of security. In this chapter, I will teach you how to harness the power of touch, trust, and connection to establish a bond that makes your child completely unstoppable.

In life, there are those singular moments that change you forever. Even as you're experiencing them, you recognize their importance. Seeing your baby for the first time, having her placed into your arms, is one of those moments. The greatest mystery of all is that we live and reproduce, and that we love this new little stranger completely. This is nature's way of assuring the survival of our species. And we are immediately caught in the split between fear and overwhelming love. Fear, because baby doesn't come with any instructions, and suddenly you recognize the overpowering responsibility of being a parent; and love, because nature has conspired to demand your self-sacrifice, commitment, responsibility, and obligation to assure baby's well-being. Soon, you will learn all about your baby. You will recognize the difference among cries of exhaustion, frustration, anger, or hunger. You will be able to distinguish between a reflex smile, a genuine smile, or a grin that indicates trouble ahead. Right from the beginning, baby responds to your reactions. In the earliest days of your baby's life, you become a master of the essentials that assure the survival of your baby. As much as you are learning about your baby, consider that the developing brain of your baby is learning a thousand times more about you. Thus, the most important voice baby ever hears, and the most important face she ever sees, from birth through childhood, is yours.

Every song you sing, every cuddle you give, every game of peekaboo, and every giggle are all creating the scaffolding for your baby's future endeavors. For example, a talent for art and music or a gift for sports or social skills is tracked by these neural pathways initiated through the interaction of you and your baby. Bonding between you and your child is the most central ingredient to the success of this process. Your child needs not only your loving presence, but also your time and attention. Today, new technology such as the PET scan (Positron Emission Tomography) and the MRI gives us a window into your baby's brain so that you can see with your own eyes the way it reacts to specific outside stimulation.

Your baby is a regular little Pac-Man, finding interest everywhere, including sounds, voices, lights, shadows, colors, mobiles, and experiences of all kinds. By responding to your baby's sense of excitement and wonder, you support a feeling of well-being as he observes that you are validating his explorations. Paying attention and actively listening to your baby fosters his sense of well-being and value. Ultimately, your baby's behavior becomes focused, as he deliberately elicits your positive responses. Your reactions are everything to him, as you are his world, and he defines himself through his interactions with you. In a sense, this collaboration with your baby will either turn on or turn off his particular genetic dispositions.

Consequently, what makes your baby unique are these very experiences crafted by you.

Neuroscience has given us hard data to reinforce the importance of early childhood experiences. The data strongly indicate that children deprived of the nurturing that stimulates brain maturation leave important areas of the brain profoundly undeveloped. We find this situation not only in orphanages in foreign countries, where babies are left untouched for hours, but also in homes where mothers are working long hours, resenting childcare, experiencing postpartum depression or other emotional or physical problems that make it impossible to connect or bond with their babies. Such lack of nurturing and care can lead to long-term health problems for baby, including posttraumatic stress disorder and failure to thrive.

5 WAYS TO BOND WITH YOUR BABY

She's finally here: your brand-new bundle of joy. Cradling her in your arms, you gaze at your new baby and feel . . . nothing. You are not overwhelmed with joy or happiness and you are not overcome with love and sweet emotions as you imagined you would be, and as you have been told you should be. You wonder: *I've been so excited about this baby, and now that she's here, I don't feel any bond at all. What's wrong with me?*

First, know that you are not alone, and that these feelings are shared by others. There are many possible reasons you feel unable to bond with your new baby, and just because you feel this way today does not mean it will be this way forever.

Bonding between mother and child from the early days of infancy can help build trust and security. Here are five simple ways that mothers can create strong bonds with their babies:

1. **Spend as much time after your child is born allowing for skin-to-skin contact.** Studies show that this contact helps you release endorphins, resulting in projecting calm and reassurance

to your baby. Soon your baby will recognize your touch, scent, and feel compared to others.

2. **Talk and sing to your baby.** Allow him to hear the sound of your voice as much as possible from the very beginning, whether singing lullabies or simply explaining how you are changing baby's clothes. Newborns can recognize their mother's voice from the time they are born.

3. **Make eye contact with your baby.** Although eyesight is still developing, newborns can see approximately twelve inches in front of them, so when you are holding your baby, be sure to also hold her gaze. Your child will begin to recognize your features and be soothed by your familiarity.

4. **Make sure you and your partner are the main people who feed your baby.** Breastfeeding can help build strong bonds between mother and child, but bottle feeding can also strengthen the bond between you and your baby, as well as your baby's bond with your partner. When feeding your baby, hold him close, make eye contact, sing or speak softly, and give all of your attention to your newborn so that he feels calm and soothed during the feeding.

5. **Respond to your baby's needs.** You cannot spoil a baby. In fact, the more you bond with your baby now, the more she will learn to trust you. If your child feels secure in her attachment to you, she will more likely grow up to be a more independent adult.

But what happens if you don't feel that you can bond with your baby?

WHY DON'T I LOVE MY CHILD?

The house is dark. You're about to go bed, and you look one last time at your sleeping child . . . the one you can't love. Even in this moment of complete vulnerability and perhaps guilt, you ask yourself, *Why?* You've been taught that all mothers love their children, would make any sacrifice for their child, including death, and yet for some reason, you can't love yours.

Based on my years of experience working in education and psychology, I discovered several reasons why parents may not bond with their children.

POSTPARTUM DEPRESSION

The most obvious reason for your detachment is postpartum depression. The chemical changes that your body goes through during pregnancy and delivery often affect your emotions and can create an imbalance powerful enough to cause depression after birth. Thankfully, if this is your problem, it can be solved. Medication, therapy, and behavior modification can all work together to help you recover and bond with your baby. On the other hand, if your problem is an emotional one other than postpartum depression, then you have to look within to find the source of your feelings. Only then can you find your way back to a healthy and happy relationship with your baby.

LOOKING BACK TO MOVE FORWARD

You come from a family of origin, and that family of origin is your history. It is here, in the early staging of your own development, that you can find the causes for your inability to positively attach with your child. Perhaps you were neglected or abused or had a competitive, controlling, jealous, demeaning, or toxic parent. Often, the very defenses you develop to survive your childhood can cut you off from intimate and loving feelings for your progeny.

THE RESENTFUL PARENT

You may be that unfulfilled mother who never reached your life goals and passions, and you may feel unsatisfied and unhappy in your life. If this is your situation, you may feel that the responsibility of raising a child is too much for you to bear. In time, this can cause resentment and ultimately cut off those loving feelings that you may have felt initially for your baby. I have found this is often the case if you married because you were pregnant and/ or your pregnancy altered the future of your goals and aspirations.

COMPENSATING THOUGH COMPETITION AND CONTROL

There are mothers and fathers who compete with their children. If you were demeaned and dismissed within your family of origin, you may suffer from low self-esteem. And if your marriage is difficult or unhappy, your child can become a pawn in your relationship. It is here that you can become competitive for your mate's attention toward your son or daughter. However, jealousy knows no bounds, and you may also feel competitive for the attention your son or daughter receives from others. If you're that competitive parent, you may still be fighting for the need to be seen from your own childhood. This may cause you to discount your child's accomplishments, as well as demean them by lowering your child's sense of self so that you can feel elevated.

If as a child you had a very controlling mother or father, it is likely that you felt out of control. Therefore, as an adult, you are likely to be controlling. This is a formula for excessive domination. If as a child you experienced a jealous parent, you often will mirror that jealousy with your own children. It is the heightened need for attention that creates those vindictive feelings that you project onto your child. As a result, if your child gets too much attention from others, including family members, you may dominate your child in an effort to squash your child's self-esteem.

THE NEGLECTFUL PARENT OR OVERPROTECTIVE PARENT

Finally, you may be that neglectful parent who is struggling to cope with your own childhood experiences of neglect. You may find yourself abusing your son or daughter through your negative interactions, both emotionally and physically. Many times, the child who grows up to be this parent was abused him/herself. If you are psychologically unavailable, unresponsive, disconnected, or demanding, your child will be not only neglected, but rejected.

One way you may attempt to self-manage the guilty feelings that accompany your inability to love your child is by becoming an overprotective parent. This allows you to compensate for your hostile feelings by overcontrolling your child's life.

SEEK HELP

If you are an uninvolved parent who is unable to positively support, value, and validate your child, you should seek professional help immediately. Nothing is carved in stone—through introspection and self-analysis, you can recognize and acknowledge your own developmental history. By catching a glimpse of your childhood patterns, you can uncover and recover your psychological resource, which will enable you to integrate your own childhood wounds. A good counselor will help define your family's characteristics as well as the triggers for stress, anxiety, and support. By becoming conscious of your own parenting style, you can deliberately learn how to take back your source of injury and heal it. This will open your heart and your mind, and by learning to love *yourself,* you can then learn to love your child.

YOU HAVE THE POWER[1]

There's no power on Earth like the power of a mother. You have the most dramatic impact on your baby's early childhood development. Innovations in technology and cutting-edge science inform us that your baby's early childhood experiences are at least as important as his gender and genetic composition.

Baby is born with approximately 24,000 genes, and it is impossible for all of those genes to express themselves. So, it is your baby's experiences that mold and influence those genes in determining how he will grow, think, learn, and process information. Before the 1990s, science informed us that baby's brain, and the processes therein, were determined by genetics. But neuroscientists tell us now that genes are only raw material, and what shapes and molds that material are your baby's experiences. For instance, you may have a baby who immediately displays the characteristics of shyness, and yet, with TLC and a lot of hugging and bonding, as well as deliberate and orchestrated exposure to others, that shy child can develop both optimism and confidence. It is clear that genetics is only half the story, and that early childhood experiences have an even greater influence over how the neural circuits in the brain are wired.

For the first time, science acknowledges that you, mother, play a vital role in the creation of your child, both before and after birth. You are the true gene therapist, fundamental to the potential design of your child. You are responsible for 50 percent of your child's linguistic, cognitive, social, and emotional development, contributing to her future achievements in life. You have a greater impact on your child's growth than simply the DNA you contributed at the moment of conception. Neuroscience tells us that we can enhance or subdue our child's individual genes through the experiences and environment we create not only after birth, but also in the womb, where it is primarily you who have control over the environment, through your diet, general health, physical well-being, and stress management. The way in which you interact with and respond to your baby will either elevate or lower the resonance of her genes. This is the way in which you can deliberately reinforce particular behaviors and extinguish others. This is how awesome your parental power really is . . . that you can actually affect your baby's gene pool, before and after her birth.

Heretofore, the overwhelming responsibility of parenting may have caused you both fear and paralysis. Yet, supported by *Your Baby's Brain,* you can breathe a sigh of relief and relax. You don't need fancy toys, flashcards, or a degree in child development to properly stimulate your baby. Your child was born curious, ready and able to soak up information. Your baby is an absolute learning machine, open to all experiences and like a sponge, absorbing all environmental stimulation. Psychologist Dr. David Reiss, author of *The Relationship Code*, asserts that your baby is a small researcher finding out about his world through his family. Testing himself against his world, your tiny scientist will use his senses to define his small sphere of influence. At first, baby is all mouth, and everything possible is placed there. Then, baby uses his sense of touch to identify and manipulate objects of various sizes, shapes, and textures, as well as dropping toys, cutlery, bottles, and so forth to elicit your response.

Expensive toys, classes, games, or books are not necessary to educate your baby. All you have to do is to create a safe environment that supports your child's natural thirst for knowledge. In the beginning, it is important to get to know your child. Pay attention to his evolving personality: what calms him, what excites him, and, most importantly, what makes him anxious. It is essential to be mindful of how your baby's brain works, and to integrate his developmental stages with appropriate parenting practices. Equipped with this information, you can intervene successfully, taking the right steps at the right time.

One crucial element to add to your parental soup is stress reduction. Only by being able to self-manage stress can your child open to the fullness of her personality and intellectual capital. It is especially important in early childhood to help your child lower her anxiety, so that she can enter that relaxed, alert state that allows her to access a larger portion of her brain's creative resources. A calm baby can process and link information better, hold images longer, and gain the impulse control necessary to focus and concentrate. On the other hand, a stressed baby will overproduce stress hormones, which will adversely affect her brain's architecture and development. Stress reduction is the single most important ingredient in child development, as it affects everything, including your child's sense of self, her ability to learn, and her desire to do so. Though you may not be familiar with stress-reduction techniques, simply because they are often eclipsed by other pedagogy, it is still one of the most important things you can do to help your child open to the complete expanse of her capacity and success. The best part is that you will see positive results immediately. Later in this book, you will learn stress-reduction techniques that can be applied in early childhood. You will be able to teach your child how to lower her anxiety and manage her stress. Once your child's anxiety and stress are managed, she can enter that relaxed place within herself where she can find her own inner voice. It is a state of consciousness similar to meditation, where she can reach the deepest parts of herself and, as a result, a greater share of her brain's natural and fertile resources. The benefits of relaxation techniques are realized immediately, leading to a bounty of creative inspiration and innovation. Once your young explorer has mastered the art of self-managing stress, an inner calm will be available to her, and like an oyster, she will be rewarded by the pearl of inner wisdom. Ultimately, a relaxed mind functions like an orchestra, and like an acorn that grows into an oak tree, your baby will sprout and grow into her potential.

According to Dr. David Elkind, "In the 1920s, psychologist John Watson espoused a concept of infant 'malleability' that is the central component of the competence concept: if infants and young children are able learners, they can also be 'shaped' by their early learning."[2] Whether it's linguistic, cognitive, social, or emotional development, the key to your child's heightened state of expansion is you. The conscious experiences that you structure for your child can amplify the ranges of her biological abilities. According to Elkind, a study at MacArthur Fellows primarily concerned with asking questions on creativity and giftedness found: "if there is a single theme which threads through the responses and strings them together it is the crucial role of home life and parental guidance in shaping these unusually creative minds."[3] The study also found that the parents of these gifted children had one thing in common: they did not pressure their children, but rather created a supportive environment that was rich in emotional bonding, social interactions, and print. Thus, when discussing the outcome of the MacArthur Fellows research, Elkind states that "it is the support and encouragement parents give children and the intellectual climate that they create in the home which seem to be the critical factors."[4] By knowing your child and paying attention to her gifts, talents, and interests, you can organize an environment that helps her to discover her true vocation. By actively listening to your child and observing her behavior, you can determine how to best affect her intellectual growth. For instance, there are certain times in brain development when your child needs specific stimulation from you in particular. If your child's age and stage are timed correctly, she will display an insatiable desire to learn and express her interests. Because your child is an individual, she will have different wants and needs from those of other children. Consequently, if you pay attention and actively listen to your child, you will recognize her gifts and talents, so that she can tap into both. Being your child's primary teacher may seem like an overwhelming task, but you really are, whether or not you consciously take on that role. Your baby will learn from you, no matter what. Whether she learns from your attention, guidance, bonding, and love or from your neglect, disregard, or absence, your interactions with her are firing up her brain's connections or synapses, either way. Each synaptic crackle and snap are forming the person that she will one day become.

Educator Maria Montessori discovered that children are born with an inner knowing that she called the "inner teacher." She, like Jungian psychologist Dr. James Hillman, believed that within your child is an inner voice, the natural self, waiting to unfold. Formal education arrives too late on the scene to greatly impact early childhood development.

Because your child is naturally curious and thirsty for knowledge, he craves stimulation. As a result, it is important in early childhood to immerse your child in a print-rich environment, containing objects that he can touch, manipulate, and observe. Early expeditions into his structured and safe environment give your baby a chance daily to expand his realm of influence and experience while mastering the skills necessary to extend out beyond his comfort zone. The well-bonded child, anchored in the security of your presence, can do this with both the competence and security that ultimately lead to good self-esteem. This is how your child learns. By extending his reach each day into uncharted territory, your child is building, second by second, day by day, his associative mass, the accumulation of ideas and images in his brain. Correspondingly, each new day, your child begins where he left off the day before, rather than from his original starting point. This is how your child advances, grasping new concepts and new boundaries with each excursion.

Each encounter stretches her natural curiosity, teaching her about her world, how it looks, feels, sounds, smells, and tastes. Maria Montessori said that "children must be free to express themselves, and thus reveal those needs and attitudes which would otherwise remain hidden or repressed in an environment that did not permit them to act spontaneously."[5] It is you whom she looks to for help to uncover the full measure of her capacity. By providing a safe space that is loving, supportive, print-rich, interesting, and thought-provoking, you build the scaffolding necessary to ensure her future trust and success.

For years, we've heard this argument of quality versus quantity, but in parenting, quantity *is* quality. If you aren't there to meet your child's wants and needs, if you're not there to be counted on, if he can't build trust based on his experience with you, then he can't transfer those feelings in a healthy way to himself and others. In that case, your child will experience the anxiety of not knowing, not feeling that his surroundings are secure and stable and something he can count on. These are the feelings that lead to fear and despair and shut down or impair your child's openness and readiness to learn. Your child needs to see you and be with you to connect and interact with you. And you need to be with your child so that you can see who he is, acknowledge and respond to his wants and needs, and help him get where he is destined to go. A few hurried or rushed moments in a day just won't cut it. Bonding is everything: it is so important that it is built into our species to ensure our survival.

There are things that your child can only learn at your side, things she can't learn anywhere else. In early childhood, you are the most influential contributor to your child's sense of security, confidence, and competence. Her entire world revolves around you, and it is her connection to you that positively reinforces her sense of self. It is that security that ultimately moves your child forward, offering her both emotional maturity and intellectual success. According to Dr. David Elkind, "the child who leaves the early years with a strong sense of security, a healthy feeling of self-esteem, and an enthusiasm for living and learning is well prepared for an admittedly rapidly changing and difficult world."[6] Elkind tells us that if your child is well-bonded, cuddled, and cared for, and if you use complex language while talking or playing in a print-rich, safe environment, filled with objects that can be manipulated, touched, inspected, and analyzed, your child will have the greatest opportunity to capture her inherent potential. Bonding begins at the beginning, from the very first moment you look into your baby's eyes. Every time you feed and nurture baby, while tending to her wants and needs, you are building up the genesis of trust. Because she can count on you to be there for her no matter what, she will relax and begin to trust not only herself, but you and the world at large. Like an alchemist searching for the philosopher's stone, your baby ventures forth into unknown territory, secure that if she looks back over her shoulder, she can count on you to be present, reassuring her that she's okay. Moreover, just as the alchemist is transformed into wholeness through the stages of his experiments, so is your baby when she crawls back to you seeking the validation and attention of your warm smile. As you get to know your baby better, you soon realize that she will do anything for your smile, anything for your attention. This knowledge fortifies the scaffolding you've built up until now, which can support your baby in the lifelong dance between emotional stability and maturity.

The value of this parental support and guidance is immeasurable. Your well-bonded and emotionally mature child will acquire specific attributes, including the ability to focus and concentrate. His ability to sit for long periods of time, pay attention, hold images, and successfully process information will give him an advantage over less emotionally mature children. A sense of self and good self-esteem instills within him a strong central core, which inspires self-motivation. Furthermore, he is more curious, risk-oriented, and willing to chance failure. While engaging in problem-solving, he can hold the tension longer and push past his efforts as he incorporates the specific characteristics needed to succeed both cognitively and socially. In other words, your valued child learns to value himself and validate others. Your securely attached child is often more mature than other children his age, not only self-motivated, but also well rounded, skillfully relating to his peers. According to Elkind, "an ounce of motivation is worth a pound of skills anytime."[7]

Estrada, P., Arsenio, F., Hess, R.D., and Holloway, D. (1987) state:

Parents/child affective relationships influence children's cognitive and social competence during the preschool years [Bretherton, 1985]. Children who are securely attached as infants subsequently approach cognitive tasks in ways conducive to cognitive development. Their problem-solving style is characterized by more curiosity, persistence, and enthusiasm, and less frustration than less securely attached infants. Securely attached children also appear to use adult direction and attention in ways that promote cognitive and social development. They are more able to benefit from maternal assistance during problem-solving tasks and to interact effectively with teachers.[8]

We seldom recognize the importance of touch. Touch is so significant that the primary sensory cortex, the part of the brain that perceives touch, actually begins to process tactile stimulation as early as four months in utero. By the tenth week of gestation, your baby develops particular skin nerves, and from the moment of birth, your baby will recognize the difference between something soft or something rough, favoring soft. Tiffany Field's research indicates that when premature babies were massaged for fifteen minutes, three times a day, their weight increased 47 percent more rapidly than the nonmassaged preemies in the study, the only variable being massage. Babies who received touch showed less stress as indicated by reduced levels of cortisol, less frowning, and less hand-squeezing. Additionally, those preemies who received massages were able to leave the hospital approximately six days sooner than the preemies not massaged.[9] According to biological psychologist Saul Schanberg, when baby rats were isolated from their mothers and therefore denied maternal licking, the pups experienced diminished growth hormones.[10] Yet when a lab technician used a wet paintbrush to imitate the mother's licking, the baby rats continued to grow. It appears that when touch occurs, the touching prompts the vegetative vagus, which stimulates the gastrointestinal tract, sending hormones such as insulin into the bloodstream. The insulin then contributes to successful food absorption, allowing human babies to develop more rapidly. Touch therapy or massage also lowers stress; babies who are massaged show decreased levels of cortisol, which when elevated can destroy immune cells. Though your baby isn't familiar with the whys and wherefores of touch, she does know how good it feels to be touched and how relaxed she is when you give her a massage.[11]

Touch also fosters your baby's happiness, health, and overall capacity to thrive. By holding and cuddling, hugging, and touching, you communicate to your baby that she is loved, valued, validated, and worthwhile. This generalized feeling of well-being, directly correlated to touch, has been shown to both lower stress and strengthen the immune system; as it is cortisol that lowers lymphocytes, weakens T-cell strength, and lowers antigen levels, which can all converge to make baby more vulnerable to illness and disease.

Your presence in your baby's life is her real gift. Not only can you nurture and encourage her emotional maturity, but you can also promote her cognitive growth. Moreover, you experience an overwhelming feeling of ease when you and your baby collaborate through each important developmental stage. Of course, timing is everything. Dr. Montessori asserted that your child's brain is receptive to specific types of learning at particular times.[12] Accordingly, there is a target window for your child to learn not just one language, but many languages without the burden of a foreign accent, as discussed in Chapter 1. There is a best time for your child to begin math, and a heightened period for your child to learn music, sports, and so on. For this reason, it is essential that you know when these windows occur, so you are prepared to integrate the correct learning tools with your child's readiness. In this way, your child will advance and perfect her linguistic, cognitive, social, and emotional development naturally. When you pay attention to these prime times of mental preparedness, your child can acquire not only an active sense of self and independence, but also a highly tuned increase in knowledge. By employing this method, you will take advantage of the windows of opportunity that integrate emotional health, social competence, and largeness of intellect. When the brain develops in accordance with its nature, it reveals optimal time frames that are most efficient for particularized learning. Working with the brain's own biological structure and ranges allows you to take advantage of the best possible teaching moments and opportunities. More than that, if you teach your child the appropriate information at the optimal time, she will be not only ready for it, but also receptive to it. Taking advantage of the right concepts and skills at the right time has the added benefit of making learning effortless. Finally, when you and your child travel down the road of discovery together, you are simultaneously introduced to the intrinsic pleasures associated with learning.

READING AND YOUR BABY

Reading begins in utero. If you consistently read the same book at the same time to your baby, he will respond joyfully to both the sound of your voice and his recognition of a familiar story. Studies indicate that when babies hear their mother's voice in the womb, they suck more rapidly.[13] They respond in a similar manner when they hear the same story read to them consistently, over regular intervals.

Because your child hears your voice through an echo chamber, from four months' gestation to birth, she recognizes your language, with its phonemes, meter, and tone. After birth, you can easily calm your baby by reading to her from that old familiar storybook she heard in the womb.

Research indicates that the most important strategy for teaching your child to read is to read, read, read to your child, early and often. Even though at first your baby will not comprehend the meaning of your story, he will respond by focusing on the sound of your voice as you formulate each word. Both are now familiar to him, especially if you consistently carry on with the same storybook, repetitively. Soon, your baby will try to interact with you linguistically, telling you his own story. As he learns to talk, storing memory and language, he will, in time, recognize the familiar letters on the storybook page.

By the time your baby is a toddler, he can read along with you, pretending to know the words and the story. It is important to not correct your baby, trusting that ultimately he will make the connection between the letters on the page and the words he has heard repeatedly.

Your toddler's responsiveness to language creates an explosion of linguistic acceleration, and now reading can really take off. Writing and reading are highly connected to language development. However, by the age of five, this language awareness diminishes, and so does your window of opportunity for ease of learning to read.

After five, reading becomes more of an effort, and though it can absolutely be taught, your child will have missed her optimal moment. Children at five are losing that unique opening offered to them by nature. Until then, reading occurs without any deliberate application and is therefore experienced with excitement and enthusiasm. In a sense, literacy emerges in the most natural way when you expose your child to reading at the ideal time. Only then will she easily connect the symbols on the storybook page with the letters read. Then, without any conscious exertion or determination, your child launches into reading.

Because emergent literacy begins before birth, literacy acquisition emerges along with, and as a result of, the environment. Thus, according to psychologist Lev Vygotsky's theory, the more successful the parent and child are at interacting socially in a literate society, the more successful the child will be in learning to read and write.[14] Indeed, emergent literacy views your child as a dynamic unity in a reciprocal relationship with her environment.[15] Within this model, literacy becomes an interactive and generative process.[16] The influence of your linguistic habits helps define the reading process itself for your child and provides the material from which she will eventually learn.[17] Since your child will model her own reading behavior on yours, your parental influence cannot be diminished.

You also want to create a "print-rich environment," a concept that has joined the constellation of terms used in reading research. The notion that the reading paradigm emerges in the beginning of life is now backed by studies indicating there is a confluence of function and form. Although "emergent" suggests that both reading and writing evolve from the child and his or her environment, it is the strategies of assimilation and accommodation that make the difference in the efficiency of this evolution.[18]

According to Jean Piaget, cognition develops through the interaction of children with their environment. He also discovered that children's thinking evolves progressively, from one stage to the next, creating a structure indicating what a child should be taught at each stage, including reading. In conjunction with this, Piaget also specified the importance of creating a print-rich environment by labeling in large and colorful print all the objects your child will come in contact with during the course of his day.[19] For example, put a big label on baby's crib, spelling out the word C-R-I-B, making letters that are distinctly formed and brightly colored to create attention and interest. You can continue this approach with objects around the house such as baby's cereal box, high chair, your kitchen table, refrigerator, and so forth. On sojourns to the grocery store with baby, make a game out of pointing to familiar objects, calling them by their printed name, for instance, laundry detergent. Even a walk down the street can be a learning experience if you call attention to the street signs along the way that he will ultimately recognize. All these associations stimulate baby's associative mass, making new connections and synapses that stimulate his brain's growth. When you intensify these experiences by modulating your voice in an animated way, you heighten baby's receptivity to the language he hears and feels throughout his whole body. It is these simple steps that excite and capture your baby's attention and readiness to read.

Elkind also stresses the importance of an enriched environment, warning us about the dangers of formal teacher-directed learning in early preschool years.[20] He indicates that during periods of rapid intellectual growth, a child will seek stimuli to enrich himself mentally. Therefore, you can serve your child best by simply providing an environment enriched with materials that he can observe, explore, manipulate, talk, write, read, and think about.[21] According to Elkind:

> Infants and young children are not just sitting twiddling their thumbs, waiting for their parents to teach them to read and do math. They are expending a vast amount of time and effort in exploring and understanding their immediate world. Healthy education supports and encourages this spontaneous learning. Early instruction miseducates, not because it attempts to teach, but because it attempts to teach the wrong things at the wrong time. When we ignore what the child has to learn and instead impose what we want to teach, we put infants and young children at risk for no purpose.[22]

In essence, by creating a print-rich environment that is safe, inviting, and engaging, you amplify your child's ability. If you create a print-rich environment filled with the enthusiasm and excitement for learning, your child will be motivated to learn. Such an environment, coupled with positive reinforcement, creates the climate necessary to inspire motivation, and when motivation is activated, reading skills follow. Reading then unfolds at the right time and in a seamless and stress-free manner.

PAY ATTENTION TO YOUR CHILD

The important thing is to know your child. When actively paying attention to your child, you will be there to guide her, recognize her stage of development, and positively affect it. Before the age of three, you have the greatest chance to influence your child's early education, as that is the age at which the basis for later development is established. You will not only catch a glimpse of your child's opportune readiness to learn, but also pick up any mild to moderate hearing losses and linguistic delays. By noticing your child's difficulties early on, you can intervene rapidly. Early intervention can both repair and compensate for such problems at a time when you can still make a difference. For example, there is a relationship between hearing loss and language deficit. This is important, because it is very difficult to remediate linguistic and intellectual deficiencies after the age of three. To observe your child's successful transitions from one learning stage to another, you have to be there. Then, when problems occur, you can recognize them immediately and intervene expediently.

Your baby's brain continues to develop after birth, creating the connections or synapses necessary for all growth. In a sense, you could say that at first your baby's brain is capable of learning anything, without the knowledge of understanding how. Neuroscience teaches us that your baby's experiences, both in the womb and after birth, in conjunction with genetics, will determine how her brain is wired. It is those earliest experiences, however, that determine how those neuronal circuits are formed. Studies in language development demonstrate that your baby's brain is neuroplastic, but that neuroplasticity diminishes over time. As a result, according to Dr. Patricia Kuhl, babies' brains establish a group of neurons in the auditory cortex, these neurons react to each individual phoneme, and separate and distinct clusters fire in conjunction with specific sounds captured by the ear. When a particular sound from a particular language is heard over and over again, the neuron that hears it will create a track, or distance, from those neurons that hear other sounds. By the time baby is one year of age, those auditory tracks are already formed, creating a complete auditory map. Now your baby no longer can hear the particular phonemes missing from her experience. That is because, lacking experience, the neuron clusters never form to react to those particular phonemes. Each birthday takes your baby further and further away from any sound not experienced, and therefore not tracked in her brain. With each passing year, she will have more difficulty learning a language other than her own. As baby grows, so do the jobs prescribed for each particular neuron. Ultimately, there are fewer neurons accessible to hear unfamiliar sounds and phonemes. Experience is so significant in language development that it even stretches into the realm of vocabulary.[23]

NINE WAYS TO ENCOURAGE BABY'S SPEECH DEVELOPMENT

Your baby is a social animal and is dependent on your reactions to his efforts at language. You can reinforce your baby's speech in a variety of ways by capturing your child's attention and engaging him in the process of learning:

1. **Play games such as peekaboo or patty-cake.** I used to sing to my grandchildren, "If you're happy and you know it, clap your hands." Activity along with words can help to advance language.

2. **Give your child items and identify them with energy.** For example, say with great enthusiasm: "Here's your spoon! Here's your applesauce!" By attaching action to words and emotion, you help your child create associations in his brain, and this can help advance his speech. Point to the light and say, "Here's the light." By pointing with your finger, you're connecting motion to language.

3. **The key to teaching and enhancing language is to talk, talk, talk** while trying to be as physical as possible when talking. Attaching emotion to language enhances linguistic connections.

4. **Be interactive.** If you're feeding your child, have a two-way conversation by asking questions. For example, "We're having applesauce. Do you like applesauce?" The synapses are connecting as you make associations. When your child's activities are interactive, you encourage him to think about

what you're saying. This is the learning process. Questions such as "Do you want to play? Do you want to eat? Do you want to take a bath?" will encourage him to think. Speaking to your child in complex language can raise his IQ approximately twenty points.[24]

5. **Remember to identify body parts.** For example, "This is your nose. These are your feet. This is your mouth." Then ask your child, "Where is your nose? Where are your feet? Where is your mouth?" Elevating your voice with emotion while doing this makes learning exciting and captures your child's attention.

6. **Sing songs, recite nursery rhymes, read stories, and have your child tell you a story.** Play with things like a jack-in-the-box, a top, or a ball, identifying each item while showing your child how it works. For example, the jack-in-the-box pops open, the top spins, the ball bounces.

7. **Take pictures and show your child what he looks like.** Let him look at himself in the mirror and ask, "Who is that in the mirror?" Then identify your child by asking, "Is that you?" This is one way to create an associative mass that enhances learning.

8. **Categorize things.** Put all the stuffed animals together. Put all the bath toys together. Put all the pots and pans together. Then you can ask your child to identify them. "Where are all the stuffed animals? Where are the bath toys? Where are all the pots and pans?" This is how she connects and expands her knowledge and uses her brain like an orchestra.

9. **Play Baroque music, 24/7, in the background.** Baroque music puts the brain in an alpha state, which is similar to meditation. It draws more blood to the prefrontal cortex and helps your child process information better, helps him hold images longer, and helps him use his brain more effectively. Baroque music, especially in the largo movements, is aligned

with your child's heartbeat, so it puts him in a calm and relaxed state, giving him a better chance to reach his full capacity.

Your toddler is uniquely tied to the strength and length of his mother's verbal communication. Toddlers whose mothers often speak to them have a vocabulary of 131 words more than those whose mothers do not.[25] By age two, toddlers with talkative moms double their vocabulary to approximately 295 words. The key here is repetition. Speaking to your child in a conversational manner, using complex language, and repeating words often is the path to language acceleration.

Because of your baby's brain neuroplasticity, he can soon distinguish and imitate the phonemes that he hears repeatedly. Not only that, but before the age of five, your toddler can learn any and as many languages as he hears regularly—the only caveat being that he hear each specific language consistently spoken by the same person. For example, if four people in one family speak four different languages, it is important that each member speak in only one language, exclusively to your baby. By twelve months, your baby can no longer identify or recognize the phonemes or sounds that he has not heard. He can only access those phonemes that he hears consistently and the sounds that are native to his own language, the language he hears each day. By the time your child is ten, however, that neuroplasticity lessens, and whatever added language he learns will now sound foreign. Like all brain development, language acquisition and the sequence and formation of neural synapses specifically correlate to the appearance of particular skills uniquely receptive at that distinct moment. Hence, exposing your child to the appropriate experiences at the prime time for learning offers your child the best possible chance to fulfill his potential.

HOW EARLY PATTERNS OF BEHAVIOR ARE FORMED IN OUR FAMILY OF ORIGIN

A number of years ago, I saw a *Nightline* interview with Bruce Springsteen. I'll never forget how I felt when I heard him express that all of his songs were about what happened to him in his childhood. Then he said that he was still trying to process the feelings that he had from those early experiences with his father, family, and friends. It's a psychological truth that in everyone's life, from birth to death, there really are only two people: Mother and Father. All your relationships are based on your early interactions with those two people, because all your patterns of connecting to others were forged in the crucible of your family of origin.

Your perceived place in the world was crafted and honed through the neural tracks those experiences created. Your sense of right and wrong, as well as your self-esteem and feelings of confidence and competence, are all wrapped up in the thread attaching you to your parents. Your willingness to risk and venture out beyond your comfort zone is a result of bonding with your mom and dad. That is how you build a strong central core, which allows you to hear your inner voice and find your true vocation. It is how you access your own resources and learn to follow your own authority. These feelings of security inspire motivation, which can be transferred to your child, and on to the next generation. It is this security that opens your child to the possibilities available to him through learning. The ingredients needed to prepare such a feast include stimulation, enthusiasm, and excitement, all enticing the senses toward the desire for involvement and commitment. The field of epigenetics tells us that such expansion in brain development, if habituated, can lead to a genetic change that can become generational.

Moreover, Dave and Wolf reported a study that examined the effects of the home environment on school learning, specifically on verbal ability. They discovered that what parents do, rather than who they are, accounts for the learning development of children in the early years of school. Through interviews with the parents as well as observational techniques, Dave and Wolf attempted to investigate the environmental process variables in the homes—that is, the interactions between children and their parents in relation to learning in the school and in the home.[26]

Dave and Wolf suggested that there is little that can be done to change the socioeconomic status of a child, but that a great deal can be done within the more influential environmental process that will improve their later linguistic, cognitive, and social functioning. In their studies on four- and five-year-old children, Dave and Wolf reviewed environmental process variables including a family's work habits, academic guidance and support, stimulation, language development, academic aspirations, and expectations. These variables correlated highly with achievement. [27]

Therefore, new questions have developed for early education that engage issues involving the entire social structure, from the family structure itself to the social hierarchy projected in miniature onto these "at-risk" children and their "super-baby" opposites. The answers to such questions will affect the social structure itself, as well as each person in it.[28] For example, it is well within the realm of possibility that businesses could construct good nursery care for their employees, offering you the opportunity to visit your child at structured times during your workday. This would relieve your baby's stress, lowering cortisol, which can a have a destructive outcome on the developing brain. Such access to your child can also relieve your stress, knowing that you can see your child at regular intervals, reassuring her that she is not abandoned by reattaching to her sense of bonding and security. On a small scale, such nursery programs already exist, but if businesses and the government partner, this childcare approach can become the norm rather than the exception.

The impact of positive parental involvement cannot be overstated. Children need time with their parents to interact, to question, and, most importantly, to have time to think creatively and reflect. A study by Estrada and others examined the correlation between the affective quality of the mother-child relationship when the child was four years of age and the later consequences for the child's elementary and secondary school-related cognitive functioning; they reported that composite scores that were indicators of the affective relationship were highly correlated with all measures of cognitive functioning. On the other hand, the affective relationship was not significantly related to the maternal intelligence quotient, socioeconomic status, or the child's sex.[29] Whether or not parental involvement in early childhood is sufficient will determine the development of both your child's brain architecture and her impulse control. Research indicates that the hippocampus, in particular, where memory and learning reside, can be altered by consistent early childhood deprivation. The amygdala, where your emotions and fight or flight can be found, also changes with exposure to ongoing stress. What happens is that the hippocampus narrows and the amygdala enlarges. Under normal circumstances, the prefrontal cortex is the captain of the ship. But when you're under stress, the process of critical thinking slows down in the prefrontal cortex, and the amygdala enlarges, thus becoming the new captain. This means that your emotions are driving your behavior rather than your executive function. If stress is temporary, the biological changes will also be temporary. However, if stress or deprivation is consistent, then the altered architecture of the hippocampus and amygdala will also be permanent. For instance, if your child is abused or disregarded and is not held, cuddled, or bonded, his brain will exhibit characteristics similar to posttraumatic stress disorder, reflecting his ongoing deprivation.

On the other hand, neuroscience tells us that positive bonding experiences in early childhood development can support and even multiply your baby's neuroglial cells, the very cells that transmit neurological signals across the brain's connective wiring or synapses. This process speeds up when your baby's neuroglial cells are increased, a mechanism that has the potential to accelerate learning. Consequently, it is easy to understand how this enhanced transmission of signals can foster not only more rapid patterns of thought, but also more complex ones. Expanded and heightened escalation of neuroglial cells is a process often found in the gifted child, another instance where parental behavior can specifically affect early childhood brain development and functioning on a cellular level.

Take the shy child. Cutting-edge science explains that shyness can actually be seen in the brain. Though shyness makes your child unique, it can create social problems for her later in life. By knowing your child, you will recognize immediately her tendency to shyness. For example, she may nestle into your neck when strangers appear, or hold on tightly to you for security. She can become fussy or display characteristics of anxiety when around strangers and in general show an elevated irritability when in the company of others. Nevertheless, you have the ultimate authority to influence your child's shyness by constructing an environment in which she is securely bonded and supported by you when around nonfamily members.

Though shyness has a strong genetic component, your child's shyness gene is a probability, not necessarily an outcome of that particular gene. If you structure specific times for social activity, never leaving your baby's side and keeping those interactions short but sweet, little by little, your shy child will begin to trust you, himself, and soon others. Because trust is based on experience, it is important to be counted on during this period, and to not let your baby down. By creating a new habit for your baby, you are desensitizing him, while fostering his interest in playing with other children. Sooner or later, your shy child will begin to outgrow his shyness and become socially functional. It is interesting to note that according to Dr. Jerome Kagan, the hearts of shy children, even in the womb, beat faster than children who are not shy, at approximately 140 beats per minute.[30] Even in utero, the shy child appears to be on high alert, especially reactive to input as he monitors his tiny world. In the past, parents were told to just play the hand they were dealt and learn to live with their child's shyness. Today, however, science has made us wiser, teaching us that though your child may have the predisposition to shyness, it is not necessarily his destiny.

As a parent, you have the power to affect and even raise your child's IQ quotients, as well. New thinking from as early as the 1960s showed that "IQ was not fixed at birth and could be significantly changed by the right stimulation in infancy and early childhood."[31] Psychologist Benjamin Bloom contended that "the environment would have its greatest effect upon a characteristic [i.e., a trait like intelligence] during its most rapid development."[32] According to Bloom, the brain develops more rapidly from conception to age four than it does from ages four to eighteen. Since your child, as a dynamic unity, is in a reciprocal relationship with her environment, you can appreciate how potent your influence is. The power of bonding cannot be overstated, and early compensation for deprivation is not only effective, but often overcomes deficits simply by exposing parents to the right information at the right time.

Supporting parents so that they can lead their children to learn is not, and does not have to be, either arduous or labor-intensive. Actually, you can see positive results almost immediately. It is irrelevant whether you are highly educated or financially well resourced; regardless of your income or educational level, you can enhance your child's learning capacity. In brain development, actions and words speak loudly, and what you do and say encourages or represses your baby's innate hardwiring to learn. Every hug, every cuddle, every story, every lullaby creates crackling impulses across the synapses of your child's brain, building that associative mass that will help determine the course of his future. It is far simpler to modulate your child's home environment than either the education or socioeconomic level of his parents.[33]

GIFTED CHILDREN

Gifted children, for the most part, have parents who make them feel special by paying special attention to them. Your gifted child would not necessarily be able to find her gift, never mind develop it, if it weren't for your involvement in her interests, whether it's exposure to science, math, languages, music, art, etc. Recognizing your child's gifts early allows you to support her on her journey to excellence. There are two common clichés: one, that "geniuses are born, not made"; and two, that "talent will out." Both of these complicate our understanding of the role parents play in recognizing talent and creating the proper environment in which it can bloom. Furthermore, geniuses, champions, and gifted children don't always display their talents early or obviously. Thus, it requires a savvy parent who's there to notice what her child is reaching for in that rich and stimulating environment she created. Elkind tells us, "The child is a gift of nature, but the image of the child is mankind's creation."[34] In a very real sense, without your special attention, your gifted child would not necessarily access the ranges of her full capacity.

Though your infant or toddler appears to be spending his day playing, he's actually using an inordinate amount of energy, time, and effort investigating and understanding his surroundings. Your child learns spontaneously, with every experience he encounters while exploring his environment. For that reason, it is essential to give active care. As Dr. Montessori reminds us, "helping the infant mind in its work of development" is your primary job.[35] She went on to state that this is the new direction for education: an approach to help the mind in its process of development, aiding its energies and strengthening its many powers. According to Elkind, one thing that many gifted children have in common is that their parents foster a strong sense of self and exceptionality by paying attention to the full spectrum of their talents. Exceptional children might never have reached their potential without this specific contribution from their parents.[36] By actively and enthusiastically participating in your child's life, you value his efforts, which supports and encourages him to achieve. By establishing a creative climate at home, filled with objects and textures that excite your baby's senses, in conjunction with your constant scaffolding and support, he will expand both his frame of reference and his scope of knowledge. Your role as a parent is crucial in cultivating the appropriate climate conducive to learning, as experience is the vehicle that compels your child to act on his surroundings. Though mental growth begins in the womb, it continues with the greatest intensity in early childhood. That is why, if you give active care in the beginning, you can guide your child in the building of his own mind. Only then can your child be merged into the fullness of his being—his destiny, capable of following his own authority and molding his own future.

Yet if you do not exert or make provisions for your child's need for attention, care, and bonding, you will not be able to discover your child's vital wants and needs or bridge together the delicate scaffold of his brain's formation. We hear so much about happiness as a choice, but I see happiness more as a condition. Following that reasoning, if you successfully integrate the patterns of brain development along with the appropriate learning experiences, your child will be set onto the path of true happiness, which will affect him for the rest of his life in everything he does and with everyone he meets.

Different learning modalities are necessary during different phases of growth, and though these phases are unique, they are linked by the importance of successfully navigating each. According to Erik Erikson, your child's aptitude and intellectual strength cannot reach their optimal possibilities if her stages of development are not passed through completely and on time. Like the caterpillar who wraps himself in a chrysalis, only to re-form into the full beauty of its complete nature, so too does your child need a secure and rich cocoon in which to mature.[37]

Your involvement in your child's development is imperative from the moment of her birth. If you don't seize the moment, you will lose your window of opportunity. Research by Dr. Benjamin Bloom gives ample support to the value of early education in relation to its effects on intelligence, telling us that it is this period of rapid brain growth that is most receptive to the environment.[38] By the age of four, your child will have reached approximately half of her IQ.

Now, with the knowledge of early childhood development, you can easily and seamlessly shepherd your child to take full advantage of the significant learning opportunities that are age-appropriate and therefore available to him. You are and will always be his first teacher, like it or not. By making your home child-centered and user-friendly, your child will be able to learn and excel with ease.

IN SUMMARY:
YOUR BABY'S DEVELOPMENT:
AGES 4 TO 7 MONTHS

Between four and seven months, your baby will go through many important developmental changes. Here is what to watch for in terms of social, physical, sensory, linguistic, and cognitive milestones:

SOCIAL MILESTONES

Some of the social milestones babies reach at this age include the concepts of action, reaction, and cause and effect. It is at this stage your baby realizes that the things she does—making faces, dropping objects, waving a rattle, crying—get a reaction from her audience. Thus, for the first time, she recognizes that she has an impact on her world. Actually, your baby is testing herself against her environment. Between four and seven months of age, you will notice your baby smiling, laughing, becoming aware of colors, and experiencing anxiety and shyness toward strangers. Socially, your baby has begun to model and imitate the behavior and faces of those around her. Now is the time to create a safe, age-appropriate, and interesting environment for your child to experience.

PHYSICAL MILESTONES

1. The ability to turn over
2. Sitting up while gaining balance
3. Holding a rattle
4. Putting everything in her mouth
5. Starting to hold her bottle
6. Reaching for objects changing hands
7. Scooting forward on her tummy while using legs for traction
8. Gaining more control of her body and head
9. Holding feet and putting toes in her mouth while at rest

By seven months old, your baby's gross motor skills allow her to:

1. Put all her weight on her legs
2. Bounce while standing
3. Support herself by holding onto her crib or furniture
4. Almost sit alone while extending her arms to be picked up

SENSORY MILESTONES

Some of the sensory milestones at this age include responding to warmth, cuddling, and all forms of affection. Your baby has an awareness of others around her, including an anxiety toward strangers. Emotions may run high. Your baby will be curious and moody. She will let you know her feelings in a heightened way. She may display assertive behavior, and she may cry if a toy is taken away or playtime is disturbed. Though stress begins to be moderated as your baby matures, anger can be easily provoked over a loss of a possession. You will begin to see humor as baby responds to funny postures and faces. And your baby can imitate your facial expressions soon after birth though she has never seen her own face.

LANGUAGE MILESTONES

Between four and seven months, your baby may begin to make vowel sounds, double syllable sounds, and join consonants and vowels. At this stage, babies pay attention to and imitate the movements of others' mouths while speaking. Your baby will also create new sounds by moving his mouth into different shapes. He will start to notice tones and the way others use inflections, and he will respond to familiar sounds by modeling what he hears, often imitating sounds in one breath. Being exposed to complex language can help increase IQ at this stage.

COGNITIVE MILESTONES

At this stage, your baby begins to recognize the permanence of objects: she is beginning to understand that if you leave, you will return; that her favorite toy will not disappear the next day; and that if she hides something, she can find it. Games such as hide-and-seek and peekaboo are age-appropriate at this stage. Also, your baby will anticipate seeing something that she may have only seen partially. She will manipulate objects and will be stimulated by color and feeling. Thus, objects she can manipulate, touch, and stack are all developmentally helpful at this stage, as your baby starts to sort toys and blocks by category.

At just about seven months old, your baby will start to challenge authority. This will become evident when he deliberately ignores or refuses to take direction. He will also display more intimate behavior. For example, he may greet you in the morning with his hands up, wanting to be taken out of his crib, hug you when retrieved, or even give you that much-looked-for kiss.

RED FLAGS

Some red flags to watch for in this age range include developmental delays, physical birth defects, hearing impairment, autism, Down syndrome, Asperger's syndrome, fetal alcohol syndrome, and congenital problems such as heart defects. Be sure to talk with your child's pediatrician about any concerns you may have.

YOUR CHILD'S BRAIN DEVELOPMENT: AGE ONE

Have you ever wondered why your toddler isn't responding to you with what you believe should be a "normal" reaction? Or why your baby keeps opening and shutting the closet door over and over again?

Humans are one of the few species on Earth born "unfinished." At birth, our brains are nowhere near fully developed. The human brain develops quite slowly over time. New technology such as CAT scans, MRIs, and PET scans all indicate that your brain is still developing into late adolescence. Therefore, the way your baby and toddler thinks is colored by his stage of development. At first, your baby will view the world in concrete terms. The way he reasons and responds is directly correlated to this particular stage. For this reason, it is important to take your child's developmental stage into consideration when speaking with your child and when placing behavioral expectations on him.

SYNAPTIC PRUNING

Your infant's brain is born with approximately 100 billion neurons; while this sounds like a lot, it is actually about half of what it will have by the end of your baby's first year. In fact, your baby's brain will increase in size by a factor of up to five by adulthood. By age two or three, the brain has up to twice as many connections as it will have in adulthood; the reason is that as we grow older, our brains perform a sort of "use it or lose it" function, effectively "pruning" unused connections over the years.

Your baby's first year on Earth is full of neuron growth as well as the pruning of synapses, which is affected by environmental stimulation (or lack thereof).

So much happens during the first year of life that many parents I know are often overwhelmed and amazed at the changes their baby makes at this time.

SOCIAL AND COGNITIVE LEARNING

The brain development that happens in your baby's social learning as well as basic problem-solving is phenomenal in the first year. Your baby goes from not knowing how to do anything to being able to speak a foreign language, following simple directions such as "pick up the book," and using items correctly, such as using a book for reading time and using a cup to drink. While your baby still may not understand the nuances of physical activity, he is learning to explore by banging things together, throwing things, dropping things, and shaking them. This is your one-year-old's way of learning how things work. He may be throwing a stuffed animal across the room over and over again, but know that this action is *not* to annoy you, nor is it done as an emotional response. Your baby is simply doing what all babies do: repeating a movement in order to understand it.

Meanwhile, your baby also begins to develop social and emotional connections during his first year. You may wonder why your normally calm baby suddenly seems scared of strangers at around seven or eight months old. This comes from a brain spurt in the frontal lobe that brings about attachment; your baby has already formed an attachment with you and with other familiar caregivers, thanks to the familiar sounds of your voices and your touch, but they may experience sudden fear when you leave and/ or when someone unfamiliar approaches.

Until your baby is one year of age, she is still lacking behavioral control. She may start to understand that hitting a sibling is wrong, but her brain is still in the process of becoming able to override the impulse to do so. Therefore, it's important for you to be aware and to react to her developmental stage appropriately.

PARENTING TIPS FOR NEWBORNS THROUGH AGE ONE

1. **Talk to your infant, sing, and listen and react** to your newborn's gurgles and mumbles as much as possible. The more bonded you are to your baby, the more he hears your voice, feels your touch, and smells your scent, the more comforted and secure he will feel.

2. **Encourage all caregivers and visitors to talk to your baby often.** This will especially help during the seven-to-eight-month stage, when he will start to feel separation and stranger anxiety.

3. **Hold your baby as much as possible during this first year.** Babies respond strongly to attachment and begin to be socialized and culturalized when accompanying Mom and Dad on simple outings.

4. **Help your baby practice and rehearse motor, sensory, and cognitive advances** by creating a safe learning environment in which she can explore. Objects that can be manipulated, touched, and observed not only enhance learning, but will help your baby to test herself against her environment. Each experience will add to her insight and understanding and stimulate her brain's associative mass. Since your baby doesn't really begin to have controlling behavior until she turns approximately one, you can understand and empathize with her if she spontaneously hits her sibling or has a temper tantrum. Here, gently changing her environment while reminding her

verbally that hitting is not okay will remediate her behavior. On the other hand, when your baby throws her toy or drops things from her high chair, she is really processing an experiment with gravity. If you participate with her instead of fighting against her by scolding and trying to control her behavior, your understanding approach will lower the decibels of her reaction, while helping her intellect expand through insight and cognition.

5. **Give your baby a safe, open space in which to learn while being supervised.** Clear out sharp and heavy objects from a living room, for example, and let your baby play on the floor with blocks, books, stuffed animals, wooden spoons, and age-appropriate toys. While this may look like mindless activity to you, this form of free play allows your child's brain to make more connections with actions.

Age 2, Piaget calls "preoperational." This is where children begin to acquire language, use mental images and symbols, and understand simple rules. They see the world only from their perspective. For example, if they cover their faces and cannot see others, they still believe that means others cannot see them.

Even by age 2, children have learned there are rules that should not be violated. They may not be rules about morality, as such. They are more likely rules about games or their likes and dislikes; for example, never let the carrot mix in with the peas on the plate. But it is the beginning of understanding the rules that will form the basis of more sophisticated moral reasoning.

Age 3, Deals with "preoperational." At this stage, children distinguish between fantasy and reality: they become more logical, less egocentric. They can concentrate and solve problems better and begin to understand the relation between time, distance, and speed, as well as other rules that govern the world.

YOUR THREE-, FOUR-, AND FIVE-YEAR-OLD: DEVELOPMENTAL MARKERS

Ages 3, 4, and 5 focus on your child's growing ability to deal with abstract ideas, understand ethical principles, and reason about rules and regulations.

Like all parents, you are concerned about your child's development. Is his development on time, advanced, or slow? If you feel concern or worry that something is wrong, it is better to confront it rather than deny it. It is important to remember that your child is an individual and will mature at his own rate of speed, within the parameters of average developmental markers. A professional can determine if a four-year-old is up to the task with cognitive development by comparing a child's maturity against the appropriate developmental markers.

STANDARD DEVELOPMENTAL MARKERS FOR THREE-, FOUR-, AND FIVE-YEAR-OLDS

1. Your child reaches for more independence while exhibiting more self-control.
2. He can problem-solve now and maintain sustained periods of focus.
3. She can hold images longer and stick to problem-solving.
4. When your child is upset or feeling out of control, he is more able to tell you how he feels.
5. Cognitive language and social development are displayed through more complicated language, vocabulary, and logic. For example, she is able to recognize abstract ideas such as time, including mealtimes.
6. He exhibits a sense of humor and delights in rhyming words.
7. She can count past ten and identify colors, shapes, and letters.
8. He may be starting to read.
9. She can perform simple tasks with ease, such as brushing her teeth, taking a bath, and getting ready for bed, as well as handling eating utensils.

10. His motor skills are developing, and at this stage, he can start to use safety scissors, while copying and cutting out shapes, and drawing a whole human figure.

Parents, it is important that you know your children. If they are not reaching these developmental markers, then your child's pediatrician should be the next line of defense. Have a good general workup by a professional to make sure your child isn't having any developmental delays.

4

AVOID THE CURSE OF OVERSTIMULATION, EMOTIONAL EQ, AND THE WORKING PARENTS' GUIDE

This chapter must start with a discussion about the importance of play. Play is a substantial part of childhood and must not be hurried or transformed into work. In fact, pure play is needed to reduce stress, to give time for creative and contemplative thought, and to experience uninhibited pleasure. Moreover, adults should not turn play into work and must not teach children during their playtime. In fact, play fosters creativity better than store-bought toys. Imagination and self-expression are essential to healthy brain development. Childhood is one of the most important parts of life and should be both respected and valued. Children are entitled to their childhood and should not be hurried through this stage.

THE IMPORTANCE OF IMAGINATIVE PLAY

The other day, my grandchild was playing dress-up and asked her grandpa and me to be her audience. She decided to have a fashion show and even asked for pencil and paper so she could write down her name and give us her autograph. This image took me back to my own childhood of orchestrating plays on the back porch, playing grocery store at the kitchen table, and playing dress-up with old clothes in the attic.

This is the magical thinking of childhood that helps the brain develop creativity. This creativity, if allowed to blossom, is the same creativity that helps the scientist discover new cures for diseases, helps companies come up with the next technological advances and inventions, and helps leaders move their countries toward peace.

When your child is little, under the age of two, he understands the world through his senses. But as he grows into his toddler years and begins to understand the way things operate, he uses his imagination to explain the mysteries of his world. Imaginative play is arguably the most important play your child will ever participate in—more important than all the toys, all the games, and all the things you buy for him to enhance his learning.

It is imaginative play that helps your child relate to his feelings and strong emotions, to gain control over his behavior, and to work through his darker thoughts and feelings of anger, fear, and guilt. You may be aware of the use of dolls by therapists and mental health professionals to help children document emotional and physical abuse. Pets and other children, and even you, Mother or Father, can become actors in your child's fantasy world. Pets give children an ally to talk to, to dress up and play with, who listens uncritically and can be manipulated freely. Moreover, imaginative play is both stress-reducing and self-soothing, two very important remedial needs of childhood.

If creative play is so important, how do you offer it to your child? Like everything else, there are rules of engagement, and you as a parent need to know the rules.

ENCOURAGING IMAGINATIVE PLAY

1. Don't discount, shame, or embarrass your child for his imagination, but rather play along and be part of his fantastical world—only if invited.
2. Let children use things that are part of the house, rather than going out and buying a lot of toys. Remember the tents you built between two chairs using a sheet, or the fort you made

under your bed? These are the things that really excite and stimulate the imagination—the simple things, the real things: old clothes, blocks, dolls, clay, pots, pans, beads, colored pencils, crayons, and paper that can be made into invitations, pictures, playbills, menus, and so on.

3. A great way to stimulate creativity is simply to read to your child in a child-directed way, meaning to use open-ended questions to provide the opportunity for imaginative outcomes to the very story that you are reading. There are so many advantages to this, including the acquisition of language and IQ enhancement.

4. The most important thing about creative play is that it should be free play; let your child take the lead. He will let you know if he needs private time, or if he wants you to be a participant in his scenario—but you should be around. You have to create a safe, rich, and contained environment, so that you can be there if needed, without interfering if not wanted.

5. Finally, bedtime is actually a wonderful time for deepening the imagination, so leave enough time in the bedtime schedule for that to occur. The bedtime ritual should include a little reading from Mom or Dad that can spur your child's imagination before he falls off to sleep. Twilight time, when a child is in that soft space between awake and asleep, is a wonderful time for him to use his imagination, and nighttime stories help direct that experience.

Now that you have some general guidelines, here are some specific ideas that you can use to spur your child's imagination based on his age:

- **Birth to three years old:** Create a print-rich environment with age-appropriate objects to manipulate, touch, observe, and interact with, including pots, pans, socks, beads, Play-Doh, and musical instruments. Don't use Play-Doh or beads until your child is old enough, since both can be choking hazards.

- **Three to six years old:** Now your child can play with little purses that are old and ready to be cast away, old hats, old shoes, plastic cups and dishes, paper, arts and crafts, clay, dolls, doctor's kits, toy cars, blocks, and large beads. If asked to join in, you can turn play into an adventure: the couch becomes a raft, the kitchen floor is your island, and so on. After age four, imaginative play becomes more sophisticated, and children are into playing house, school, and other fantasies using dress-up costumes, including tiaras and magic wands, and sheets for superhero capes, tents, and forts. Legos, blocks, clay, cars, paints, crayons, and other school supplies are useful tools. Provide your child with arts and crafts materials that allow him to color his dreams and write his stories, bringing his imagination into his conscious world.

You will be creative until the day you die. Whether it's simply daydreaming, writing, painting, listening to music—all of the inventions that have brought us to this place and time are a result of someone's imagination. So, it is important to give your child a safe place to foster the associations in his brain that allow for the development of inspiration, the stimulation necessary for problem-solving, and the a-ha moment when complicated ideas take form.

MAKE FREE PLAY A PRIORITY IN YOUR CHILD'S LIFE

Today's kids are immersed in a laundry list of activities and classes even before they reach school age. As a parent, you want to give your child the best advantage in life as possible. However, overscheduling and overstimulating your child may be hindering his intelligence rather than helping him.

Free play is critical to your child's development. Many of the world's greatest discoveries occurred during relaxed states. Albert Einstein reportedly came up with the theory of relativity when daydreaming while doing repetitive work at a patent office. James Watson claims his sudden insight during a good night's sleep led to the discovery of the double helix, or DNA molecule, Isaac Newton is said to have come up with his theory of gravity after seeing an apple fall from a tree while lounging in his mother's garden.

Our natural state is peaceful, and by calming our minds, we distract ourselves from our distractions. This helps us organize our environment to allow creativity to blossom. Therefore, you need to give your child time to access her natural state and find her gifts.

While your child is young, you should provide free play opportunities in safe print- and material-rich environments. These environments help foster elements of observation, manipulation, communication, and creativity.

By age four, 50 percent of your child's IQ is in place; by adolescence, 80 percent. Instead of constantly making sure your child is "doing something productive," give her time to be herself . . . and watch the amazing ways she will use that time. At least once each day, set aside free play time for your child.

INCORPORATING FREE PLAY INTO YOUR FAMILY LIFE

- Give your baby or toddler a safe space that is confined and secure. Let him explore his play area, for instance, while you are nearby reading a book.
- Before giving your baby or toddler free play time, be sure to remove potentially dangerous items such as hot tea and coffee, toxins of all kinds, choking objects, glasses, knives, and other sharp objects from the area.

You can choose to start with one of these practices at a time, starting with one that you feel best works with your family structure and schedule.

THE POWER OF OUTDOOR PLAY

In this age of technology, it is important to understand the power of outdoor play in children's lives.

As a social animal, participating in outdoor play helps socialize and cul-turalize your preschooler through peer-group socialization. Games teach your preschooler how to know the rules and follow the rules. He learns about instructions, teamwork, camaraderie, collaboration, competition, and motivation as he pushes past his efforts to win.

Outdoor play can help your preschooler develop her motor skills and strengthen her muscles and bones. Not only does your preschooler get a chance to lower her stress and anxiety through physical activities outside, but she also has the opportunity to connect to her natural self: that part that responds to nature.

Cognitively, your preschooler can learn a great deal from spending time outdoors and trying things out, rather than simply hearing about them. In fact, outdoor play is a step toward your preschooler's independence. Through games, both collaborative and competitive, your preschooler can develop confidence, competence, and self-sufficiency. This all transfers to your preschooler's sense of self and intrinsic motivation. Further, your pre-schooler is socialized by his peers and when playing with others is taught to share, collaborate, and be tolerant.

Furthermore, your preschooler learns to think critically as he strategizes and plans how to compete and win not only for himself, but also as part of a team. In a sense, outdoor activities and sports can teach your preschooler how to test himself against his environment. Your preschooler can expe-rience cognitive and language strides simply through outdoor games that have rhyming, complicated language, grammar, and syntax. When exposed to other children, friendships, and social interactions, your preschooler develops phonology, complex language, and the comprehension necessary for peer-group interaction.

To make the most of outdoor playtime, all outdoor activities should be age-appropriate and parentally supervised. Here are some ideas for games that can teach your preschooler valuable skills: hide and seek, in which your child can learn counting; spy games such as Clue; story games, like telling a story and having each child add to it; memory games, such as the Telephone

Game; rhyming games, such as childhood rhymes recited during jumping rope; Red-Light, Green-Light; ball games of all kinds, including pee-wee baseball; Red Rover; and Statue.

Activities that involve nature—such as riding a bike with training wheels; collecting leaves, shells, and rocks; and building forts and castles from sand, leaves, twigs, shells, and stones—require cognitive skill, planning, and execution, which can all help your preschooler mature and learn about healthy social interactions and relationships.

When your preschooler is physically active outdoors, she has the opportunity to reduce her stress and anxiety. In fact, you are teaching your preschooler to cope and manage her own stress. Outdoor games can lead to better immunities and feelings of well-being, as well as a healthier, happier preschooler, both mentally and physically. Outdoor play can also give you the opportunity to teach your preschooler about safety and danger, including stranger-danger.

When I was a child, my parents told me, "Don't talk to strangers," though I was allowed to play with other children in the backyard and ride my tricycle in the neighborhood. This allowed me to interact with my surroundings, to explore, to try out new things, building on my experiences. This is how you develop the confidence and competence that lead to maturity. Today, however, children have helicopter parents who satisfy their guilt about too many hours away from their children by overprotecting them. When children are given theoretical information about their world, while being forbidden to enter that world, they remain inexperienced and immature. This is where your children find themselves today.

A friend once asked me which parental warnings my children would remember. Would it be like my mother's "don't talk to strangers"? Or would it be something like "don't go with strangers," or "if abducted, scream 'Stranger!'" and so forth? In our new normal, children are exposed to violent and threatening information that they are not old enough to cope with. Yet media will remind them of such danger daily. Whether it is an AMBER alert, a 24/7 news cycle, or kindergartners sharing information overheard at home, children all too soon become aware of school violence concerns. Especially little children, who are by nature narcissistic and fear that whatever is happening in the outside world will happen particularly to them.

The tragic events of Columbine, Paducah, Santana, and, more recently, Palmdale, Parkland, and Santa Fe have evoked a fear psychosis that permeates all school populations from early childhood on. The one place most occupied, other than home, no longer feels safe.

When children are frightened by such information, it is often helpful to gather a group of parents together and organize one morning a week, preferably Saturday, where you can practice and rehearse age-appropriate safety measures with children who are of the same age:

- Teach children not to go to a car parked near a curb, no matter who calls them or what they say.
- Don't help a stranger find a puppy. Explain to your children a stranger is older than they are and capable of finding a pet by himself.
- Teach your child that if someone grabs him, start screaming "Stranger! Stranger!" while flailing his arms and legs like a windmill.
- Teach your child to grasp onto anything that can stabilize him if someone tries to carry him off. This is called Velcro, a mental image of sticking onto something stationary.
- Teach your child never to open the door to anyone, whether a stranger or not, unless you, their parent, have given them specific instructions in advance.
- Finally, the key to having your child be on alert is to practice and rehearse these very techniques.

There is now a new normal in our culture, a very dangerous one, and though we tell children to respect their elders, we must counter that rule, teaching them that strangers can mean danger, and they are not to obey other people—no matter their age—unless specifically directed by their parents.

Another constant source of angst, other than school safety, is the limitation of time. It used to be that only older people talked about time moving more quickly as they aged, but now we are all conscious of the pressure of time. With modern technology and conveniences, you can accomplish more in less time, by squeezing extra activities into fewer hours. And we expect the same from our children. Many of your technological conveniences such as television, computers, phones, email, and the Internet are all organized to give you more quality time with yourself and your family. Unfortunately, it has accomplished just the opposite.

Children are paying a high price for being hurried through childhood. In 1960, fewer than half of all toddlers went to preschool prior to kindergarten. Today, children are entering preschool earlier than ever before. Now, 85 percent of all toddlers in the United States currently have a preschool experience. They also begin sports activities earlier than ever before, with children as young as two years of age already being signed up for summer camps that specialize in tennis, golf, or both. This hurrying children through childhood can have a deleterious and crippling effect on not only a young child's emotions and feelings of competition, but also on growing bones and joints, causing hip and arm fractures as well as rotator cuff injuries.

Each day children are being stressed for success. Just like their parental counterparts, their schedules are filled to the brim, bulging with activity. Not only are children separated from parents too early, but they are also away from home for most of the day, busy with school and extracurricular activities that may last until dark, often past suppertime. If you stop to think of all the opportunities you want for your child, such as sports, ballet, lessons in piano or other time-consuming instruments, afterschool practices, and clubs, you can understand why children have little time for any contemplation, inner work, or creative free play. Consider that it is during free play that your child has the opportunity to access the deepest parts of his own resources, where he learns best because his stress is reduced, and he can experience a state of calm and quiet. Sadly, children often communicate more with their pets and their toys than they do with their parents. Every child knows that pets and toys love them unconditionally and listen to them with complete acceptance and validation.

THE BENEFITS OF GROWING UP WITH PETS

My dear friend Susan is a horse whisperer who has helped many children with PTSD heal. One day while having lunch together, I asked her to explain why animals, and horses in particular, help children with PTSD recover. She explained that children of abuse and domestic violence, as well as children who have physical and emotional challenges, respond to horses (and other animals) because they intuitively recognize that they can trust them.

Children who are emotionally and physically injured and abused have no voice and often are emotionally and physically paralyzed, unable to express themselves. These children are frozen, and yet, as they sit astride a big, powerful horse, they learn once again to trust, relax, and surrender to the movement of their new ally. A horse neither judges nor criticizes but loves unconditionally. Not only does he respond with nonverbal cues, such as sound, nuzzling, and pricking up his ears, but he is also honest and will not let your child get away with anything—no deception, no deceit. Further, because a child burdened with either physical or emotional challenges or abuse is often cloaked in dishonesty, he may encounter, for the first time, a friend whom he can count on to not let him down.

When a horse carries your child, who feels small and powerless, his very movement relaxes your child and restores control through action. When riding a horse, your child can find a safe place of unconditional acceptance and love with her best friend and therapist—her horse.

The history of mankind's initial connection with domesticated animals has long been debated, but a discovery in Israel of a man buried with his arms around a pup, dating back 12,000 years, may be evidence of just how long ago humans discovered the benefits of having pets.[1] Today, many people love their pets and consider them to be members of their own families. Whether you choose a cat, a dog, a gerbil, a bird, a horse, or a rabbit, the benefits of raising children in a home with pets are great:

- **Pets give unconditional love.** They are nonjudgmental, and especially for only children, lonely children, or children who have sibling rivalry or emotional distress, a pet gives them someone to talk to. A pet can comfort, give support, and listen to a child's troubles without judgment or consequence. When playing, a pet can become your child's partner and best buddy.
- **A pet can teach a child that he doesn't have to take out his anger or fear on others.** Some children become bullies, and if they don't have a safe place to share their truest emotions, they may project those emotions onto other children. Because a pet will love your child no matter what he says, a pet gives him a confidant, a safe place in which to verbally pour out his fears and his anger, and a safety valve to inoculate him from acting out.
- **A pet can teach empathy.** Caring for a pet that is so dependent on you teaches empathy. Your child learns to read your pet's needs: Is he hungry? Does he need to go outside? Maybe the pet is scared of the wind, rain, or snow and needs to be comforted. Moreover, empathy is the one skill that can be taught, a skill that bullies often lack.
- **A pet can teach confidence and responsibility.** Children can gain confidence by having the responsibility of caring for a pet. Children as young as three years old can manage simple tasks such as filling a pet's water and food bowls. As your child gets older, he can groom and walk the pet.

- **Animals can help socialize children and increase verbal skills.**
  You've likely seen even little kids who are still learning to talk attempting to chatter away with pets. In this way, pets give not only social and emotional support, but also cognitive and language support to children. A pet's simple presence provides verbal stimulus to help your child practice talking and socializing with another living being.

- **Pets (and animals in general) can be very therapeutic for children.** Studies have shown how pets can help lower blood pressure, speed up recovery time, and reduce stress and anxiety. We see this with troubled children, autistic children, and children with Asperger's or PTSD: when children are with animals, they can immediately relate, because they sense the animals are unconditional in their love and affection.

THE IMPACT OF TELEVISION AND INTERNET VIDEOS ON CHILD DEVELOPMENT

Though print media is less problematic than television or the Internet to a growing child, it still has an impact, as magazine covers and books for children are filled with inappropriate and oversexualized language and pictures. Nevertheless, it's much easier to protect your child from unsuitable and overly sophisticated print material, as young children do not usually have the reading skills to comprehend such information.

According to Elkind, "Television, however, engages our senses immediately and does not always require the verbal mediation of a broadcaster to be conveyed or understood. Even young children don't need to understand the verbal description of tragedy taking place on television—the horrible images speak for themselves. Because television information does not require verbal encoding or decoding to extend our experience, it is very accessible to young children and sometimes hurries them into witnessing terrifying events never before witnessed by this age group."[2] What is so disturbing about this is that your child doesn't have to read or understand what is being said on television; she only has to observe. Her brain simultaneously captures both her emotions at the time of viewing and the image, creating an imaginary experience. Then, your child casts herself into the character on television, as her brain stores the memory of the violence or abuse on the screen as if it were real and actually happening to her.

Moreover, very young children become knowledgeable, not only about crimes, violence, and divorce, but also highly sexualized experiences, which they could never have imagined without the exposure to television. Yet there is a lack of understanding and a sense of guilt when children find themselves viewing such confusing and disorienting material. Here, children develop what Dr. David Elkind calls pseudo-sophistication. Though they can talk about grown-up things in a childlike manner, and imitate adult behavior, they don't really understand what's going on. The superficial insight into complicated and complex relationships on television causes children to seem more knowing than they in fact are. Emotional maturity and physical maturity do not follow a parallel path. Consequently, precocious children can easily be hurried, and therefore pressured, into an older paradigm before they are ready. In a sense, television has become the third parent in the room, exposing children to unsuitable images of violence and sex. Even cartoon-like programming for children features girls and boys who use loose and inappropriate language and dress in an overly sexualized and provocative manner. According to a Tufts University study, as discussed in Elkind's *The Hurried Child*, toddlers as young as one not only pay attention to highly charged and graphic displays on television, but also react to them. Even babies recognize the difference between happy and sad, positive and negative emotions portrayed during a thirty-second TV spot, and react emotionally. When watching cruelty and abuse on TV, children as young as six weeks and as old as ten years experience that violence as their reality. This is because children are both narcissistic and egocentric, and because the brain stores memory with both experience and emotion.

GAIL GROSS

Children relate to television as if it were real and can react to programming by becoming anxious, having nightmares, and behaving as if they've experienced the abuse they've seen.

Some children's television is inappropriate in its design and scope—and so are some children's toys. Encouraging children to grow up too soon, manufacturers have developed highly sexualized dolls and inappropriate toys for both boys and girls. Just consider the latest Barbie or Ken doll, BRAT doll, Descendants doll, and so forth. The girl dolls are provocatively dressed with oversized and stylized lips and breasts, while the boy dolls often have an exaggerated and bulging crotch. Then there are the board games and video games, kicking it up a notch to a whole new level of unacceptable fare for children. And parents and children are following along, wearing clothing that is modeled for them on TV, in the movies, and on toys. It's time to pause and think about what we're doing to our children and to their future. And it is time for toy manufacturers to become more responsible, thinking at least as much about their consumers as they do their bottom line.

JUST A WORD ABOUT MULTIMEDIA FOR TODDLERS

You're on a lunch break at work talking with other parents about the question of exposing your child early and often to multimedia. As with everything else in parenting, you want the best for your child, including having him up to speed on new technology. Feeling pressured, you seriously begin to weigh the pros and cons of whether high-tech viewing is as important as imaginative play. Software for toddlers is moving toward the norm in our culture. Those parents who hold out and wait until their child is four or five years of age are questioned by peers, as well as their children. Even public libraries now have sections devoted to PC software for toddlers. Toddlers whose parents brag about how PC-savvy their children are only serve to add to the tension. On the other hand, there are those PC-savvy parents who are concerned that it is too early for their offspring to be indulging in computer viewing, and they worry about the best age and stage in which to start. So what's the best time to allow your child to interact with computer technology?

PROS AND CONS

Pros:
- Computers have become a part of our culture and therefore our education, as well as job preparation.
- Your child will ultimately pick up computer skills simply through osmosis, by playing with other children.
- When children should be first introduced to computers is still up for grabs, though the general consensuses is about three years old.
- Parents who allow computer access in early childhood think of computers in terms of a book, and therefore see that computer as an educational advantage.

Cons:
- Those parents concerned about the use of early childhood computer usage point out that your child's growing brain can be overstimulated from such exposure.
- Worried parents point out that computer usage can be addictive.
- Finally, anxious parents believe that children should be engaging in creative play rather than being exposed to hyperactive patterns and dialogue online that heighten and accentuate normal interactions in order to entertain.

In a report written by parent and child development experts, titled "Fool's Gold: A Critical Look at Computers in Childhood," researchers state that "early computing has no proven positive effects and may even be physically and intellectually harmful, especially for the youngest users."[3] Sadly, the danger of computer usage is so new to our collective psyche that it is difficult to find any longitudinal research that measures, over time, the impact of computer usage on toddlers.

Advocates of toddler software often cite the success of programs such as *Sesame Street*, but what they fail to mention is that when *Sesame Street* was evolving, they took into consideration the developing brain and responsibly changed their programming accordingly.

Early childhood development specialists, as well as educators, are deeply concerned about this new trend. Moreover, there is no credible study to date to indicate that access to computers accelerates learning. As we discuss often in this book, the explosion of language directly correlates to a leap in cognitive development. Further, language requires interacting with others so that your baby can practice and rehearse speaking while simultaneously building his brain's associative mass. So, as in all early childhood brain development, children need to relate to others, rather than just be passive viewers.

Another point of contention over computer exposure is the concern that flashing patterns, images, and cartoons can affect the brain's ability to pay attention, as the brain receives flashes and short bursts of program content. According to Dr. Sandra Sexson, another troubling aspect of computer usage is that it short-circuits children's use of imagination and creative play, so essential to learning. Introducing children to computer-game characters limits their ability to organize their own imaginative character in creative play. This is especially true when children repetitively watch the same programming that includes repeated, and often redundant, familiar characters.[4]

SUGGESTIONS FOR TODDLER PC VIEWING

- The magic number to begin PC viewing is three years of age. At that point, your child has already developed language and the ability to focus and pay attention. Also, your child will not fall behind if introduced to computer usage as late as age six. When tablets are used in preschool and kindergarten, it is important to be certain that they are supervised with scheduled time for viewing.

- Be aware and pay attention to make sure not to overstimulate your child with computer usage before the age of three. Consider how overwhelmed your child's growing brain can become from exposure to images and games developed for the precise purpose of engaging them and the injurious effect that hyperstimulation can create.

- After the age of three, direct your child to computer content that is interactive, paying attention to the effect that such programming has on your child's speech, values, and so on. Remember, your child is a social animal, and he will imitate what he sees, early and often, including behavior and gender biases.

- Whenever possible, coview with your child so that you are seeing what your child is doing. Never use the computer as a babysitter.

- Monitor not just what your child is watching, but for how long. Children should not be on a computer for long periods of time—thirty to forty-five minutes should be the daily maximum.

- Remember the importance of creative play. There's nothing more important to your child's brain development than his imagination, his own fantasies, and his free play time. Don't compromise it with technology—you will find it is no substitute.

FAMILY STRUCTURES

Heretofore, recognized family constructs were relatively traditional, but our ever-changing family compositions have created a new vehicle for stress. Fifty percent of all families with children under one have two working parents, indicating that parents are detaching from their offspring way too early. Also, 50 percent of all marriages in today's society end in divorce—this statistic is so common that it has become a cliché. The crippling effect of divorced parents on the psyches of their young children takes its toll, leaving children in the wake of divorce with a terrible sense of loss, a deep feelings of insecurity, and the anxiety that accompanies grief. By blurring the boundaries of what children believe to be irrevocable and everlasting—their family—divorce fractures a child's sense of self and trust in his place in the world. Parents are everything to a child. In a child's eyes, his parents are like appendages, not seen as separate from him, which is why children are so possessive of their parents. "My mother," "my father" are often heard bandied about in the conversations of children. But when divorce is imposed upon children, they are left in the debris, with loss of trust and connection with others. Such feelings of fear make children of divorce display problems in relationships, particularly with intimacy and commitment.

LOVING TIES THAT BIND—HOW YOUR BEST EFFORTS ARE PUTTING YOUR CHILD AT RISK

You think that preparing your child for success means teaching him how to stand on his own two feet. While that's true, most modern parenting swings between damaging extremes: either you throw your child out of the nest before he can fly, or shield him so much that he never sees the sun. Throw potentially toxic familial relationships into the mix, and you've already littered your child's path to success with obstacles before kindergarten has even started.

I repeatedly explain throughout this book that we detach from our children too early. That even a late adolescent male, as old as twenty-four, still wants and needs a hug from his mom. In the West, we tend to push our children out of the nest too soon—ironically, before they've learned how to fly. Instead of accomplishing what we set out to do, which was to make them more independent and self-sufficient, we create the inverse by pulling the rug out from under them prematurely, leaving them feeling insecure, stressed, and anxious. This all leads to needy, dependent children.

Along with feeling insecure and needy, children who are not well bonded have difficulty with trust. These children have a sense of free-floating anxiety, feeling on some level that they have been rejected and abandoned. Because they feel let down by their parents, they don't feel that they can count on them to be there no matter what. And because trust is based on experience, such children have a problem feeling that their parents are reliable. To compensate for these feelings of abandonment, they often turn to outside groups, cliques, and gangs, creating a substitute family and looking toward the gang leader as a surrogate parent. By not getting the parental bonding and approval needed for healthy personality development, children reach for their peers to bond with, depending on their peer group for socialization. We are seeing this more and more in urban settings, as witnessed by the gang violence in large metropolitan cities, such as Chicago.

We must decide if this is the future we want for our children. The answer of course is that you must take your power, you are the only one who can move your child into a healthy direction. Here is how you do it.

HOW CHILDREN LEARN

Throughout each stage of early childhood development, you will find a common thread. Your presence is needed at every stage to sew together the fabric of your child's future. Educators know that though there are many influences on your child's linguistic, cognitive, and social development, the most basic truth is that *you* are the most important one.

Bonding is the most crucial word in parental involvement. It is the key that unlocks the door to your child's capabilities, and it begins with creating a safe and secure attachment between you and your child. This bonding starts the first moment you hold your baby, continuing all through childhood. Ultimately, in adolescence, your child will begin the long and arduous process of separating from you. Until now, your child has been securely attached to you, but at early adolescence he will begin to separate so that he can integrate emotionally and intellectually all that represents his mother and father. Only then will he be able to individuate and, through a mysterious alchemical process, become a complete human being, reattaching to his parents while maintaining his own individualism.

Preparing your child to walk successfully in the world is not as complicated as it seems. In the following chapters, you will find three steps that are easily incorporated into your child's daily schedule. You will discover how to use the right techniques, at the appropriate time, to help your child access the full force of his capacity as you watch your child blossom and grow into the person she was meant to be. Also, you will experience the greatest joy in your life: watching your child revel in the excitement of learning. I will discuss these three steps in conjunction with the applicable exercise for each in Chapter 6. But for now, here is an overview:

Step A. Bond well with your child while nurturing her emotional maturity.

Step B. Positively affect your child's cognitive, linguistic, and social development.

Step C. Practice and rehearse stress-reduction techniques, including creative visualization.

THE REWARDS WILL BE GREAT—FOR YOU AND YOUR CHILD

At this point, it is important to note that the rewards for parental involvement in early childhood are great. When children are well bonded and securely attached, they do better at everything. They process information better, they problem-solve better, they stick to their efforts longer, and they develop a strong central core that allows them to stay calm in a sea of chaos as they resist pressure. Children who are well bonded are more likely to be emotionally mature, to have friends, to get along with others, and to be self-motivated.

Charles Silberman explains in *Crisis in the Classroom*, "To be practical, an education should prepare a man for a work that doesn't yet exist and whose nature cannot even be imagined. This can be done only by teaching children how to learn and by giving them the kind of intellectual discipline that will enable them to apply man's accumulated wisdom to new problems."[5] Likewise, you are preparing your child to walk in the world of tomorrow by exposing her to the appropriate learning models at the critical times of her development, which allows her to process information effectively and experience a love of learning. This will move your child from theory to practice as she integrates the way in which she processes accumulated knowledge with the intellectual discipline to solve new problems.

By helping your child discover his gifts, you create a legacy for the world at large. Children who reach their highest potential become those adults we count on to create the next preventive vaccine, cure for cancer, beautiful concerto, great work of art, or solution to address climate change.

When a child is relaxed and stress-free, his brain is just waiting for outside input. To that end, you have the power to awaken your child's creativity so that his brain can be used as an orchestra, open to all possibilities. When children are relaxed, cortisol stands down. It is only when your child is anxious or fearful that cortisol is summoned, bathing the brain and affecting its function. Only you have the capacity to inoculate your child against stress, by protecting him through the elixir of your love and bonding.

By being there and paying attention to your child's personality, you have the opportunity to plan her experiences in advance so that you can deliberately and successfully influence her behavior. For example, if you have a shy child, you can prepare him for social exposure and control the exposure so that he remains within his comfort zone. Then, little by little, you can enlarge and expand his social interactions so that he can ultimately become socially secure and functional. In addition, if your child has a favorite object of affection, toy or otherwise, and he doesn't want other children to touch it, put it away so that when he plays, he doesn't feel challenged to share it. Sharing is highly overrated in young children. When children are forced to share their toys, they are often made to feel discounted and insecure. Just as adults want their options, so too do children deserve to have their feelings respected.

HARDWIRED TO LEARN

Parents exert a powerful influence over child development; *you* can help your child become the best that he can uniquely be. But to do that, first you have to understand how your baby's brain develops.

YOUR BABY'S BRAIN CELLS

The core component of the nervous system and the brain is the neuron (brain cells), and your baby is born with roughly 100 billion of them. They don't divide, they don't die, and they aren't regenerated when they are lost. When they are lost, they're gone forever.

Neurons play important roles in processing and transmitting information. They do this through the synapses, or synaptic connections, that connect them with one another. Your baby is born with over 50 trillion synapses, and by age one, he will have more than 1,000 trillion of them! Some experts have estimated that this is like having a computer with a one trillion bit-per-second processor. That is some impressive thinking ability![6]

A typical neuron fires or sends information to other neurons five to fifty times every second. The more signals sent between two neurons, the stronger the neural connection grows.

These connections, and the increased activity they enable, make possible faster and more complicated patterns of thought—the very patterns associated with gifted children. Unlocking your child's gifted potential comes down to stimulating these patterns during optimal windows of growth.

THERE IS ONLY ONE YOU

Unless you're cloned, it takes an egg and a sperm to make a child. And you have to be present to raise one. That means you have to be there so that you can bond with your child and support his needs. You are your child's touchstone. Even more than that: your baby sees you, the parent, as part of himself; he doesn't think of you as a separate person.

Every experience, including simple acts of love, kindness, bonding, and touch, as well as the ways you stimulate him (by playing with him, talking to him, reading to him, and so on), influences the way your child's brain grows. In fact, you can enhance your child's intelligence and cognitive development simply through the environment you create and the way you interact with your child. In her book *The Handbook of Child Psychology*, Florence Goodenough says that parents can affect their child's IQ (a measure of intelligence) by 20 to 40 percent.[7]

THE IMPORTANCE OF PHYSICAL AND EMOTIONAL ATTENTION

On the other hand, if your child is deprived of physical and emotional attention, he will fail to thrive cognitively and emotionally. In the most extreme cases, he can even die.

Animal researchers discovered this as early as eighty years ago. Researchers in the 1940s found that primates who were deprived of their mother after birth fixated on any available object as their mother. When they were deprived of further social interaction, they developed mental illness and depression. Mice who are isolated from their mothers and are denied their mothers' instinctive and constant licking overproduce cortisol in their blood, which distorts the natural expression of their genes and changes the structure of their developing brain. This not only negatively affects their IQ, but also makes them more high-strung and less able to handle stress.

A thirty-year longitudinal study examined thirteen borderline cognitively disabled toddlers, one to two years of age, who were placed in an orphanage. Each day, a cognitively disabled teenager was assigned the same toddler and, under supervision, was just asked to hold and cuddle the baby. At the end of one year, all thirteen children were no longer borderline disabled and exhibited average intelligence. Eleven were adopted out and their progress was followed. Many of them went on to white-collar careers such as teaching, accounting, and others. Meanwhile, the two children left behind in the orphanage slipped back into cognitive disability.[8]

These studies demonstrate that inadequate nurturing can inhibit critical areas of the brain from developing, which can lead to a disastrous outcome for your child's mental and physical growth. These studies also demonstrate that you have to be present to respond to your child's needs and to bond, to frame and form the smart connections so needed for emotional, moral, and academic success. A few minutes a day won't cut it and won't get the job done. Focusing on quality over quantity just won't work.

When it comes to bonding, more simply is more. If at all possible, it is far preferable for your child to be with you throughout the day. In Kenya, for example, most babies under six weeks are at home with their mothers. Even after that, rather than hand their babies off to nannies or daycare centers, mothers or fathers thoroughly wrap their babies and strap them to their own bodies. Due to the utter closeness of their children, parents are keenly aware of their needs, and, as a result, Kenyan babies are said to rarely cry. This parental attention meets baby's needs leading to a well-bonded and emotionally secure child—something that modern Western culture has not yet figured out how to accomplish successfully.

But what happens when both parents work, as is common in the West, and must leave their baby in another's care? Since your baby sees you as inseparable from herself, being handed off to daycares, babysitters, or nannies—and apart from you—can trigger separation anxiety. This anxiety sets off a biological storm of stress hormones, including cortisol, causing the fight-or-flight response.

Studies have used saliva tests to demonstrate rising cortisol levels in children detached from their mothers too early. Although cortisol is necessary for proper body functioning and can be helpful in short durations, when it is produced to excess or persists over a long time, it bathes the brain in a destructive amount of stress hormones.

Studies in rats have shown that excessive amounts of cortisol actually kill neurons. Raised levels of cortisol for prolonged periods also impair functioning of the immune, digestive, circulatory, and reproductive systems and affect the growth response. In short, excessive or prolonged stress can affect your baby's brain in destructive ways with dire consequences.[9]

But the answer is not only to have your baby always with you. A secure bond doesn't just happen. Instead, it must be created—deliberately, consciously, and skillfully—through the commitment, obligation, and responsibility of parenthood.

The good news is that regardless of your own background or current situation, you can be what your child needs. For example, researchers have shown that your socioeconomic status accounts for only 10 percent of the variance in your child's academic success. It is what you *do*—supporting her, cuddling her, interacting with her, and reading to her, among other things—that has far more impact on your child's development than which degrees you've earned or how much you have in the bank.

NURTURE YOUR CHILD'S EMOTIONAL GROWTH

As parents, we often talk of child development as it pertains to intellectual growth. There are certain things parents can do to help give their children the best possible opportunities for increased IQ and to further learning capabilities. But what about emotional growth? Once your child can relax and focus, she is then in the best frame of mind to proceed with the two areas of growth most critical to reaching his or her full potential: emotional *and* intellectual development.

Emotional and intellectual skills go hand in hand. Without healthy emotional maturity, your child cannot achieve anywhere near his full cognitive capacity. Emotional intelligence affects moral development, as well. Emotionally mature children can make better use of their brains than immature children of the same age. It's that simple.

Maturity enables a child to sit, concentrate, learn, and so much more. It is the foundation of self-motivation, self-confidence, and a sense of competence. All of those qualities are essential to making use of your child's talents and knowledge in order to interact in a productive way with other people in the world.

The study of emotional development in infants and children is a relatively new science. It is only in the last few decades that educators have come to realize how important the emotions are to cognition, morality, psychosocial development, and all other areas of proficiency.

Howard Gardner was one of the first to point out that there are "multiple intelligences" beyond intellectual intelligence. Though it is intellectual intelligence, as measured by IQ, that is valued most in the West, Gardner identified seven intelligences. The first five are linguistic, logical-mathematical, spatial, musical, and bodily-kinesthetic. The remaining two deal even more directly with emotional growth: interpersonal and intrapersonal intelligences.

After 1980, Gardner added additional forms of intelligence to his list, except emotional intelligence.

Psychologist Daniel Goleman furthered the understanding of how interdependent our various forms of intelligence are with his book *Emotional Intelligence*. Goleman writes: "One of psychology's open secrets is the relative inability of grades, IQ, or SAT scores, despite their popular mystiques, to predict unerringly college achievement. . . . At best IQ contributes about 20 percent to the factors that determine life success, which leaves 80 percent to other forces."

Goleman, along with the majority of educators, now believes that it is *emotional intelligence* that enables a child to make the most of his or her cognitive skills and knowledge. Goleman presented a summary of neuroscientific research to demonstrate that the prefrontal lobes of the brain, which control emotional impulses, are also where memory is established and learning takes place. He showed that if a child is emotionally immature, and therefore more likely to be emotionally volatile, the child's frequent feelings of anger, upset, and anxiety can get in the way of his ability to learn and remember what he has learned.[10]

Thus, guiding your child in how to develop emotionally and engage socially, in a calm and relaxed way, is important to the establishment of self-confidence and self-esteem. It is also key to helping your child feel motivated and to make the best use of his or her talents and other forms of intelligence.

Psychologists have determined that there are many different types of intelligence. Healthy emotional growth begins with successful bonding between parent and child. Children master the social skills that are critical to emotional maturity by watching the behavior of parents and modeling their behavior after them.

If your child is emotionally well-adjusted, she will have a secure sense of herself and self-worth. She won't have to wear the right jeans or a nose ring to get peer approval. She will also have developed an understanding of right and wrong, "good and bad" behavior, ethical and unethical choices, that enables her to develop morally, as well.

Your child will be motivated to take her meaningful place in adult society because she has the scaffolding in place to support her. It is the *you, her parent,* who has helped put that scaffolding there.

In the future, as we continue to shift from an industrial to a service-based and technological economy, the importance of mastering social skills, especially interpersonal intelligence, will only increase. "People skills" are at the heart of "service" jobs. Furthermore, without healthy emotional maturity, it is very difficult for a child to integrate and implement intellectual advances and adjust to the world. With emotional security, the sky's the limit.

HOW TO COMPENSATE: THE WORKING PARENTS' GUIDE

Women today make up half of the workforce in America. As a result, working mothers are asked to oversee both home and career. Because no one can either have it all, or do it all perfectly, full-time working moms often carry the burden of feeling that they're always letting some part of their life down, which leads to free-floating guilt and anxiety. But there is a way to restore balance to a working mom's life; it requires organization and a plan. First and foremost, you need to identify your parenting plan. The following is applicable to all parents, whether working or stay-at-home.

YOUR PARENTING PLAN[11]

Here are some strategies to help you lighten your burden and free you of guilt:

- **Nowhere is the old Girl Scout adage "be prepared" more necessary than for the working parent.** Research tells us that the most significant part of parenting is bonding. As a working parent, you must find ways to connect with your child throughout the day. When I was a working mother, I left tape recordings of my voice, making up stories incorporating my children's names, reading bedtime stories, singing, and saying prayers. It was successful in many ways and helped my children feel secure, calm, and quieted. Today, you can use Skype, FaceTime, and other technology to achieve the same ends by making your presence felt throughout the day. You can also assign a special toy as a comfort toy for your child, to be used as a substitute in your absence, to soothe and calm your baby. Furthermore, having a picture of yourself that your baby can see, whether over his crib or on a wall in his room, reassures him that he has not been abandoned. During a coffee break, lunch break, afternoon break, or bathroom break, if possible, call your child so that he can hear your voice letting him know that though you can't see him now, you will soon be together. Knowing you are nearby, and that you will return, lowers your child's anxiety and his cortisol levels. Hearing a parent's voice is a huge release of tension, similar to stepping into a warm bathtub or having a massage, allowing your baby to relax, soften, and lower his anxiety.

- **Don't Waste Time.** As a working parent, you have to compensate for time away from your child. Therefore, you can't waste time and must try not to get distracted. Self-discipline is a huge support for working parents, so set predetermined units of time for phone calls, shopping, emails, and so on, limiting these types of connections and distractions to correspond with your child's bedtime. Limit your time spent on social media, watching television, reading, and socializing during the week. Reserve your evenings for your mate and never multitask when interacting with your child, who needs your full attention to compensate for time away. Concentrate on your work at work and try to use your break and lunchtime to reunite with your child, whenever possible. If you can do this consistently, you will create a pattern in which she will learn to expect to see you at regular intervals; this alone will keep her cortisol output level.

- **Family Time Is Bonding Time.** Weekends should incorporate your child whenever possible, even though it's also a time for laundry, grocery shopping, and catching up with friends. Try to keep a balance, overriding your need for extracurricular activity with the greater need of your child for you. It is during the weekend that you can nurture your child, and if you make it into a family affair, the whole family can bond and reconnect. Even if it means waking up early, having breakfast together is both important and beneficial. Studies show that children who consistently have their meals with their parents perform better academically than children who do not. Also, organize age-appropriate activities so that your child knows what to anticipate and expect. Regardless of which activities you engage in with your child, it is essential to be present. Don't talk about work-related issues or coworkers and don't spend time on your phone.

Children want their parents to see and hear them, so practice active listening, caring touch, and eye contact during family outings. Concentrate on the things that are important to your child, practice my empathic process so that you can hear your child's worries, thoughts, and feelings, and get to know your child by paying attention to his needs and wants. Your child, no matter how young, can participate in my empathic process (see page 21), which will invest him in the foundation of boundaries by empowering his developing sense of self. No matter what you do during the weekend and family time together, the key is to be actively engaged, involved, and present.

- **Make Time for Your Mate.** Children are the most secure in families where parents are happy together. Your significant other is the one person that you can count on, no matter what, whether you are right or wrong. He is that head on the pillow next to you, who is there for you, in your corner, unconditionally. It's important for working parents to make time for one another. Practice my empathic process (page 21) one night a week, which will give you a safe space to share your thoughts, feelings, and emotions about everything, including each other. It gives you a chance to check in with each other, to touch base and see how you are both doing. This conversation must happen without defense, where each person gets to speak for equal amounts of time, with an equal parcel of time used talking together to problem-solve. This approach requires active listening, touch, and focus. Once a month, a date night can be just what the doctor ordered, restoring and revitalizing the intimacy so important in a distracted and stressful life. A date night does not have to be expensive; it can be a picnic in the park, a walk down the lane, or a candlelit dinner at home. The point is to reconnect with each other by reestablishing your relationship. And when leaving baby with a babysitter, follow the same criteria as you would when hiring a nanny; in that way you can enjoy your night out with confidence.

- **Make Time for Yourself.** Whether it's a ten-minute meditation, a warm cup of tea, writing in your journal, a warm bath, or a massage, it is important to restore and recharge your own vitality. By taking care of your personal needs, you renew the balance needed for a sense of well-being. Since your time is spread thinly between home and work, your personal needs can too easily get lost, as we often put off what is important to us to serve others. It's well to remember that to be a good parent or mate, you have to first take care of yourself. If you're tired, or sick, or stressed beyond repair, you won't be able to be there for yourself or anyone else. When I was working on my PhD, a colleague of mine gave me a wonderful insight: she stated that no matter what her obligations were during the day, she always saved some time for herself at night to read a favorite book. Not only that, but she gave herself a spa day once a week, awakening early on Sunday morning to practice yoga. And, no matter what, she made sure to get a solid seven hours of sleep each night. Though these seem like little things, they add up to a pattern of self-love, which you are modeling in a positive way for your child. Be what you want to see. Finally, good nutrition is paramount in securing strong energy levels, emotional stasis, and clear thinking, reminding us of the renewed focus on "clean food."

- **Partner with Your Employer.** Working parents need to have an open line of communication with their employers, so that they know there are children involved who might require an emergency plan. Discuss what is acceptable if your child falls ill during the day or has an emergency. A written request is always best, as you and your employer can reread the needs, wants, commitments, obligations, and responsibilities required, preferably before employment or at the onset of a family. In a large company, it's worthwhile to ask your colleagues what considerations they have negotiated. This will help you fine-tune your own request. It's important when talking to your employer to be prepared to be authentic and never defensive. Furthermore, there is always more than one way to solve a problem, so be willing to consider alternative ideas and possibilities, including your willingness to make up lost time and productivity. If you are starting a family, it is valuable to know what, if any, accommodations are possible for maternity leave, remembering to ask about pay and time. Other questions should include vacation time, disability, and sick time. Knowledge is power, and every working parent needs to know the answers to these questions before they accept a position.

- **Give Up Guilt in Search of a Transgression.** We are the only animals on the planet that engage in guilt. By burdening yourself under the weight of guilt, you can find yourself unable to function effectively. Guilt can paralyze and stymie your performance at home, as well as at work. Though it is easy enough for working parents to find things to feel guilty about, it serves no purpose. The better approach is to continue to try to problem-solve. None of us can change the past; all we can do is try to do better in the future. Instead of feeling guilty for fulfilling the demands of a working parent, you would be better served to think about the good things that your work provides. For example, beyond the obvious food and shelter are the benefits of good education, childcare, medical care, and so forth. Ironically, being successful at both parenting and work requires a similar paradigm, including setting priorities, choices, concentration, and compensation for time away. If you are feeling overwhelmed by the prospect of a career and a family, you can either seek outside professional help or participate in a support group, which can often be found online. By reaching out to people with similar problems, you may find common ground and solutions.

- **The Importance of Good Childcare.** Ask experts, other parents, your pediatrician, and family members to give you suggestions for good childcare. Whether it's a nursery school, a babysitter, or a nanny, the criteria are the same: childcare professionals have to share your values and your discipline style. And if your choice is a nursery school (daycare), they have to have proper security measures, a good teacher-to-student ratio, teachers who are licensed in childcare, cleanliness, secure and clean inside and outside spaces, and a program to facilitate early childhood development, rather than just being organized around conduct and control. Always interview a nanny, a babysitter, or a nursery school's director and teachers. If your choice is a nursery school, you should visit more than once, making sure to make at least one unannounced visit so that you can see for yourself the way a particular nursery school program is facilitated. Be prepared for your interview with questions that are important to you. If you are hiring a nanny or a babysitter, you want references, a drug test, and a background check, so that you know not only her experience, but also her history. Never hire a nanny or babysitter without trying him or her out first, watching to see how he or she interacts with your child or children, and letting other family members have an objective voice in your decision.

- **Keep Mornings Peaceful.** Keep mornings peaceful, as they set the stage for the whole day. Do as much as you can the night before, including laying out your child's clothes, bathing him, and packing his lunch and snacks, so that you can focus on him each morning as you prepare your child to face the day. Get up early enough to have a calm and quiet stress-free breakfast with your child. Your child will take his cue from you, and if you are peaceful and calm in the morning, that's how he will start his day. In the same way, it helps to put your clothes, keys, and wallet in a designated place each night, alleviating the stress of having to search for them in the morning. Try to divide your domestic obligations with your significant other. When you divide your workload, not only do you feel part of a team, but you feel valued and appreciated. Whenever possible, create a schedule for dinner meals, determining whose responsibility it is to cook which meal each night. As a working parent, I found it helpful to create a menu, shopping only for that menu and cooking each week in advance over the weekend. That way, I avoided a lot of waste, and my meals were prepped and ready to go. And I always kept a to-do list so that my spouse and I didn't repeat responsibilities or jobs already completed. Try it—it works!

- **Keep a Calendar.** The more organized you are, the easier your life will be. If you keep an up-to-date calendar, you can stay ahead of any scheduling problems or changes. Take time each week to sit down with your significant other to review your calendar, making sure that the two of you are in sync, not only with each other, but with your children. Your nursery school and nanny should be apprised of your daily schedule, so that if an emergency arises, they know where you are and how to reach you. Of course, they should also have a current list of all doctors, emergency telephone numbers, and safe family members, or friends who are available when you are not.

STRATEGIES FOR THE WORKING PARENT

One way to avoid the guilt of compensating for time away from baby is to focus on strategies that can work for you to help you meet your child's parenting needs. I was a working parent, and I know how difficult it can be to juggle three lives simultaneously—home, work, and school—never mind the guilt that goes along with just not being there. In the best of all possible worlds, it would be better if moms were there for the formative years, bonding and not separating prematurely. We know, for instance, that children learn something from their mothers that they cannot learn anywhere else, and that is security. Furthermore, a well-bonded child does better at many things, including processing information, focusing, problem-solving, and sticking with a problem longer, as well as developing cognitive, linguistic, and social benefits.

However, this is not an ideal world, and mothers do have to work to make ends meet—sometimes holding down more than two jobs at a time. Whatever your specific family situation may be, there is a lot that parents can do to turn a potentially stressful experience into a win-win situation for the whole family. As in all of life's situations, it is important to know the rules.

RULE 1: INVEST IN FAMILY MEETINGS— THE EMPATHIC PROCESS

Sit down as a family in a neutral space and have an empathic family meeting where the entire family, including the children, brainstorms how to create ways to participate in the family so that the family system works and is on a positive course. This requires authenticity from all members involved, including parents. This family meeting works for all family structures, including the single parent. It is based on the premise that each member gets an established and equal amount of time to speak and to listen actively, which is the best way to communicate. Make eye contact while actively listening to one another, and whenever possible practice a gentle touch to demonstrate intimacy and focus. Now, each party is invested in the outcome, has a role in creating the rewards and consequences for appropriate behavior, and thus learns positive ways to solve family problems. Since all members of a family are a part of the whole, it is important to reinforce their membership by being both respectful and mutual. When employing the empathic process, never be defensive, regardless of what is said. Without defense, you will create a safe space in which parents and children can return again and again to problem-solve.

Rules of empathic conversation include:

1. No humiliating, shameful, or embarrassing statements
2. Listen with your full attention
3. Invest each participant in the conflict-resolution process, with rewards and consequences for appropriate behavior
4. Employ mutuality
5. Use trust, based on experience
6. Teach that each member of the family can be counted on, no matter what—reliability is key

The empathic conversation should take place at least once a week, in a neutral and safe space. I always recommend the kitchen table—the alchemical heart of the house, where all things mix together for nurturing and transformation, such as baking and cooking food. It is important not to have this discussion in anyone's office, study, or bedroom (someone's power place). This approach teaches role modeling of the highest order—valuing yourself and others—and it reconnects us to our family so that we can check in once a week and see where everyone is, how they are doing, and how they are feeling. This process can also be used to reassign and rotate chores. By investing your children in the process, they are more likely to follow the rules.

RULE 2: STRUCTURE IN AS MANY THINGS AS POSSIBLE

For example, get enough sleep and give up on being a perfect parent or keeping a perfect house. Relationships are much more important and much more flexible than those goals. If you make mistakes and are easier on yourself, you open up a space for others to be more human and misstep every once in a while. On the other hand, it is important to give yourself the best chance for the least stressful day.

Set an alarm clock, allowing you time to wake up both yourself and your family, making sure that everyone has enough time for personal hygiene, to prepare breakfast, to take necessary vitamins and meds, and to get to school or work on time.

Grocery shop with a weekly list, including the lunch preferences of your children. During the school year, pack lunches the night before. Invest your children in deciding what they may like for lunch. Don't force-feed them—it may contribute to eating problems later.

Lay out younger children's clothes by mutual agreement the night before, allowing children choice to build confidence and competence. In some cases, you may even want to dress younger children in things that won't wrinkle. This can save a lot of time in a busy morning.

Print up an activity sheet and pin it to your children's doors, giving them a heads-up so that they have the freedom to plan personal time. Add a list of chores to the activity schedule, attached to a weekly calendar for rewards and consequences. Use a visual form of awards, such as stars posted where all can see.

Finally, schedule play time for yourself and your family—not always together.

RULE 3: IF CHILDCARE IS A MUST, DO YOUR HOMEWORK

As discussed, if you are enrolling your child in a childcare center, check out not only the facility, but also their schedule, their curriculum, their discipline strategies, and their emergency policies—noting especially whether it fits your personal discipline and emergency style. The better the job you do in the beginning, the lower your stress level later.

If your child doesn't go to nursery school or a childcare center, make sure you carefully check the references of those you hire to be caretakers. See tips in the following section for more info about hiring an in-home nanny or babysitter. If your child must stay home alone after school, be sure you teach them how to safely do this, including keeping doors locked, not letting anyone but immediate family in, and not playing with fire, the stove, toxic cleaning supplies, or dangerous implements. Have an emergency plan and a responsible adult checking in with your children at regular intervals, if only by phone. Most important, be sure your child is old enough and responsible enough to do this. I don't recommend leaving anyone under thirteen years of age home alone, and certainly no one with a mental challenge.

CREATING A SUCCESSFUL ENVIRONMENT WITH A NANNY OR A BABYSITTER

Congratulations! You've hired a wonderful nanny or babysitter to care for your child. Bringing someone into your home to care for your child can be a challenging task, one that is fraught with emotions and conflict. After all, you are opening up not just your home, but also your lives to a stranger, and you are entrusting this person to essentially be *you* in your absence.

As a parent, there are some steps you can take in order to create a successful environment in which you, the nanny or babysitter, and your child can feel comfortable and secure. Here are some tips to help create a smooth transition and successful environment for everyone:

1. **Create a contract that includes a comprehensive agreement of services.** This contract should clearly outline what the nanny is expected to do, specifically, on a daily basis. It should also include issues such as scheduling, tardiness, goal-setting, annual raises, one-on-one meetings, and required employment termination notice. This will help alleviate any confusion and set up clear expectations from the very beginning.

2. **Try to create a warm, welcoming work environment for your nanny or babysitter.** Consider your nanny's or babysitter's preferences, such as dietary likes, dislikes, and allergies—after all, this person is working in your house and, in many cases, living there.

3. **Do not attempt to compete with your nanny or babysitter or be jealous of her/him.** If children bond with their nanny or babysitter, as they usually do, there can be moments where they accidentally call her "Mommy" or him "Daddy" instead of by

her or his name. Know that this occasional slip is natural and does not mean that your child loves you any less.

4. **Be careful not to blur the lines of your professional relationship.** It is important to value your nanny or babysitter, but also remember that she/he is an employee. Therefore, your nanny or babysitter should always be treated professionally, with respect and affection. If your nanny or babysitter becomes your confidant, those professional lines can blur, and it can become difficult to maintain a working relationship.

5. **Set weekly one-on-one meetings.** This weekly evaluation is important to both you and your nanny or babysitter. Use this time to let your child's nanny or babysitter know how she or he is doing. She or he can give you feedback, as well. Setting regular meetings helps further establish trust between the two of you, creates a safe space in which to express emotions, and ensures expectations are being met on both sides.

Remember: your nanny or babysitter is not you, and he or she will never truly take the place of a parent. Feel comfortable in your decision, and be sure to show respect and kindness toward your nanny or babysitter in front of your children; they will, after all, model your behavior, and treat the nanny or babysitter as you do. By taking the simple steps listed above, you can help create a nurturing environment for your child in your absence and build a successful relationship between you and your child's nanny or babysitter.

RULE 4: KNOW THE HOUSE RULES

Create house rules with your family that can be adhered to and make life easier for the entire family. These should include common courtesy, respect, reliability, responsibility, and fairness.

Chores that gain rewards should be added to the house rules, and tokens that can be cashed in for personal wishes can be established weekly. These reward tokens should not include money, but rather private time with Mom and Dad; objects desired (such as a new lunch box, a new bike, a new art kit); an outing with friends or a movie, etc. Children are part of a family, and you don't want them to feel that they are paid for their membership. On the other hand, allowances should be established for each child, because, as a part of this family, there is consideration for their special financial needs. This teaches responsibility in money matters. There should also be a specific bedtime, study time, and computer/tablet schedule.

Whenever possible, be present for as many school-related and extracurricular activities as possible. Children need you be invested in them, and you need to know what is going on in their lives—school and social. Scrutiny is not spying. Parents are entitled to parent, and they need to know where their children are, when, and with whom. But this must be done in a respectful way by maintaining healthy boundaries between you and your children.

Finally, create ways to bond and be there even when you are not, recording bedtime stories on phones or tablets and even being creative in making up bedtime stories by using your children's names as characters in a recorded adventure.

RULE 5: WORK TOGETHER TO REDUCE STRESS

There are plenty of ways to take stress off of you, your partner, and your children:

- Meditate, using progressive relaxation techniques. This can be a lifelong practice to reduce stress and, by so doing, enhance learning.
- Take a warm soaking bath. Gift yourself with a timeout.
- Ask for help when needed. Kids love to chip in when asked. Learn to delegate. No one can do everything all the time.
- Be the adult and create quality time with your children, giving each child private time whenever possible.

- Communicate, connect, listen, and pay attention—know your child. Value yourself, and you will value your child.
- Don't burden your children with your problems—let them have their childhood. If necessary, seek professional help from a counselor.
- Be reliable so that your children can count on you.
- Most important, have empathy for yourself and for your children—this will teach them empathy, the best protection for getting along in the world.

You and your child are on a journey together—honor the process. Recognize that while no family situation may be perfect, as working parents, you always have the power to create the best possible scenario for you and your children. Remember as you are following these tips that the only thing you really have to do is meet your children's needs, nurture them, and be there by being reliable.

Some advice about how to stay calm with a difficult child:[12]

1. Let biology be your ally. Take time in, instead of time out, by focusing on your breath, and calming yourself. Be sure to teach this breathing technique to your child.
2. Don't react. Be proactive and stay ahead of the problem, remembering that emotions are illogical and reactive. If you see tension rising, like the rumble of a volcano, change the focus by changing the environment.
3. Don't project or fall back to your child's level. Keep being the adult, stay conscious, and stay in control.
4. Change your attitude. Try to keep in mind that your child is a child and sometimes acts out.
5. Don't let feelings control you or push your buttons. Parents must parent.
6. Whatever discipline consequences you and your child create should be carried out consistently.

7. Teach that all emotions are okay, though not all behaviors are. Help your child recognize his feelings and the source of his anxiety by giving him immediate feedback.
8. Teach your child how to transition emotionally. How to breathe and pause so that he can release his tension without acting out.
9. Keep an eye out for trigger situations so that you can be prepared. Help your child role play, so that he can confront difficult situations when they arise. In this way, he will learn how to move easily from one emotional state to another.
10. Finally, don't worry. Focus on the good stuff. Remember to promote positive imagery and verbal cues to your child daily.

WHAT IS YOUR PARENTING STYLE?

The other day I was listening to my grandchildren play with their friends. They were discussing whose parents were the easiest, and whose were the most strict. It took me back to my own childhood, when my friends and I would compare our parents' parenting styles. From a young age, children of every generation are very aware of the importance of different parenting styles.

While each parent (working or stay-at-home) is unique, there are four main parenting style categories that most of us fall into. Ready to find out what kind of parenting style you have? Read on.

PARENTING STYLE #1: AUTHORITATIVE

Authoritative parenting is actually what we consider the optimal approach, because it fosters traits of open communication, rules and consequences, boundaries, maturity, and the necessary social skills for healthy relationships.

You might be an authoritative parent if you:

- Hold high standards and expectations for your child, while also being empathic and kind

- Advocate for your child
- Establish safe, positive, success-oriented environments that encourage strong bonding with your child
- Have clear expectations for your child
- Structure your child's environment with consistency, follow-through, and clearly communicated potential rewards and consequences regarding chores, homework, mealtime, and bedtime
- Communicate regularly with your child, checking in to see how they are feeling and using my empathic process (pages 21) to invest them in the process of rules and consequences

PARENTING STYLE #2: AUTHORITARIAN

This is the strict parent who could be defined by the biblical phrase "spare the rod and spoil the child."

You might be an authoritarian parent if you:

- Maintain a strict approach to parenting that lacks communication and the possibility of negotiation
- Spend a lot of time punishing your children for not following your rules compared to time spent communicating both your expectations and potential consequences if those expectations are not met
- Believe you need to always project the image of being in charge
- Are somewhat aloof around your child. Not wanting to appear "soft" around your child, you do not allow him to see you as vulnerable

PARENTING STYLE #3: PERMISSIVE

The permissive parent is overly lenient and is unable to teach rules, create structure, or be consistent with consequences.

You may be a permissive parent if you:

- Allow your child to disobey rules regularly, without any consistent follow-through or consequences communicated ahead of time
- Would rather compromise than confront conflict
- Believe it is most important to be your child's best friend
- Find yourself spending a lot of time overnegotiating, overcompromising, and bribing your child

PARENTING STYLE #4: UNINVOLVED

The uninvolved parent is neglectful to the physical and emotional needs, safety, and care of his child.

You may be an uninvolved parent if you:

- Are often gone from home and leave your child to take care of himself on a regular basis
- Find yourself preferring to be in places other than with your child
- Are unaware of the other people in your child's life, including not knowing your child's friends or teachers
- Make excuses and rationalize why you are away and disconnected from your child in order to network for business, social connections, and maintain your public image

Did you find yourself relating to one of these parenting styles more than another? If so, it will help you, in the long run, to regain a sense of balance in your parenting life.

WHEN PARENTING STYLES CLASH

You've grounded your child, taking away television privileges. You come home from running errands, only to find your partner and your child watching television. "Dad said I could!" exclaims your child. "You're being unfair," says your partner, in front of your child. "What she did was no big deal, and *I wouldn't have handled the situation that way.*"

What is "no big deal" to one parent may be a big deal to the other, but nevertheless, it is never appropriate to sabotage another parent's discipline in front of your child. Even though, as a child, you said that you would never parent like your parent, you and your mate bring to your marriage those very parenting roles that you each experienced, good or bad. These are the patterns that you know, that make up your comfort zone. And because you didn't turn out so badly, you reach for this parenting style when you become a parent.

WE DO WHAT WE KNOW

You instinctively parent your children the way you were parented; you've been brought up one way and your partner another. This truth inevitably leads to differences in both the expectations and the methods of parenting. *Even if you didn't like a lot of what your parents did, you reach for what you know.*

In our minds, we feel justified; you've never been a parent before, so you project onto your new family all of the expectations, feelings, and values from your family of origin. After all, that is who you are and that is what you bring to your partnership. So, when you look down that long tunnel of parenting options, you pull out the familiar. Our expectations often hit a wall, called the Other Parent, and we don't understand why our partner can't see things our way. Conflict in child-rearing can not only cause chaos in your relationship, but, in fact, is one of the greatest causes of divorce.

WHAT TO DO IF YOUR PARTNER'S PARENTING STYLES CLASH:

1. **Communicate regularly and openly with your partner.**
   Communication is the key to everything.

2. **Know your child.** Different children require different parenting styles at different times. For example, you would discipline a shy child much differently from the way you would an aggressive child.

3. **Educate yourself.** Make sure you are fully aware of what is going on in your children's lives currently rather than just guessing or basing your knowledge on your own childhood experience. Talk with other parents and know what your children's peer groups are doing.

4. **Engage in the empathic process.** Set up neutral space, such as the kitchen, for you and your mate to communicate regularly about family problems. The kitchen is the heart of the house where alchemy happens. Here, you're creating new traditions and new education styles, *together*, that fit your new family. Be honest and do not get defensive when your mate is speaking. This gives you a chance to reflect on the good, the bad, and the ugly of your own upbringing, and your partner has chance to do the same.

5. **Come up with a parenting plan that will work for your family and the kind of children you have.** You bring to the plan one parenting rule of your choice that is of utmost importance to you and is nonnegotiable, and your partner does the same. Then, work together to negotiate the rest until you have a new plan that reflects your combined parenting styles.

6. **Once you have a combined parenting plan, stick with it.** Once you've settled what you're willing to do, merging two different families, sit down with your kids and verbally lay out the new plans together. Be consistent, so your children know what to expect and what the rules and consequences will be. By investing your children in the discipline process, they will be more likely to follow the rules that they have taken part in creating.

7. **Always present a united front before your children.** Do not disagree with each other or question each other's parenting decisions in front of your children; if you disagree, have that conversation with your partner privately. United you stand, divided you fall.

8. **Seek help.** If communication breaks down—for example, if you or your mate sabotage each other in front of your children—you may need to explore the reasons behind your behavior. Perhaps anger and dysfunction are being projected into your parenting roles. Then it's time to see a therapist. Seek professional help to bring you and your partner back to a middle ground where you can learn to communicate and support each other.

HOW DIFFERENT PARENTING STYLES AFFECT CHILDREN

Regardless of which parenting style you choose, it's important to note that each parenting style has the possibility of affecting children in different ways.

CHILDREN OF AUTHORITATIVE PARENTS

Authoritative parents regularly communicate expectations and potential consequences, thereby raising a child in an environment that provides both security and confidence, which helps build his self-esteem. Because of the example his parents set for him, he learns valuable social skills and is able to have healthy relationships with others.

CHILDREN OF AUTHORITARIAN PARENTS

The child of an authoritarian parent (who offers too much structure and too little communication) often feels insecure, performs for approval, and connects approval with love. He may have low self-esteem and have difficulty in social relationships. Further, he may break out when away from Mom and Dad by misbehaving.

CHILDREN OF PERMISSIVE PARENTS

A child who is raised without structure may have difficulty self-managing her behavior. Freedom without limits can be destructive to child development; without consequences, children don't have a sense of boundaries. As a result, the child from a permissive home will seek structure to help her feel valued, validated, and secure. She may have problems with relationships and lack the self-discipline necessary for social interaction with her peers. Her schoolwork may suffer from lack of organization and motivation. This child often lacks responsibility; has difficulty with boundaries, responsibility, obligation, and commitment; and is unaware of the importance of significant consequences.

CHILDREN OF UNINVOLVED PARENTS

This kind of neglect can be very dangerous to a child because it affects his sense of self, self-esteem, and well-being. This impacts a child's ability to trust. It also makes him take on responsibilities far too early, as he parents himself, robbing him of his childhood. Children of uninvolved parents often have problems with intimacy and friendship with their peers.

At the end of the day, parents must parent; you should be what you want to see. From a very young age, your child will mimic you and your conduct. We may have "off" days and we all make parenting mistakes from time to time, but remember: your child is always watching you. What you teach him through your parenting style has the potential to affect every aspect of his life, from academics to his relationships with others.

THE DISCIPLINE TO-DO LIST

- Pay attention to your patterns of parenting from your own family of origin so that you can consciously decide how you want to parent.

- If you have a partner, discuss how you can create a new style of parenting, merging the best from each of your familial experiences and transforming them into something that works for you both.

Finally, all parents (working and stay-at-home) know that you are only as happy as your least happy child. The journey through childhood is often filled with unseen and unexpected minefields. The question is how to navigate them effectively. Each road map has a key to unlock the heart. And it is through the heart that you can find your way to happy parenting.

6 REASONS PLAYDATES ARE GOOD FOR MOMS AND DADS (NOT JUST KIDS!)

You're having one of those weeks when you feel like your life is run by a pint-sized dictator. The toddler of the house has consumed your every waking hour, commandeered your schedule, and dominated your thoughts. You know you need a break, but your partner is traveling out of town for work and your babysitting options have just run out. What's a desperate mom to do?

Try scheduling a playdate. Yes, playdates are fabulous opportunities for your child to learn social skills and make new friends, but there are also many benefits for Mom, as well:

1. **Playdates give you a chance to reconnect with the non-mom side of you.** Sure, you're there with other moms and other children, but this is your chance to chat about non-mom topics and flex those non-mom brain muscles. Whether talking about politics, finance issues, work, or the latest bestselling novel, you can give your brain a workout by engaging in conversations that don't involve diapers and sleep schedules.
2. **Think of playdates as Parenting 101 crowdsourcing.** While they are a great chance to talk about non-mon issues, playdates

are also the place to get some answers from those who have been there, done that. Got a child with night terrors? Can't get your child to eat anything other than cereal? Chances are, another mom in the group has gone through the same thing and can offer up advice from experience.

3. **Playdates are a great chance for you to get some exercise.** We all know how challenging it can be to fit in a workout when you are busy raising children. Planning playdates that involve stroller walks or jogs, family-friendly hikes, and fun activities like roller-skating or riding bikes can give you a chance to catch up with other moms while also getting some exercise, which can help you feel better and more prepared to take on the rest of the day.

4. **Playdates can offer much-needed pats on the back.** You work hard as a mom, and at the end of each day, you don't get a medal. But playdates can offer you reassurance that you are, in fact, doing a great job, Mom! Mothers have no greater cheerleaders than other mothers, and as much as we may selflessly love our children and do whatever it takes to raise them well, it's still nice to have the support and encouragement from fellow moms that we are not the parenting failures we sometimes see ourselves as being.

5. **Playdates get you out of the house.** Sometimes, especially in those early days with an infant, it can be a challenge to take two steps outside of your front door. As moms, I bet most of you have had those days where suddenly you look up and the sun is already setting, but you are still in your pajamas. Scheduling playdates gives you a reason to get dressed and get out of the house, and once you are out, it's much easier to then stay out and run errands or attempt other fun adventures with your little one.

6. **Playdates can help you de-stress.** In addition to a chance to exercise, catch up with other adults, and work your brain, playdates can help bring your stress level down. Motherhood can be a very stressful time, and bonding with other moms gives you a chance to alleviate some of that stress in a safe, supportive environment.

PARENTING WITHOUT INSECURITY

Parents should parent, which requires them to assess situations and, when needed, to step into their adult. We are all social animals and we learn through imitation. If you've ever watched your toddler imitate you while playing with dolls, trucks, or peers, you can see what an impact your behavior has on him. *Be what you want to see.*

You are always teaching your child. From birth to death, all of the patterns your child learns while interacting with you will inform his relationships forevermore. Remember when you said, "I'll never do to my child what my parents did to me"? And then, once you had your child, you heard yourself repeating the same dialogue, as an echo from your past? That's how it works. Your child will take all of his cues from you. If you're calm, don't panic, and stay balanced in your interactions with your child, he will develop that same behavior.

Let your child tell you what she needs from you. This requires you to listen actively and have empathy for her. Never discount her feelings when either her body or her pride is hurt. Be her support, her home team. If you're insecure, you will absolutely pass on your insecurities. Empower your child to honor her own feelings by being her reliable touchstone. If your child trusts you, she will trust herself and therefore the outer world. Moreover, relaxation techniques can help you stay in balance and not overreact emotionally to your child's experiences, whether she's suffered an injury, a fight, or an illness.

Help your child realize that you are there for him, and you will support him to be there for himself. Thus, you are teaching your child to be independent by allowing him to feel bonded, safe, and secure. This will help him extend out and explore his world.

Nurturing is not smothering. Give your child the room to grow and to make mistakes. As a conscious parent, you can choose how to override your own fears to build a strong and healthy child. If necessary, seek professional help for your emotional problem so that you don't pass them on.

If you have a new baby at home, you may feel overwhelmed and amazed at the changes your baby experiences in his first year. His brain development, including basic problem-solving, is phenomenal, occurring simultaneously with the development of his social and emotional connections.

It may seem like so much is happening all at once, but there are many things you can do to help nurture your baby's development during his first year of life (see tips in on pages 93).

PARENTING WITH PATIENCE

Your child wants to be seen and heard. When you demonstrate patience, you are also giving your child the message that she is prized and appreciated. However, when you lose patience, you can create a sense of stress and frustration in your child, that can undermine her sense of self.

THE BENEFITS OF MODELING PATIENCE

Children copy what they see, so when you parent with patience, you model respect, empathy, security, and good self-esteem. These are the characteristics you want to foster in your child. These are the experiences that teach your child how to be present and intimate, not only with himself, but also with others.

When you stop, look, and listen to your child, you show her that she is important, that you believe in her, and that you have empathy and compassion for her feelings. Active listening is based on patience and leads to the confidence needed for self-mastery. Finally, patience encourages not just empathy and compassion, but also self-reliance and skill.

CONSCIOUS PARENTING

Patience is a virtue. By becoming a conscious parent, you can override your reactive behavior and impatience deliberately, so that you can be present for your child when he needs you. By not projecting your inner discord or stress onto your child, you learn how to choose your behavior, rather than being a victim of it. This is conscious parenting, and it not only helps you integrate your compulsions, but also models for your child what it is to be a proactive, healthy adult.

BE WHAT YOU WANT TO SEE

Children are social learners, and they learn through experience, environment, modeling, and imitation. I've mentioned this a few times already, but it holds true: be what you want to see. This will help you be present in your child's life, as well as your own. By paying attention, being an active listener, making eye contact, and touching his hand when talking with your child, you lower his frustration and give him the message that you are with him and you are present for whatever it is he is doing. This teaches him that patience is really listening and being present in a relationship.

My empathic process (pages 21) is a perfect working tool to teach patience, because it gives a safe environment in which to allow your child to practice and rehearse what it means to be patient, present, and invested in the process of relationship.

THE NEW NORMAL: NONTRADITIONAL FAMILIES

Throughout the years, we've seen family structures move to less *Leave It to Beaver* and more *Modern Family*. In fact, a recently released Pew Research

Center study shows that now, less than half (46 percent) of all children in the United States live in a home that falls under the former description of a "traditional" family, a.k.a. households that consist of two heterosexual partners in a first marriage.[13]

Today, more and more children are being raised by single parents (34 percent, up from 19 percent in 1980), same sex parents, unmarried parents, parents with partners, two parents in a remarriage, grandparents, and so on . . . and for the first time in documented history, these "nontraditional" home settings outnumber the traditional. Not only that, but research today indicates, for the first time, the importance of grandparents and how they act as allies for their grandchildren. This relationship can give your children the necessary stability and grounding so important in families where Mom and Dad must both work outside the home.[14]

HOW DOES THIS "NEW NORMAL" AFFECT CHILDREN?

I believe that no matter which family structure children grow up in, all children have the same opportunities for successful, happy lives as long as their caregivers meet the following four critical needs:

1. **You must meet your children where they are.** No two children are alike, and just because something worked for you as a child or worked for another child does not mean it will work for your child. I believe that when you acknowledge your child's individuality, when you truly listen to her, see her, and meet her where she is emotionally, mentally, and physically, then she will be ready for whatever steps he must take to grow and flourish.

2. **You must keep your children safe.** When children feel safe, they are more likely to try new things, to grow, to make mistakes, and to learn on their own within the cocoon of your security. By being there for them when they need you, you are

showing them that they can rely on you, no matter what. This builds a relationship of not only love, but of trust, respect, and security. When your children feel safe and trust you, they are more likely to talk about their problems with you, come to you when they need help, and share the happy and sad parts of their days with you.

3. **You must socialize and culturalize your children.** It is your responsibility to teach your children about the appropriate rules for life. In addition to teaching them manners, show them what it is like to be a good citizen of the world, to have empathy for others, and how to navigate society by following generally accepted behavior while still maintaining their unique identity.

4. **You must shower your children with love and affection.** You can never love your children too much. Show your children you love them by telling them each day, by showering them with hugs and kisses, by reading with them at night. When children know how much they are loved, they feel safe and less anxious. They are learning from you how to show love and affection to others, so that they can be intimate and trust their relationships with friends and partners.

These four pillars are common needs that must be met by all families in order for children to have the greatest opportunities in life. As long as there is a lot of love in your home, and you meet your children's needs by socializing and culturalizing them and keeping them safe . . . you've succeeded.

Yes, the definition of a "traditional" family is changing. That doesn't mean the definition and importance of *family* is changing. As a society, we have to get real and relate to what is, which is a very diverse range of family structures. We must operate within the "new normal," not discriminate against it. We should embrace it and move forward with a focus on our future: our children.

THE SLEEPLESS SOCIETY: THE IMPORTANCE OF A GOOD NIGHT'S SLEEP FOR STRESS REDUCTION AND CORTISOL CONTROL

HOW TO HELP EVERYONE SLEEP BETTER

Are you getting enough sleep? The CDC recommends that adults get at least seven to eight hours of sleep, while school-aged children should get at least ten hours of sleep each night, and teens should get nine to ten hours of sleep.[15] The following sections discuss some things you can work on during the day that will help you and your child get a better night's sleep.

SLEEP SUCCESS TIPS FOR PARENTS

Parents lose a tremendous amount of sleep—up to 50 percent—in the first year of their child's birth, especially breastfeeding moms who can be on call as often as every two hours. Nevertheless, there are many things that parents can do together to help share the sleep burden and lighten their load.

For example, partners can take turns feeding, and alternate night shifts with baby. If Mom is breastfeeding, she can pump in the day, and her spouse can feed in the night. The point is teamwork and collaboration. If Mom or Dad has an important meeting in the morning, their partner can fill in the gap and compensate. At the end of the day, this is how we build intimacy and mutuality, the cornerstones of a good relationship.

SLEEP SUCCESS TIPS FOR CHILDREN

It is important to set a structure for bedtime with standards and rituals. Then, your child knows what to expect and can rely upon you to follow a set procedure that helps him feel valued, secure, and bonded—three very necessary feelings for a good night's sleep.

First, create a quiet ambience by lowering lights and turning off all technological devices. An hour before sleep is the deadline for television, radio, computers, phones, tablets, and games that are stimulating. The atmosphere should be one of calm and quiet, helping your child wind down at the end of the day and prepare for sleep. Baroque music in sync with your heartbeat in the andante movement will automatically relax your child. Structured routines, such as brushing teeth and a warm (but not too hot) bath will help relax both your child's body and mind, while lowering the decibels of her stress. A regular story time, with a book read by a parent, also helps your child feel cozy, positively attach, and relax.

The idea is to lower the anxiety level of your child and support him through the rituals of preparing for sleep.

CHORES AND WHAT THEY MEAN TO YOUR CHILD

In the beginning, we want to be sure that we teach our children the life skills that will allow them to take care of themselves when we are no longer around, or not wanted around. But a lateral benefit is that not only is your child learning good housekeeping skills, but also dexterity, task mastery, and self-sufficiency, which builds to a self-actualized child. Think back to your youth. Can you even recall when or where you first learned to make a bed, wash a dish, or launder an article of clothing? Probably not, yet the knowledge of how to take care of yourself is part of the preparation for adulthood.

While handing out chores, be realistic with your expectations. You want your child to succeed and have a feeling of accomplishment, a job well done. Be careful and skillful in your job assignments and see to it that they are both age-appropriate and safe. The aim here is teaching, and what you are trying to develop is a secure, self-actualized child who is equipped to go out into the world and make a life that is, in essence, modeled after yours.

Each member of a family should be responsible for different tasks around the house, regardless of outside work.

Here are a few guidelines to follow when chores are created:

1. **Chores should be fair.** Rotate chores so that one child or another does not get stuck always doing the same chore.

2. **Make sure that all chores are safe and age-appropriate.** You don't want a three-year-old washing dishes.

3. **Be reasonable in your expectations.** While it is important to follow through and give children feedback so that they know that they have your attention, you also do not want to crush any young or fragile egos. This is all about building a sense of competence. Keep in mind: it is not what you say, but how you say it. Home should be a safe haven in which to make mistakes, make adjustments, and learn.

4. **Whenever possible, find a reward system other than money.** I prefer tokens, which can be accumulated and traded for things that each particular child holds dear. In this way, children don't develop a feeling of entitlement—that they should be paid for every favor they do around the house. It is better to help your children realize that they are an integral part of a team. On the other hand, there are times when a money reward is warranted, such as a period in which you are teaching your children how to manage money, value it, save it, and spend it responsibly. The approach here, as in all other forms of conscious parenting, is a balanced approach.

5. **Always set a mastery level (a standard) for excellence and keep it within your child's reach.** Don't make the mistake of being too hard to please. We all have memories of jobs not taken for fear of failure. This is all about teaching life skills. Maria Montessori got it right when she built chores into the daily curriculum of her school. She realized that love and work build a centered child who transfers that feeling of self-worth and trust into the outer world.

6. **Engage your child in the discussion.** Come together as a family and share intimate time together while planning which chores need to be done around the house so that it runs smoothly for the whole family—who should do what this week

and what the reward tokens will be worth when they are cashed in.

PARENTING SOLUTIONS FOR CHILDREN WHO ARE WETTING THE BED

1. **First and foremost, let your child know: it's not his fault.** The brain needs to develop enough to put brakes on the bladder, and this happens at a different age for each child. Wetting the bed, in most cases, is not something a child chooses to do purposefully. Rather, it is a neurological development that stops when the brain is developed enough to send the right signals to the bladder. Make sure your child understands this, and that he knows that he can count on you to love and support him unconditionally, while explaining to him that bed-wetting is not intentional and therefore not his fault.

2. **Contact your child's pediatrician.** Get a physical and neurological workup to make sure there is no physical problem. If necessary, and only if under the advisement and supervision of your child's doctor, consider prescriptions for medicine that can help, such as nasal sprays that can help make less urine.

3. **Engage in my empathic process (pages 21).** Talk openly with your child and create a plan of action together. This proactive, nonjudgmental team approach can help restore your child's sense of control by allowing him to invest in his own solutions.

4. **Reward your child for dry nights.** During the empathic process, have your child give input as to which sort of rewards might be appropriate for having dry nights.

5. **Change the bed together after nights he wets the bed.** Approach this with love and support, and this action can help

your child feel like he is doing something proactive to help himself. This can help your child regain some sense of control that was lost by wetting the bed. It is important to NOT use this as a punishment.

6. **Consider trying a bed alarm.** These have been proven to be quite helpful for some families, as they help train the brain to wake up when the bladder begins to go.

7. **Give your child a journal.** Let him know he can write out his true feelings about his experiences in this journal, that it is a safe place for him to release any frustrations, feelings of inadequacy, shame, and also feelings of pride and relief when he has dry nights.

8. **Try meditating with your child.** Meditation can give your child a sense of stabilization. It can help alleviate anxiety and help him feel centered.

As the parent, you are your child's advocate as well as his safety and security. Bed-wetting usually does not last for very long, and if you offer your child support and positive reinforcement during this time, he is more likely to be able to come out of it without lasting trauma.

5

GAINING MOMENTUM— COORDINATE YOUR CHILD'S EMOTIONAL, SOCIAL, AND MOTOR DEVELOPMENT

Intellect alone does not guarantee a child will be a prolific learner. If you want your child to succeed, you have to coordinate her emotional, social, and motor development.

In this chapter, I'll teach you how to sync the timelines of your child's multifaceted development to maximize her potential. I'll explain the ins and outs of your child's emotional processing so that you can ease transitions and arm your child with powerful coping strategies. You'll learn when your child is really ready to be a buddy and how to help her build meaningful, lasting friendships. And to assuage the fears of every mother, I'll spell out a no-fuss guide to your child's motor skills to help you understand how to foster and boost physical intelligence.

Your baby's first test of child development occurs at the moment of birth. Your doctor will give him a series of tests, including:[1]

1. Moro Reflex—more commonly called the startle reflex, where baby is placed on his back and thrashes out his arms and legs while extending his neck.[2]
2. Walking/Stepping Reflex—If baby is held upright over a surface, he'll automatically alternate one foot in front of the other.[3]

3. Rooting—occurs when baby is touched on the cheek and turns toward the hand or finger in an effort to find Mother's nipple.[4]

4. Tonic Neck Reflex—when baby is laid on his back and his head is turned to one side, his arm will reflexively straighten on the same side, while his opposite arm bends or folds. The Tonic Neck Reflex is often called the fencing reflex, for baby's posture imitates a fencing stance.[5]

5. Palmar Grasp—when baby's palm is touched and closes immediately on the finger or instrument placed there.[6]

6. Plantar Grasp—a test that requires stroking the soles of baby's feet and watching to see if baby flexes his feet and closes his toes.[7]

By one year, baby begins to lose his Moro reflex. By the time he's two months of age, the same is true for the walking/stepping reflex. The rooting, however, can last until four months, while the tonic neck reflex extends to the fifth month. The palmar grasp can still be observed at about six months of age. And finally, the plantar grasp is still observable at one year.

An average chart tracking baby's achievements from 0–3 includes:

AGE (IN MOS.) ACHIEVED BY PERCENTAGE OF CHILDREN[8]

	50%	75%	90%
While lying on his back, baby can move his head easily, reaching side to side, though he typically keeps his head centered for the majority of time.	2	2½	3
Baby lies on his tummy—he can raise his head and look out.	2	2½	4½
Baby rolls over to either side.	2½	3½	4½
When baby's on his tummy, he can lift both his head and his chest while holding himself up by his arms.	3	3½	4½
Now baby can sit with help and can keep his head straight and stable.	3	3½	4½
Here, baby can sit unaided for over 30 seconds.	6	7	8
Baby can raise himself up to a standing position using any available support.	7	9	10
Baby is now preparing to walk by crawling, scooting, and hitching across the floor.	7	10	11

Baby can sit up from a lying down position independently.	8	9½	11
Now, baby can stand up without support for at least 10 seconds.	10½	13	14
Baby can walk without help.	12	13 ½	14

Creative play is essential for baby's emotional and psychological growth. In fact, it may be the most important tool in your toolbox.

HERE ARE IDEAS TO INSPIRE YOUR BABY AND SUPPORT HER NEUROLOGICAL DEVELOPMENT.[9]

0–3 Months	Baby is completely captivated by geometric patterns, colorful mobiles, cuddly soft animals, toys that make sounds such as rattles and squeaky animals, music, reflective light mobiles that cast shadows on the ceiling and wall, black-and-white geometrics, and circular objects that she can grasp and hold onto.
4–6 Months	Baby is highly interested in textures: soft, smooth, scratchy, and so on; engages in games such as peekaboo; and gravitates to round objects such as balls. At this stage, baby is all mouth and uses her mouth to distinguish and interpret games and toys. Thus, toys that make noise, books, and paper of all sizes and shapes are all fascinating to baby.
7–9 Months	At this stage, baby becomes attached to toys, stuffed animals, dolls, blankets, and shapes of all kinds. If a particular blanket accompanies baby to sleep, it may become her security blanket, carried everywhere. Also, rubber animals and toys fill baby's bath with delight. And now, games such as patty-cake, catch me if you can, how big is the baby, and where is the light become highly pleasurable.
10–12 Months	As baby becomes more mobile, so do her toys. Now her interest moves to pots, pans, and spoons in the kitchen that can make noise; toy cars, trucks, and boats; pull toys that can move with a string; and stacking toys of all kinds such as squares, circles, and triangles. Now baby can participate in moving objects such as rolling a ball and pushing a toy.
13–15 Months	By 13 months, baby has become a really good mimic. You see this as she make-believes that she is talking on a phone; play-eating from plastic plates and cups; talking with her imaginary dog, cat, cow, chicken, or horse; and simple objects in her favorite toy box, Mom's kitchen.
16–18 Months	By 16 months, baby shows more enthusiasm for music boxes and all things that create sound such as drums, xylophone, and pots and pans. She's also highly attracted to color and colorful things such as balls, beads, and ribbons. Now baby is more interactive and enjoys toys that pop up. For the first time, we see baby creating things with clay, bubbles in the bath, and blowing bubbles.

19–21 Months	Now, baby shows a high level of creativity and imagination. As a social learner, baby imitates making food with clay or mud, riding an imaginary horse with either a rocking horse or pogo horse, pails and shovels, as well as plastic cars large enough for her to ride. She's still interested in balls and pull-apart toys. Additionally, she now likes to play with snap toys that come apart and can be put back together, as well as puzzles. She's also still highly attracted to color and enjoys playing with colored chalk or crayons. Interactive games are more interesting to her as she continues to participate with peekaboo, catch me if you can, and hide and seek.
22–24 Months	At 22 months, baby's imagination is an explosion of creativity as she copies all obvious adult behavior. She may imitate cooking with plastic pots and pans as well as eating with plastic dishes and cups. Clay is useful for fake food and the creation of circles, triangles, and squares. Baby becomes interested in building sets, blocks, cars, trucks, planes, and phones, as well as household objects such as grown-up pots and pans and spoons that substitute for drums. Paper cylinders, plastic bowls and tops, and plastic stacking toys all capture baby's interest, and baby is still captivated by interactive games.
2–3-year-olds	Now, baby's motor skills are so refined that she can push a baby in a baby carriage, swing on a swing, swim in a pool, and ride a tricycle. Here, baby's creativity is in full bloom as she plays dress-up and treats her dolls as her babies. Still interested in music and interactive games, your toddler is now expanding her independence and expresses herself artistically through the use of coloring, painting, and drawing.

In the back of every parent's mind is an unconscious calendar designating the approximate guidelines for child development. You have a general idea of when your baby should roll over, sit up, stand, talk, walk, and so on. And as these markers approach, you may experience anxiety, hoping that your child makes these milestones on time. Neuroscience tells us that children do not develop according to a specific timeline, but rather through systematic increments, with each maturational advancement building on the one before. In a sense, a form of scaffolding occurs, which allows your baby to practice specific skills that are later integrated into an ever more complicated system of movements. This gives him an expanded radius of action and dominion over his surroundings. For instance, your baby will first grasp objects using his entire hand, which is called the ulnar grasp.[10] Then, he moves to the pincer grasp, in which he involves only the thumb and index finger, touching at the tip, which helps him navigate small objects.[11] Consequently, before baby can walk, he must gain mastery of the independent actions of his arms, hands, legs, and feet. Ultimately, he will incorporate all these pieces into his first step. Your baby's physical skills are defined as gross motor skills, while his more precise motor movements such as those involving his small muscles, including eye-hand coordination, are considered fine motor skills.[12] Screening tests such as the Denver Developmental Screening Test help parents assess whether their children are developmentally on target. It is important to note that babies develop from head to tail, a stage called cephalocaudal, as well as from inner to outer, called proximodistal.[13] From the beginning, babies can move their heads from side to side, and they can lift their heads as well when placed on their tummies. By three months, baby may actually be thrown off balance by lifting his head too high. This helps him roll over, a stage that will ultimately lead to sitting.

Your baby can grasp things at birth, including Mom's or Dad's finger, and if baby's open hand is touched, she can close it. By four months, she can hold objects. Soon, she can move objects from hand to hand and pick up items of interest. At age one, your baby can navigate small objects and use her pincer grasp to obtain them, and by a year and a half, baby's eye-hand coordination is so good that she can build buildings out of blocks. In fact, your three-year-old's dexterity is such that she can use a pencil or a crayon to draw a circle.

With the assistance of crib railings, furniture, toys, and pets, your seven-and-a-half-month-old can soon stand up. By eleven months, he can stand alone. These are the stages of development that prepare baby's eye-hand coordination and muscle groups for walking. From eleven and a half months on, your baby's motor development has moved him down the path toward mobility. Also, your baby may crawl before he walks, but not necessarily. In his second year, your baby will be climbing couches, chairs, and stairs as he masters putting one foot in front of the other. Now, he has the motor skills to run and jump, and by age three, your toddler has already gained enough balance to stand on one foot and hop. Though as a newborn your baby exhibits a walking reflex when held upright, it is not until his cortical control frees him that he can actually walk. All of that kicking and body movement is strengthening his neural connections and muscle development, allowing baby to support his weight as he prepares for mobility. Even when placed in warm water, infants imitate walking.[14]

However, a developmental time clock is not the sole contributor to his physical milestones. According to Esther Thelen, "infant and environment form an interconnective system, and development has interacting causes; such as his desire and motivation to do something (for example, pick up a toy, or get to the other side of the room). The infant's physical characteristics and his or her position in a particular setting (such as lying in a crib or being held upright in a pool) offer opportunities, and constraints that affect whether, and how, his goal can be achieved. Ultimately, a solution emerges as a result of trying out behaviors and retaining those that most efficiently reach the goal."[15] As a result, baby is all about problem-solving in relation to maturation. Here, once again, the nature-nurture partnership is evident and explains why babies walk on different timelines. Every parent is familiar with the stories of late walkers and late talkers. Though it is worthwhile to pay attention to loose developmental timetables, it is also valuable to recognize that each child matures at his own rate of speed. As it is baby's own neuronal and muscular maturation, in conjunction with his environment, that will determine the speed at which your baby walks and talks.

When you consider that our species is born completely helpless, without the capacity or physical strength to survive alone in the world, the real miracle is that we do. In the beginning, your baby has little muscle control, and therefore her capacity is measured by her early unrefined reflexes such as sucking, rooting, and grasping. In fact, it is because the brain stem develops earliest that baby has some control over her survival reflexes. From 0–3 months, your baby experiences an intense period of synaptic development in her brain, which leads to physical, social, and intellectual growth. She begins to build an associative mass, recognizing that when she cries, she will be held. Little by little, her reflexive movements will be substituted for more deliberate ones. From the fourth to sixth months, your baby's brain cortex matures, so that her more primitive activity slows down, replaced by her motor skills. Simultaneously, the neurons in your baby's brain are coded by myelin. This coding acts as an insulation, protecting the electrical pathways of each neuron. Thus, the neuron's signal is kept on target, so that it doesn't crisscross with the electrical signals of other neurons. Your baby's brain is developing all along, becoming so efficient that it discards or prunes synapses or connections not being used. This myelination and pruning will ultimately establish clear and precise pathways from billions of cells. A baby will be two years old before this process of myelination and pruning is completed.[16]

Your newborn's sensory capacity is as limited and vulnerable as her motor skills. Her ability to differentiate and focus on people or things is limited. Yet from the very beginning, the one voice and face she recognizes, and prefers above all others, is yours. Baby's vision range is approximately thirteen inches. In an effort to protect your baby, nature conspires to place her viewing range at thirteen inches, the precise distance between mother and baby when breastfeeding. And though baby can follow an object with a range of eighteen inches, the object of her fixation is Mother. Little by little, baby's vision is getting stronger until at approximately six months she can see things binocularly, while simultaneously gaining muscle mastery.[17]

At this stage, baby begins to prepare himself for further mobility. While lying on his tummy, he tries to raise his head off of his blanket and elevate his chest. Though still struggling with balance and the synchronization of his eyes and hands, your baby practices daily the first skills he'll need to walk. By three months, baby can balance himself on his arm, moving his constellation of control down to his feet. As baby continues to strengthen and lengthen, he moves his body from side to side, until lo and behold, one day he reaches that next milestone and rolls over. He's as surprised as you are. This happens somewhere between two-and-a-half and six months. This is no small task, but he's been practicing it all along by moving his hands and feet and turning his back. His effort exhibits cortical power, including the motor cortex, basil ganglia, and the cerebellum. Your baby is a quick learner, and once he figures out what he did accidentally, he becomes a roll-over master. While exercising his whole body in this one supreme effort of rolling over, he continues to stretch and strengthen, contributing to the maturation and control of his nervous system. Soon, his movements become deliberate as he begins the subtle dance of muscle memory, moving his body in concert toward an ever more nuanced elaboration of task mastery. Now he's catching on, and before long, he will confront his next challenge: sitting on his own.[18]

Each achievement is a watershed moment as your baby synchronizes both her muscle strength and balance, consciously manipulating her body toward her goal. Crawling is next, though in some cases baby may skip this stage altogether, while others invent variations of the typical crawl. It is at this time that baby becomes more social. Though she may still be afraid of strangers, she exhibits delight when around little children. At this stage, your baby is thinking and working out, little by little, the steps needed for advancement. According to neuroscientist Bruce Shapiro, babies "reach for their function threshold."[19] Of course, this may require that they miss various stages of development, such as crawling. For example, an early walker may synchronize a low body weight with strong muscle capacity. As a result, your baby may stand up at nine months old and just take off. Nevertheless, somewhere between nine and eighteen months, she will begin her very first steps toward walking. The range of 9–18 months is simply measured by the necessary collaboration between the mind and the body. In the beginning, baby will use any prop available to give her both mobility and balance, including your family pet. When you realize that every muscle and every digit, both fingers and toes, are moving in coordination to assist baby in her first steps, you can see how central maturity is to mobility.[20]

Between eighteen and twenty-three months, baby starts trying to run, hide, tumble, and climb. She may even try to hit or kick a ball and begins to cup her hands in order to hold fluid. Now baby is responding to color and light so that brightly tinted crayons become one of her favorite toys.

Your baby is unfolding at her own rate of speed. She is not social learning. She's simply moving beyond her comfort zone to explore her environment, as soon as her body can support her journey. Thus, the idea of a normal range of development is filled with exceptions for every rule or milestone.[21]

However, there are things to look for that may give you cause for concern. If baby hasn't started walking by eighteen months, or can stand but not sit, a visit to the doctor may be warranted. On the other hand, if things seem to be moving along at approximately the right pace, remember that it's not only baby's biology that is controlling her development, but also her environment.

Every marker reached by baby is enhanced by experience, and each experience creates new brain associations and connections. These encourage baby to further expand his frame of reference by extending and trying more complicated endeavors. As baby builds his associative mass and gains mastery over each developmental marker, he experiences confidence in himself. It is this confidence that leads baby toward independence and competence. With each step, baby is becoming self-actualized, reaching for his own authority. His growth has been from head to toe as he evolved from helplessness and primitive reflexes to an advancement of motor control and brain development.

Each time your baby masters a new stage of development, he may for a time forget a recently learned behavior. In a sense, the brain is reordering itself to accommodate the new task. This developmental loss is not permanent and will only last for a limited time. In the past, the brain was thought of as a machine that advanced in skill as it matured. However, today neuroscience tells us that a partnership exists between your baby's brain and his environment. Somewhere in the first year of your baby's life, he will already have trillions of synapses or neural connections, and some of those connections will be discarded or pruned by the time he is grown. What decides which synapses live and which die, which are turned off and which are turned on? The synapses that are the most used will be activated, and those that are not stimulated by experience will simply fade away. In this way, your baby is hardwired to learn, for it is the interaction of experience, stimulated by emotional gratification, that reinforces baby's synaptic connections. The brain is so efficient that it prunes those synapses not used and activates those that are. Every time your baby acts and receives a positive reaction for his behavior, that reaction strengthens his brain's synapses. Thus, the response for each experience is coded or stored in the brain.

By a year and half, your toddler will demonstrate that she has a sense of herself. She can recognize her face in a picture or mirror and is beginning to understand that she is separate and unique from the world around her. She is still parallel-playing with little interest in being social. In fact, if placed in social environments with other children, your two-year-old may become anxious. In addition, she is expanding her vocabulary and is beginning to use sentences. She can understand simple games and simple directions . . . though her new surge toward independence may keep her from obeying. Your toddler is now moving, moving, moving as she walks, runs, and climbs everywhere. Simultaneously, fine motor skills are allowing her to begin to feed herself, hold a cup, and use utensils. Moving through the continuum from seven months toward three years, your baby masters rolling over, sitting, crawling, standing, walking, running, dancing, galloping, and tumbling. Ultimately, she achieves the autonomy that goes along with her hard-earned independence, as she experiments with the boundaries of her environment, through the use of her body and mind. No longer parallel-playing, your three-year-old has become more social, though she will still experience times when she prefers to play by herself. Storytelling is now essential to your three-year-old toddler, for her memories of past events find their way into her stories. In her efforts to exert her autonomy, your three-year-old toddler will also start asking you the proverbial question: "Why?"[22]

By age three, your toddler has made huge developmental leaps in his gross motor skills. Not only can he run and jump about 15–24 inches and hop on one foot, but he can also walk up and down a staircase independently, using both feet. Coincidentally, all of these advancements are the requisite skills needed to play games. He can't, however, stop short or turn quickly. This motor skill explosion is due to both his environment and the development of the sensory and motor areas of his cortex. His body is cooperating with him as his muscles and bones get larger and stronger while his lung capacity expands, giving him all he needs for both coordination and acceleration. As a result, it is his genetic imprint in combination with his environment that will direct both his interest and skills. By age four, your toddler can jump 24–33 inches, go up and down a stairway with alternating feet, hop approximately six times on one foot, and is able to turn, stop, and start quickly. Your five-year-old can jump 28–36 inches; walk up and down a staircase without help using alternating feet; hop approximately sixteen times; can easily turn, start, and stop short; and can now participate successfully in games.[23]

Your three-year-old's fine motor skills are getting more precise each day as he exerts his autonomy trying to dress himself, button his clothes, feed himself, and draw faces. His eye-hand coordination is strengthening, and your toddler now can participate in his own personal care and personal hygiene. For example, your three-year-old can feed himself; pour juice, water, or milk; use cutlery; and, most important, go to the potty alone. He can draw a circle and make a face as a complete body, minus limbs. At four, your toddler can dress himself independently, use plastic scissors, cut a line, draw a person, begin to copy letters, make paper into triangles, and take care of his personal hygiene. By five, your toddler can copy squares and triangles, and draw a more complete person. He is in complete charge of his personal hygiene, including washing his hands and face, brushing his teeth, and combing his hair. As his fine motor skills and gross motor skills mature, your toddler refines his capacity more precisely, integrating his abilities. This merging of skills is referred to as a system of actions.[24]

As your toddler develops physically, she becomes more in control of her body. Now she can ride a bike and use scissors, cutlery, and even chopsticks. It is now, at around age three, that your toddler begins to favor one hand over the other. Most children are right-handed, as the left hemisphere of the brain has authority over the right side of the body. On the other hand, if both sides of the brain are symmetrical, the right hemisphere is in control and your toddler will be left-handed. There are those cases, however, when a child is ambidextrous. This is often the case with a left-handed child. In addition, more boys are left-handed than girls. In fact, there seems to be a genetic component to handedness, and 82 percent of the population inherits the gene for right-handedness. If your toddler did not inherit the right-handed gene, she has a 50-percent chance of being right-handed anyway. If not, she will either be left-handed or ambidextrous. If your toddler does not inherit the right-handed gene, her handedness may just be randomly determined. Even if you and your partner are both right-handed, your toddler still has an 8 percent chance of being left-handed. Nevertheless, your three-year-old will express a preference for one hand over the other in coordination with the advancement of her motor and fine motor skills.[25] Never, never try to change your child's dominant hand, as it can lead to both stress and anxiety . . . not to mention terrible handwriting.

By age five, half of your child's IQ is in place. Now, she is ready for kindergarten.

THE ABCS FOR PEAK PERFORMANCE
THE THREE MOST IMPORTANT STEPS FOR EACH AGE AND STAGE

In this book, I unlock the scientific data and open the door to the mystery of accelerated learning. By understanding the developmental stages of early childhood, you will master the art of expanding your child's potential and performance through the experience of your daily interactions, and it is as easy as ABC.

We will identify every important milestone in your child's life, and I will chart a course for you and your baby toward complete linguistic, cognitive, social, emotional, and moral maturity.

Step A: The most important step, of course, is bonding. Yet it is so simple that it is often left out of child development books. Bonding is the one essential element needed in the alchemy of healthy brain growth.

Step B: By participating in the exercises provided for each stage of child development, you will learn how to create age-appropriate experiences to foster and enhance your child's intellectual and emotional growth. You will also build a scaffolding of information, which helps you to support Steps B and C.

Step C will explain in greater detail how to help your child relax and reduce stress while enhancing her focus and concentration. You will uncover the value of the ancient arts of meditation, yoga, qigong, and creative visualization, as well as the importance of music in the science of learning. By the end of this book, you will be prepared to use the critical strategies and skills necessary to create a healthy, happy, and academically advanced child. More than that, your child will now be able to successfully self-manage whatever life has in store.

Not only are the activities and practical exercises enjoyable, but they also lay the foundation for each successive stage of your child's maturation. When you interact with your baby at every age and stage, you actively listen to him, see him, and get to know him more each day. With you by his side, as an active participant in his life, he is able to unite his emotional, spiritual, moral, and intellectual ontogeny.

In education, every ending signals a beginning. According to psychologist and psychoanalyst Erik Erikson, it is important to navigate and resolve each stage of child development successfully before moving on. There is an ancient Inca myth that you can only get back into the garden by eating the fruit, because the fruit of the past holds the seeds of the future. The same is true in child development. Therefore, if your child passes through each stage of development successfully, she will be ready, intellectually and emotionally, to open to the next stage enthusiastically. If she completes one stage before moving onto the next, she won't carry with her the unresolved issues and residue of the stage before; she will begin each new stage afresh, open and ready to learn. First, however, you must know what's needed at each stage of growth, what is age-appropriate, and what the consequences are for not successfully completing each stage. Here is the way to positively affect your child's development, for in the process of creating a strong scaffolded foundation, you will also create a strong and healthy child.[26]

In the following chapter, you will see that I separate the exercises for emotional and cognitive advancement. Though those two categories overlap, they are still in some ways interdependent. Emotions and intellect do not unfold in a parallel manner, but rather in a spiral movement, similar to the DNA molecule helix. If you could envision a DNA molecule or a rising scaffold, supporting intertwining paths of emotional growth and intellectual achievement, you would see that each advancement supports the next on an upward trajectory.

THE POSSIBLE HUMAN

We are the only species born underdeveloped. It is our extralarge prefrontal cortex that separates us from all other animals and makes us human. Because of our large prefrontal cortex, where our critical thinking and executive function live, we have rapid brain growth that parallels the continued growth of our heads. If, on the other hand, we were born fully developed, our heads would be too large to pass through the birth canal. So, we humans have an unusually prolonged period of helplessness, as our brains rapidly fire to organize the trillions of synapses, the connections that build our life. Although this process continues until the day you die, you will use more energy from birth until age ten than you will use from age ten to age 100. Hence, the importance of early childhood, when your child's young and vulnerable brain is creating all of those connections in conjunction with her earliest experiences. For this reason, I cannot emphasize enough how critical bonding is to early childhood: it is everything. Because the well-bonded child has most of her needs met, she feels safe and secure, and therefore calm and content. If your baby is not well bonded, she will be anxious and insecure, overproducing stress hormones including cortisol, which will bathe her brain, changing its structure permanently. In fact, this child may experience a failure to thrive and as a result face problems not only with you, but with all of her other relationships, forever. It will be difficult for her to connect with others, to follow instructions, to deal with anger and aggression. School will present a greater challenge for her, as her temperament and behavior can make it difficult for her to form friendships, making it challenging for her to hone the interpersonal skills necessary for social interactions. She will carry these insecurities with her throughout all of her life, missing opportunities because of her emotional immaturity. Can this dire situation be remedied? Yes, but only if it is recognized, acknowledged, and remediated during the first three years of life. Therefore, the importance of parental involvement and bonding cannot be overstated.[27]

Yet there is a bright side to your influence, which is that you can make the difference. By knowing your child and paying attention to her wants and needs, you can build the trust and security needed to help her access the range and scope of her full abilities.

In this chapter, you will find an overview of early child development, differentiating between emotional, moral, and cognitive growth. In addition, I will explain the role of parents and their effects on optimal performance in all those realms. You will also find information on the most effective stress-reduction techniques available to help your child manage his own stress and anxiety, thus processing information at an optimal level. Later in this chapter, we will discuss in further detail how your child thinks and feels at every age and stage. You'll get a clear picture of his development of mind and body along with the appropriate tools, exercises, and activities necessary to guide him toward his full potential.

Once you can interact with your child in a stress-free environment, you will both open to a relaxed and happy state of mind. Both you and your child will experience a sense of an open and complete relationship, where knowledge and independence can bloom and grow. Moreover, you will have helped to create a self-actualized, self-possessed, confident, and independent child who can muster his own resources to be self-motivated and independent. It is this child who can focus, concentrate, and problem-solve.

You will become your child's true gene therapist, showing her the way toward her own inner voice, where she can find her true vocation and happiness. Sigmund Freud summed up his work with a simple phrase, describing a successful life as one that is fulfilled in work and in love. By giving your child your time and attention in early childhood, you will maximize her chances to achieve a joyous and productive life, and that is the greatest gift of all.

STEP A: HOW TO NURTURE YOUR CHILD'S EMOTIONAL MATURITY
A LOOK AT SKILLFUL SOCIAL AND INTERPERSONAL COMPETENCE

Emotional and intellectual development are two of the most critical areas for building a happy, healthy, and academically advanced child. Though these skills develop on parallel paths, without the element of emotional maturity, your child cannot achieve the full magnitude of his cognitive potential. Since EQ or emotional intelligence affects motivation, it is essential for supporting your child's ability to master his own intellect. For example, if your child is emotionally mature, all things being equal, he will outperform other children of similar ages. He'll process information better and in a sense use his brain better than a child who is emotionally immature. Why? Because emotional maturity enables your child to focus and concentrate, sit still for long periods of time, and open to new and exciting material. Therefore, it is the foundation of self-awareness, which fosters motivation, morality, and good self-esteem. It is this feeling of self-confidence that makes your child feel capable, and it is that feeling of capability that leads to his sense of competence. These are the fundamental qualities that your child needs to access the full thrust of his talents and knowledge. Your emotionally mature child feels at ease and comfortable, not only with himself, but also in the way in which he interacts with others. He can tap into his own emotional and intellectual productivity, guiding others to a more rewarding life.

Many years ago, I was privileged to hear a lecture from the nationally renowned educator Howard Gardner. He was one of the earliest educators to recognize the existence of "multiple intelligences."[28] In the West, we are most familiar with IQ or intellectual intelligence, but Gardner identified many more intelligences, including but not limited to interpersonal, intrapersonal, linguistic, logical-mathematical, bodily-kinesthetic, spatial, naturalistic, and musical. Then, in the 1980s, Gardner presented even more types of intelligence, except emotional. Though emotional development and its importance in infancy and early childhood has only been studied over the last few decades, most scientists today recognize the significant role that emotions play in linguistic, cognitive, social, moral, and emotional development.[29]

EIGHT INTELLIGENCES, ACCORDING TO GARDNER[30]		
Intelligence	Definition	Fields or Occupations Where Used
Linguistic	Ability to use and understand words and nuances of meaning	Writing, editing, and translating
Logical-mathematical	Ability to manipulate numbers and solve logical problems	Science, business, medicine
Musical	Ability to perceive and create patterns of pitch and rhythm	Musical composition, conducting
Spatial	Ability to find one's way around in an environment and judge relationships between objects in space	Architecture, carpentry, city planning
Bodily-kinesthetic	Ability to move with precision	Dancing, athletics, surgery
Interpersonal	Ability to understand and communicate with others	Teaching, acting, politics
Intrapersonal	Ability to understand the self	Counseling, psychiatry, spiritual leadership
Naturalist	Ability to distinguish species	Hunting, fishing, farming, gardening, cooking

In his groundbreaking 1995 book *Emotional Intelligence*, psychologist Daniel Goleman stressed the importance of emotional intelligence while explaining that there was an interdependence throughout all multiple intelligences.[31] I interviewed Dr. Goleman in 2012 and was particularly interested in his position that success in life relies on many factors and is not exclusively dependent upon your SAT scores or GPA.

He explained that our natural intelligence quotient accounted for approximately 20 percent of the variables that determined performance, while 80 percent of our success can be attributed to other factors. It is EQ, or emotional intelligence, that Goleman and contemporary educators recognize as contributing to most of your child's knowledge and cognitive ability.

In a neuroscientific research study by Goleman, he indicated that memory and learning are established in the prefrontal lobes of the brain. Thus, it is the prefrontal lobes that control your emotional impulses. If your child is emotionally immature, he will be vulnerable to emotional outbursts of anger, anxiety, and volatility. Under normal circumstances, the prefrontal cortex is the captain of your child's ship, controlling his executive function and helping him think critically. But if your child is emotionally immature, his emotions can take over, grabbing the controls and inhibiting his ability to think while overriding his executive function, making it much more difficult for him to access his memory and learn.[32]

Bonding well with your child establishes his confidence and competence, thus enabling him to develop his emotional maturity. Then, he can interact comfortably under all circumstances, and on all occasions, in a calm and relaxed manner. These are the characteristics that heighten your child's self-esteem and motivation so that he can discover and expand his talents and intellect.[33]

LET'S BEGIN AT THE BEGINNING

According to social scientist Albert Bandura, we are all social animals and learn by imitating and modeling behavior. Keep in mind that your child is watching you, always. You are the center of her universe, the focus of her attention, and everything you say and everything you do will be copied by this tiny actor. It stands to reason that your child will adopt your ideas and prejudices while mastering her social skills. The sum total of your actions will inspire and direct her to and from emotional maturity.

An essential part of bonding is the development of trust, so when your child crawls out of the room to play, looking over his shoulder periodically to make sure that you haven't left, he is learning how to trust. If he finds you where he left you when he returns from his foray, then he is well on the road to trusting. Each encounter away from you is counterbalanced by the knowledge that you haven't abandoned him, until ultimately he can relax, knowing that he can count on you to be present when he returns. This is how you build a relationship with your child, creating the intimacy of knowing you can be trusted to always be there for him. When your child learns to trust you, he learns how to trust himself, and if he learns how to trust himself, he learns how to trust others. Trust is the foundation upon which your child builds his sense of self, not only with you, but also with the world around him. This is how he becomes self-actualized.

According to Vygotsky, this scaffolding allows your child to focus and concentrate.[34] When you bond with your child, you are providing her with the scaffolding needed to support her ability to learn and process information effectively. There are several pertinent aspects that must be incorporated in scaffolding, including a safe, secure, and accepting environment at home, as well as a preponderance of parental interactions, both emotional and social. Your child needs to be loved, not judged, so that she can be motivated to override any and all obstacles that obstruct her path. Obstacles such as poverty, disabilities, etc., can be compensated for by a well-bonded child. Nevertheless, it is important to know your child's history, both physical—was she full-term? did she have a traumatic birth?—and emotionally—is she shy or unusually aggressive? Here is the intimate information that only you can provide, and it is this very information that creates a bridge between your child's past and present. Only then can you meet your child where she is, giving her the security to strike out on her own and explore her surroundings. In keeping with the idea of scaffolding, it is also relevant to organize a structured environment. Children need and want order, and they like consistency above all things, not very different from wanting to be cared for after birth. Your child wants to know the rules, what to expect, and what is permissible, so that she can have freedom within the limits of knowing what is acceptable. Now she is traveling on the road toward emotional maturity. By having a structure that is consistent, your child can align herself with her emotional world and widen her range of maturity.

TALKING WITH YOUR CHILD

Your child's first social interactions are the conversations he has with you throughout the day. It is the give-and-take of listening and talking that socializes your child, teaching him requisite social skills. I like to tell parents to talk, talk, talk. Talk about everything and anything, often and always. Language builds your child's associative mass and increases those ever important connections in your child's brain. More than that, talking engages and stimulates your child's interests and feelings of joy and well-being. It is indispensable to bonding, as it grows the atmosphere of intimacy. It is here where a sense of being valued and validated originates, creating a lifelong practice of establishing and solidifying the child-parent bond, which will be transferred to your child's adult relationships. By forming a habit of open and empathic communication, you clear the path for the difficult and emotionally charged problems that occur during the natural separation of adolescence. In Chapter 2, I discuss my empathic process and how you can use it effectively to communicate in your family.

As a parent, you are the most important person in your child's life, so he will mimic and imitate everything you do, the good, the bad, and the ugly. When you relate to your child and interact throughout the day, he is learning important social skills that he will later transfer to his own social sphere of friendship. Through your actions, you are teaching him how to advocate his feelings, how to voice his opinion, and how to express anger and hurt in an assertive but nonaggressive manner, always showing respect for his peers. These are the behaviors that will set your child on the path to healthy social interactions, relationships, and emotional growth. On the other hand, if you bully, control, discount, oppress, or dominate your child, you will see him imitate those behaviors with his friends and schoolmates. You must be what you want to see. Only then will your child learn the lessons of your successful social strategies. Once your child models your behavior, he will adopt, apply, and transfer those behaviors to all his social encounters.

TIMING IS EVERYTHING

Emotionally immature children have a problem settling down and getting themselves ready to learn. Regardless of their IQ, if their emotional development is delayed, it affects all other development. The good news is that there is help for these children, and it is simply accomplished and near at hand, because it is you. You can make the difference by getting involved, paying attention, reinstituting structure, and practicing the particular kind of parental nurturing and bonding necessary to build your child's interpersonal skills. Remember, time is of the essence.

By remedying emotional underdevelopment, you have the opportunity to help your child cultivate a strong central core, the foundation for his emotions. When life happens and your child is confronted with family problems, peer-group pressures, or typical struggles with temper and temperament, he will be able to stay calm and adjust rapidly to change. Here, your well-adjusted child will act based on his own internal and intrinsic values, rather than be vulnerable to social tensions and peer-group socializations. He will have a strong sense of himself, which leads to self-confidence and self-worth. He won't have to follow the herd, because the herd is relatively unconscious. Rather, he can follow his own authority and in the end lead the herd. Your support and loving feedback validates his choices and understanding of good and bad, positive and negative conduct. Here, you can see the role that scaffolding plays in your relationship with your child. By knowing your child, you build the bridge that supports him through his growth and development. If you ever doubt how relevant you are in your child's life, recognize and acknowledge that it is you who built the scaffold.

Many years ago, there was a worldwide survey studying successful people, asking what they all had in common. You may be surprised to know they were average students who had very high emotional EQ, meaning that they were friendly and knew how to get along with people from all walks of life. Knowing that they couldn't be experts in all things, they were comfortable in hiring the A students—the experts—to work for them. What was unique to them were the social skills that allowed them to manage other people successfully. They had mastered the art of interpersonal intelligence, which increased their people skills. These skills will be most significant to our future high-tech, industrial, and service-based economy. So you can see how important it is for your child to develop emotional maturity. It is almost impossible for your child to both integrate and implement his social skills if he is unable to approach his own thoughts and ideas without distraction. On the other hand, if he can find his way back to his own resource, that strong central core, anything is possible. By mastering his emotional intelligence, he will find his inner voice, his true vocation, and his destiny.[35]

STEP B: HOW TO INFLUENCE YOUR CHILD'S INTELLECTUAL GROWTH

Your child's view of the world, her perspective and understanding, evolve over time. Just as an artist uses local color (the color of the plain air motif and its surroundings) to enhance his painting, so does your child use her surroundings to enlarge her reality, day by day, week by week, month by month, and year by year, thereby increasing not only her knowledge, but also her ability to process that knowledge, linking to already-stored information and crossing a threshold of neurons to create something new. Each new experience builds on the one before in accordance with and relevant to her stage of development. By matching her intellectual readiness to her chronological age, you can support and encourage her intellectual expansion, keeping in mind that the main point is to know what the pivotal windows of opportunity are for each particular skill, those moments when your child's brain is activated and ready to go. Your child's social and emotional development follows the same pattern of integrating, of matching the right activities and exercises with her appropriate age and developmental stage. In this way, your child will progress by leaps and bounds, naturally, without tension or stress. But first, it is important to know just how children learn. Though different theories come and go, we now have the advantage of technology to clarify a number of misunderstandings.

THE WAY CHILDREN UNDERSTAND THEIR WORLD

By becoming actively involved in your child's growth, both intellectually and emotionally, you will reinforce his courage to venture out of his comfort zone. Thus, by creating a print-rich space with objects that stimulate his senses and can be observed, manipulated, smelled, and touched—including textures, rough and soft, colors, and age-appropriate toys—your little adventurer will happily learn about his surroundings and return to you to tell you all about his discoveries.

The confidence that you'll be there, that you're reliable, and that he can count on you frees him up to play creatively. Through manipulating everyday objects, including both familiar and unfamiliar items, your child learns not only how things work, but also why they do what they do. Everything in the realm of your child's experience is new and interesting. Like a detective, your naturally curious child is motivated to investigate everything. Whatever you place in his vicinity, he will reach for and play with. For him, task mastery is its own intrinsic reward, for it is with that mastery that your little detective gains the tenacity and proficiency that leads to a greater sense of self and self-esteem. For example, when your child learns how to pour a glass of water or successfully places the right peg in the right hole, he feels successful and self-actualized. This offers him the intrinsic value that inspires motivation. In the beginning, your little toddler performs for your approval, always looking back to make sure you are watching. But he will soon become self-motivated, performing for his own inner satisfaction. By learning to trust his own authority, your child feels the internal rewards that make him feel good about himself, rather than anxious and fearful of failure.

There are many styles of learning—visual, auditory, verbal, kinesthetic, and so on—so it is not surprising that children often favor one or two of these modalities. However, if you expose your child to an environment that encourages the use of different styles of learning, her brain will process information laterally. According to Donald H. Schuster and Charles E. Gritton, in their book *Suggestive-Accelerative Learning Techniques*, children can learn more rapidly and process information better if they can relax and thus use their brain more harmoniously, like an orchestra.[36] Furthermore, when you expose your baby to more than one learning modality, you engage more than one of her senses, introducing her to the full thrust of her intellectual capital. Keep in mind that when interacting with your baby in creative play, it is important to excite her senses by pointing out the collateral sights, sounds, feelings, and smells that accompany each and every new experience.

The importance of creative play cannot be overestimated, for it is in the state of creative play that our brains relax and process most effectively. Here is where most discoveries come from, where thoughts can be linked to create new ideas. In chapter 6, I will show you the strategies and tools to use with your child to help her achieve her greatest intellectual potency. In this relaxed state, new data can be understood and processed, so that associative information can be accessed to problem-solve.

STEP C: THE EFFECTS OF STRESS-REDUCTION TECHNIQUES ON COGNITIVE, LANGUAGE AND SOCIAL DEVELOPMENT

TEACH YOUR CHILD TECHNIQUES TO HELP THEM RELAX, FOCUS, CONCENTRATE, AND PROBLEM-SOLVE

The stress-reduction techniques you will find here are the result of my many years of practice and experience. Through my own exploration into matters of mental, physical, and spiritual techniques, I have over time developed my own approach, one that I feel is the most effective and efficient for children, and which begins at birth. Through my travels, I've discovered that there's a core principle running through all stress-reducing activities. First and foremost is the idea that relaxing the body prepares it for a state of mindfulness, in which more blood is thrown to the prefrontal cortex, causing the body to relax and the circulation to improve. The simplest form of relaxation for baby, of course, is massage, and nothing soothes and comforts baby more than being close to her mother, hearing her voice, and feeling her touch. Ancient cultures have always known that relaxation techniques can heal the body and expand the mind. Children who learn these relaxation techniques can hold images longer and process information better. Moreover, when your baby's stress declines, her memory improves, and in the end, your happy baby performs easily at her optimum level. So, by reducing your baby's stress levels, you are preparing her to learn.

I've studied stress-reduction techniques and learning for forty-five years and have conducted a number of studies on stress and learning in the Houston Independent School District. What I have learned is that children of all ages experience stress and anxiety. Yet there are simple ways to alleviate stress that are easily taught and quickly mastered. Simply focused breathing can take an anxious child to a place of calm. Activities such as listening to Baroque music, mindfulness meditation, qigong, creative visualization, and so forth are now considered mainstream and therefore have found a place in the curricula of many schools. All of these disciplines enhance your child's learning by allowing her brain to expand exponentially, opening her to her own resources and creativity. This relaxed state stimulates the endorphins that are responsible for joy and happiness while lowering cortisol. Now your child can easily focus and concentrate in the most seamless way without effort. As your child's mind focuses on a particular thought, word, or object, it becomes still and peaceful. This is actually the natural state of the mind, and it will give your child the sense of control that is needed for calmness. This feeling of control leads to security, which then finds its way into self-management. By teaching your child how to manage her own stress, you are giving her the tools she needs to develop the self-discipline necessary to learn and achieve in life.

Measured breathing is the easiest way to relax the body and the mind. Because breathing is something we all do, and therefore know how to do, it is the easiest way to teach mindfulness. If you hold your baby to your chest, calmly and quietly, so that you can feel her little heartbeat against yours, you can slowly, slowly sync your breathing with hers. As your child gets older, she'll learn to synchronize her breathing to her own heartbeat, placing her into a calm alpha state. The alpha state achieved in relaxation lowers both breathing and heart rate so that your child will experience a feeling of peacefulness, calm, and quiet. There are many positive outcomes that originate from the alpha state, and almost all of them are transferred into everyday life. Once you and your child learn how to enter the alpha state of relaxation, you become more aware of the subtleties around you, including your own behavior toward others. Most important, studies show that a still, quiet inner nature can stimulate both accelerated learning and performance.

ERIKSON'S STAGES OF PSYCHOSOCIAL DEVELOPMENT

Erik Erikson was a psychoanalyst and a student of Freud in Vienna. Because of the threat of Nazism, he left Germany for America in 1933. Analyzing his own childhood and professional experience, he developed a psychosocial model that stressed the influence of social interactions on the developing personality.

In a sense, he modified Freud's idea that early childhood experiences shape the developing personality by contending that ego development continued throughout life.

Erikson's theory of psychosocial development covers eight stages across the lifespan: "Each stage involves a 'crisis' in personality—a major developmental issue that is particularly important at that time, and will remain an issue to some degree throughout the rest of life. The crisis, which emerges according to a maturation time table, must be satisfactorily resolved, for healthy ego development. Successful resolution of each of the 8 crises requires the balancing of a positive trait, and a corresponding negative one. Although the positive quality should predominate, some degree of the negative is needed as well. The crisis of infancy, for example, is (basic trust vs. basic mistrust). People need to trust the world and the people in it, but they also need to learn from mistrust to protect themselves from danger. The successful outcome of each crisis is the development of the particular 'virtue' or strength—and in this first crisis, the 'virtue' is *hope*."[37]

ERIKSON'S PSYCHOSOCIAL STAGES[38]

Erikson's psychosocial crisis stages		
Basic Trust versus Mistrust	12–18 months	Baby develops sense of whether world is a good and safe place. Virtue: hope.
Autonomy versus Shame & Doubt	12–18 months to 3 years	Child develops a balance of independence and self-sufficiency over shame and doubt. Virtue: will.
Initiative versus Guilt	3 to 6 years	Child develops initiative when trying out new activities and is not overwhelmed by guilt. Virtue: purpose.
Industry versus Inferiority	6 years to puberty	Child must learn skills of the culture or face feeling of incompetence. Virtue: skill.
Identity versus Role Confusion	Puberty to young adulthood	Adolescent must determine own sense of self ("Who am I?") or experience confusion about roles. Virtue: fidelity.
Intimacy versus Isolation	Young adulthood	Person seeks to make commitments to others; if unsuccessful, may suffer from isolation and self-absorption. Virtue: love

Generativity versus Stagnation	Middle adulthood	Mature adult is concerned with establishing and guiding the next generation or else feels personal impoverishment. Virtue: care.
Integrity versus Despair	Late adulthood	Elderly person achieves acceptance of own life, allowing acceptance of death, or else despairs over inability to relive life. Virtue: wisdom.

In Erikson's psychosocial model, your baby's first crisis is *trust vs. mistrust*, which occurs from birth to 18 months, a time in which your baby realizes that his well-being depends on the reliability of those around him. To resolve this crisis, your infant hopes that he can count on his primary caretakers to be there for him consistently. Thus, the virtue for his first crisis is hope. If the people and objects in his sphere can be trusted to meet his needs consistently, then your baby will transfer his feelings of trust from you to himself, and to the outside world. The most important thing you can do for your baby, to help him successfully navigate this first psychosocial crisis, is to help him develop trust by being present when he needs you to show up, whether it's to feed him, diaper him, comfort him, or care for him when he is ill. Because your baby lacks certainty about his environment, he looks to you for stability. If you can be trusted to be there, he will trust you. This is how your baby develops security, by feeling that if threatened, he will be protected by you. And that is because, at first, his limited emotional repertoire makes his physical needs the most pressing.[39]

However, if your care as his primary caretaker is unpredictable, and if your child feels that he cannot count on you to be there no matter what, he will develop mistrust. That mistrust will transfer into his own feelings of insecurity as he begins to doubt his capacity to influence his environment. That mistrust puts your baby on high alert, with feelings of anxiety and fear, doubting the safety of the world in which he lives. Not only that, but that mistrust will follow him throughout his life and will forever influence the way he relates to others. If you aren't trustworthy, and can't be relied upon to meet your child's needs consistently, you will evoke in him fear and mistrust, which then causes him to bring those feelings into the next psychosocial stage. The remnant of whatever isn't resolved in each particular stage is not left behind, but rather brought forward into the new psychosocial developmental stage and crisis.

HOW PARENTS CAN INFLUENCE ERIKSON'S FIRST CRISIS STAGE OF TRUST VS. MISTRUST:[40]

1. It is critical for you to be consistent in caregiving, sensitive to your baby's needs, and responsive at every turn.
2. Bond with baby. You can't spoil your baby with love, and "tough love" is an oxymoron.
3. Be reliable. You are your child's primary representative in his universe; if he can count on you, he will trust that he can count on himself and others.
4. Be actively and warmly responsive to your baby. It is important to note here that baby directs the majority of his attachment behaviors such as smiling, clinging, crying, and sucking toward you, his mother, hoping that you will respond to him in a warm and positive manner and be there when he needs or wants you.

Your baby's second crisis in Erikson's psychosocial model is *autonomy vs. shame and doubt,* which occurs from 12–18 months to three years. As your toddler develops and matures, she will start to strike out toward independence. Every baby has a singular goal in mind: freedom. It is at this stage of autonomy vs. shame and doubt that your toddler moves with urgency from the control of others to self-control. If she has successfully navigated her first crisis of basic trust vs. mistrust, she will now be entering her second psychosocial stage with a sense of trust in her own experience. Here, she becomes more self-aware and more self-reliant, valuing her own judgment above that of others, including you.

It's not surprising, therefore, that the virtue of this psychosocial state is *will*. When your child develops a wider range of skill sets, such as picking out special toys or putting on shoes and articles of clothing, he is illustrating his thirst for knowledge and independence. You may notice him moving away from you, resisting foods he doesn't like, or resisting people he is uncomfortable with. Here is where your toddler begins to investigate the range of his abilities, and thus it is important to create an environment that is both encouraging and noncritical. For example, rather than forcing a particular food to eat, or outfit to wear, or toy to play with, it is more productive to demonstrate patience and allow your child to try out new activities without help, all the while knowing when to step in and protect him from either danger or too much failure. It is a delicate dance to give your child the freedom to try things out for himself, not criticizing him if he fails, while helping him avoid constant failure. Potty-training is a perfect example of this delicate balance. Here, you're trying to teach self-control without injuring your child's sense of self. If you encourage and support your child through autonomy vs. shame and doubt, you will reinforce the virtue of his will, leading to the independence necessary to survive the outer world. What you're trying to develop in your child is good self-esteem; however, if he is either overprotected or not allowed to assert his independence, he will come up short, questioning his own ability to succeed, and will feel inadequate.

What is important about this stage is that a careful balance be struck between your child's striving for independence and accepting his boundaries. In this way, he will learn through trial and error when he is ready to be self-sufficient. This is where shame appears, amplifying the atmosphere that encourages your child to disown things he wants to do by learning the rules and following them. It is mother and other primary caretakers who must establish those rules, while being consistent in making sure they're followed. This period, called the Terrible Twos, is the first time your child attempts autonomy. Having felt out of control up until now, and dependent on others, your child, for the first time, is driven to control. In fact, your child's need for independence manifests itself when he resists authority. Therefore, his new sense of power and self-awareness translates to a form of negativism, and his favorite word during the Terrible Twos is *"no!"* But don't be disheartened, because at around 4–6 years of age, this drive for complete independence softens.

HOW PARENTS CAN INFLUENCE ERIKSON'S SECOND CRISIS STAGE OF AUTONOMY VS. SHAME AND DOUBT:[41]

1. It is imperative for you to be both clear and consistent when setting limits and consequences.
2. Concise language and consistency are most important now, so that you can gently guide your toddler away from unacceptable behavior. This will create the balance needed between autonomy, shame, and doubt.
3. You are trying help your child develop self-control, self-confidence, and competence.
4. It is best not to exacerbate your child's conflict, which could easily lead to his self-doubt. If self-doubt is not resolved in the psychosocial stage of development shame and doubt, it will automatically move into the next stage rather than being appropriately resolved.
5. On the other hand, if you create acceptable opportunities for your child to exert his independence, such as picking out an article of clothing to wear or choosing between one vegetable or another or one toy or another, he will have freedom within limits, experiencing the potency of success.

Your child's third crisis in Erikson's psychosocial model is *initiative vs. guilt,* which occurs from three to six years old. Your child is striving to balance her desire to follow her own goals with the moral dilemma that some of those goals may be unacceptable. At the core of the initiative vs. guilt stage are the opposing feelings of the self. The virtue therefore is *purpose*, as your child learns to regulate or balance her goals against her moral sense of right and wrong, which can prohibit her from acting on her own desires. Though your preschooler continues to push out, testing herself against her environment, wanting to add more and more to her repertoire, she is also being met by the need to receive approval from others. This is a time when your child asserts herself, a time of action that you may interpret as aggressive. Most important to the initiative vs. guilt stage is play, as it allows your child to use her interpersonal skills by planning activities such as games involving other children. Here is where your little leader is born, as your child develops the security and initiative to make decisions and direct others. Now is not the time to squash your child's independence by either too much control or disapproval. This could lead to an exaggerated sense of guilt, which could make your child feel less capable and more likely to depress her self-initiative and become a follower. Of course, it's important to protect your child from danger, as children can often push the envelope. However, if you overcriticize or constrict your child's initiatives, you will impair her sense of self. Also, at this stage your child will show a heightened state of inquisitiveness. So treat your child as you would a friend, showing respect for her thoughts while valuing her questions. Otherwise, your child will feel guilty or devalued, either feeling interfering with the healthy resolution of this stage. If your child feels guilty, it will negatively influence her social interactions and suppress her creativity. Though a little guilt is necessary for conscience and moral development, controlling your child too much can inhibit her natural unfoldment. Balance is the key to this stage of initiative and guilt, so that the virtue of purpose can develop.

The reconciliation of these two opposing interests, initiative and guilt, can create a split in your child's personality. On one hand is your child who is filled with joy and excitement to try out new things, and on the other hand is your child who is trying to understand what is and is not appropriate behavior. How your child balances or reconciles these two drives can lead to the virtue of purpose, which requires the necessary courage to strive for goals without the pressure of guilt.

As in all other stages, if this crisis of initiative vs. guilt is not resolved, your child will carry the unresolved conflict into the next stage of psychosocial development, causing him to race to succeed, brag, boast, bloviate, exhibit narrow-minded behavior, or experience psychosomatic illnesses.

HOW PARENTS CAN INFLUENCE ERIKSON'S THIRD CRISIS STAGE OF INITIATIVE VS. GUILT:[42]

1. At this stage, it is important that you create an environment in which your child can have the time and space to do things on his own, while still under your supervision.
2. Once again, freedom within limits is the best possible model for the development of balance between the need to over-compete and overachieve without feeling guilty.
3. Don't overcriticize your child's initiatives.
4. Respect, value, and validate your child's thoughts and questions.

Your Baby's Brain is concerned with children from birth to five years of age, though the chart at the beginning of this chapter includes all eight stages of Erikson's psychosocial development model for your perusal.

LAWRENCE KOHLBERG'S THEORY OF MORAL REASONING[43]

In the 1950s, American psychologist Lawrence Kohlberg created stages of moral development that were similar to Piaget's moral model, expanding on Piaget's ideas. Both Kohlberg and Piaget used a storytelling approach that incorporated stories with a moral crisis. At the end of the story, Kohlberg offered several solutions to the dilemma. The story that best describes the moral conflict that Kohlberg presented to his research participants was about a man named Heinz.

The theme of the story is that Heinz's wife was dying of cancer. There was a new drug available that could save her life. A local chemist created the drug, so Heinz went to the chemist and asked to buy the drug. The chemist, on the other hand, had just invented this new medication and wanted to make a large profit, so he raised the price of the drug to ten times higher than the cost to make it.

Unfortunately, Heinz did not have enough money to buy the drug. No matter what he did, even receiving help from his family and friends and finally raising half the money, he still couldn't meet the chemist's demand for payment. He told the chemist his story, asking for help, explaining that his wife was dying and offering various ways he could pay for the lifesaving drug.

Nevertheless, the chemist said no. He explained that he had created the drug and that this was his golden opportunity to make money. Heinz was bereaved, and exhausting all possible means for payment, he made the desperate decision to break into the drugstore and steal the lifesaving medicine.

After telling this story, Kohlberg asked ten questions similar to the ones below: [44]

1. Should Heinz have taken the drug without paying for it?
2. Would his behavior have been different if he didn't care for his wife so much?
3. Would it make a difference if it wasn't his wife that was dying but someone else?
4. And finally, if Heinz's wife died, should law enforcement arrest the chemist, charging him with murder?

The study included seventy-five boys, 10–16 years of age. Kohlberg continued this as a longitudinal study covering thirty years. The questions evolved around the idea of justice. By reviewing the children's answers for each question, relying on their different ages and stages of development, he discovered that the way children reason morally changes as they age. He concluded that children consider moral problems differently depending on their cognitive development, reaching a choice or moral decision independent and distinct from the adults or peer group in their orbit.

In his study, Kohlberg created a final sample of fifty-eight boys whom he reexamined in three-year segments for approximately twenty years. Each boy was interviewed independently and confronted by ten moral problems. Kohlberg wanted to understand the thought process of the sample population—not if the boys judged the behavior, but rather the thought process behind their conclusions. In the end, he established that the reasoning power of the sample population changed according to the boys' cognitive development.[45]

As a result, Kohlberg created three stages of moral reasoning, each stage separated into two parts. His theory was that moral reasoning progressed gradually from one stage to the next. As your child moves into a new stage of reasoning, that new stage replaces the reasoning of the level before it. Kohlberg believed that the last level of moral reasoning was for all practical purposes theoretical and rarely, if ever, reached. Moreover, he stated that it was his opinion that most adults are realistically operating at level two, which he called conventional morality. It is at this stage that a majority of Americans conform to social norms without question.

Stages of Moral Reasoning[46]		
Level and Age	Stage	What determines right and wrong?
Preconventional: Up to age 9	Punishment and Obedience	Right and wrong defined by what they get punished for. If you get corrected for stealing, then obviously stealing is wrong.
	Instrumental—Relativist	Similar, but right and wrong is now determined by what we are rewarded for, and by doing what others want. Any concern for others is motivated by selfishness.

Conventional: Most adolescents and adults	Interpersonal concordance	Being good is whatever pleases others. The child adopts a conformist attitude to morality. Right and wrong are determined by the majority.
	Law and order	To this end, we obey laws without question and show a respect for authority. Most adults do not progress past this stage.
Postconventional: 10 to 15% of the over-20s.	Social contract	Right and wrong now determined by personal values, although these can be overridden by democratically agreed laws. When laws infringe on our own sense of justice, we can choose to ignore them.
	Universal ethical principle	We now live in accordance with deeply held moral principles that are seen as more important than the laws of the land.

LEVEL I: PRECONVENTIONAL MORALITY

It is at this first level of moral reasoning that children are controlled by external rules. Your child from infancy to ten is too young to have developed his own moral compass—rather, his personal code is created by the rules and consequences established by the adults in his sphere of influence, especially you. These external controls are most often obeyed, not because of moral reasoning, but rather to escape punishment or gain rewards. Thus, the preconventional stage of morality is really one of self-interest, where your child has not yet found his own authority and reasoning is based on the authority of others. At this stage, your child understands right from wrong behavior in terms of rewards and punishments.[47]

Age: 0–9 years

Stage 1: Orientation toward Punishment and Obedience. "Will I be punished?" Your child will know the rules and follow the rules to escape punishment and possibly gain a reward. Further, she will disregard the reasons for a behavior and instead concentrate on the physical form. For example, the size of an infraction or consequence. Authority figures have the power in your child's life, and they should not only know the rules, but obey the rules to avoid punishment.

Your child believes if punishment is executed, something bad must have happened.[48]

Stage 2: Instrumental Purpose and Exchange. The basic idea of stage 2 is self-interest: if I do this for you, what will you do for me? Therefore, a behavior is deemed as good if it helps satisfy both your child's need and the need of another. The motto here could easily be value for value, or an even reward exchange. Behavior is seen in relation to what is needed, while separating out the value from the consequences. Your stage 2 child will say that there is more than one way to solve a problem and begin to appreciate that different people have different opinions.[49]

LEVEL II: CONVENTIONAL MORALITY (OR MORALITY OF CONVENTIONAL ROLE CONFORMITY)

At this level, your child internalizes the rules of those in authority. They are interested in pleasing others, being viewed as "good," and following social norms. Though it is hard to believe, this level is reached by ten years of age, and most people never go beyond this point.[50]

Age: 10–20 years

Stage 3: Maintaining Mutual Relations, Approval of Others, the Golden Rule. Your stage 3 child considers that if he follows the rules, she is entitled to a reward. At this stage, your child wants to please you and others, and by internalizing the rules while still observing the standards of adults, she begins to internalize those standards. It is at this time that she starts referring to herself as "good" to people she holds in high esteem. Now she can model authority figures and determine for herself whether behavior is right by her own personal code of morality. For the first time, she looks for a motive behind the behavior, as well as the person acting out. Thus, she considers not only the act, but also the circumstances behind it. Additionally, your stage 3 child is moved to respect social norms by following and obeying the established rules of authority.[51]

Stage 4: Conscience and Social Contract. Stage 4 respects the social order, considering a behavior wrong, irrespective of reasoning, if it breaches human rights and causes harm. According to Kohlberg, this is the pinnacle of moral development, and most people can never get there. In this stage, morality hinges on justice and the rights of others, while personal judgment is founded on personal principles, as well as individual reasoning. Kohlberg tells us that only 10–15 percent of people are able to operate on such a high moral level, as it requires a solid core that is based on critical thinking. However, because most humans are social learners, they find their moral ground linked to societal norms; to think independently, through the prism of ethics, is an amazing feat, requiring a giant leap into the possible human.[52]

LEVEL III: POSTCONVENTIONAL MORALITY (OR MORALITY OF AUTONOMOUS MORAL PRINCIPLES)

Level 3, according to Kohlberg, is as high a level as most people can reach. Moral reasoning is an internal affair, based on intrinsic beliefs of justice, fairness, right and wrong, and an overall moral code. At this stage, moral dilemmas can be resolved through moral standards.[53]

Age: 20 years and up

Stage 5: A Social Contract of Morality. Includes protections for the right of the individual through the mutual acceptance of democracy. Though society recognizes that the democratic will of the people serves the best interests of the people, there are still times when your needs and the law are in opposition. Then, the laws of the greater good and the laws of the individual are not always clearly defined, as for instance in the Heinz problem. Nevertheless, in the long run, it is best to know the rules and follow the rules of your community.[54]

Stage 6: The Universal Principles of Ethics and Morality. In stage 6, people listen to their own inner voice rather than being influenced by the opinions of others. Regardless of peer pressure, the constraints of others, or the laws of society, individuals in stage 6 follow their own authority. These individuals are self-actualized, acting in alignment with their own internalized moral code, and willing to take the consequences for their own actions, recognizing that if they violated their conscience, there would be an emotional cost.[55]

INFLUENCING YOUR CHILD'S MORAL DEVELOPMENT ACCORDING TO KOHLBERG'S SIX STAGES:[56]

1. Most important, be what you want to see. Children are social animals and they imitate social behaviors, especially yours.
2. Talk, talk, talk. From the moment your baby opens his eyes, his most valued experience is the sound of your voice. By talking to your child and referencing your thoughts about your experiences in relation to him, he will begin to catch a glimpse of the principles under the patterns of your values.
3. Invest your child in the development of his own moral compass by actively involving him in the small moral dilemmas of his daily life.
4. Be an active listener. As soon as your baby starts to talk, he will want to tell you about his world and how he stretches and tests himself against it.
5. Even in the nursery, children seem to demonstrate altruism. If one baby cries, another will follow. Observe your baby's sensitivity to the feelings of other infants and take every opportunity to model empathic behavior. In this way, little by little, you can build his central core and moral code.
6. Keep in mind that your young child will interpret and respond to moral dilemmas relative to her age and stage of development.

7. When building your child's moral reasoning and conscience, it is important to socially interact with her by talking about moral dilemmas throughout the day. Use story time for stories, myths, and fairytales, with a moral to the story, so that she starts to recognize and even anticipate how good prevails in the end.

8. Children show the greatest progress in moral development when their parents actively listen to their opinions and ask them child-centered questions. Ask your child clarifying questions so that you can be certain that he understands the issues at hand. Use humor and praise while talking to your child and actively listen to him when asking his opinions.

9. When modeling moral reasoning for your children, guide them to a higher level of thought, following a scaffolding approach.

10. Never lecture, challenge, or contradict your child's thoughts and opinions. Ask child-centered questions to help your child come to a conclusion that exposes him to a higher order of thinking.

11. Use every opportunity to pose a moral conflict, so that your child will have a chance to think about these questions during the course of a day.

12. Role-play with your child, raising moral dilemmas that the two of you can solve together.

13. Create a safe and understanding space so that your child knows that she can ask you anything without fear of retribution.

14. Use my empathic process to teach your child empathy, so she can learn what it feels like to walk in another person's shoes.

15. Make a game out of creating stories with your child involving moral dilemmas. In this way, your child can be the architect of the story, following the course of human conflict toward a positive resolution.

PIAGET'S FOUR STAGES OF COGNITIVE DEVELOPMENT

Intellectual development, the faculty by which young children acquire knowledge, was often addressed by Jean Piaget in his discussions about the development of children. Of Piaget's work, Friesen says:

> His work has had a dramatic effect on our understanding of the characteristics of children's thinking and their acquisition of knowledge. It is Piaget's work that has helped us understand how young children learn. Through his research, educators have come to realize the importance of providing appropriate experience matched to the developmental level of the child.[57]

Piaget (cited by Teale, 1982) argued that "the child builds up his knowledge through interaction with the world," and that "intellectual growth is a process of assimilating new experiences to the current state of the child's cognitive organization."[58] According to Piaget, "this is a process that requires an accommodation of existing mental structures, and that, in turn, stems from part of the mental organization, which allows for the intake and the assimilation of the new experience."[59]

Piaget (cited by Biehler and Snowman, 1986) was able to state broadly that cognition develops through the interaction of children with their environment. Piaget's stages of mental development:[60]

- In **Stage 1 (birth–age 2)**, infants are concerned with "sensorimotor" achievements—they use their senses to inspect the world and begin to see a distinction between themselves and other objects. They have no concept of "object permanence," meaning that when their mother or anyone else disappears from sight, the infant believes that person is gone forever.[61]
- **Stage 2 (ages 2–7)** is "preoperational." This is where children begin to acquire language, use mental images and symbols, and

understand simple rules. They see the world only from their perspective. For example, if they cover their faces and cannot see others, they still believe that means others cannot see them.[62]

- **Stage 3 (ages 7–11)** deals with "concrete operations." At this stage, children distinguish between fantasy and reality: they become more logical, less egocentric. They can concentrate and solve problems better and begin to understand the relationships between time, distance, and speed, as well as other rules that govern the world.[63]

- **Stage 4 (ages 11–adult)** is called "formal operations," which focuses on the child's growing ability to deal with abstract ideas, understand ethical principles, and reason about rules and regulations.[64]

As seen above, Piaget created a model to illustrate that thinking develops in this progressive movement through a series of stages and applied this paradigm to education. A specific educational model was constructed to differentiate what should be taught to children at various stages. For example, preschool, kindergarten, and primary grade children are all in the preoperational stage, while children in grades five to nine are in the transition from concrete operations to formal operations.[65]

Piaget was the founder of today's cognitive reformation, recognizing the significance of mental processes through his observation of children. By observing and questioning children, Piaget discovered a comprehensive theory of cognitive development. He believed that children had an inborn capacity to adjust to their surroundings, and it was that adaptation that was the beginning of cognitive development. In a sense, when a baby is rooting for his mother's breast, or investigating the perimeters of his environment, he creates an ever more precise understanding of his space, and a better capacity to relate to it.[66]

In Piaget's theory of cognitive development, he defined a sequence of qualitatively unique and distinctive steps. At each one of these steps, your child experiences a new way of thinking.[67]

From early childhood through adolescence, cognitive development evolves from sensory and motor behavior to critical, abstract thinking. These mental operations develop gradually, following three connective ideas:[68]

1. Organization
2. Adaptation
3. Equilibration

According to Piaget, *organization* is the ability to integrate more complicated cognitive systems of thinking that organize more effective views of reality. He called these organizations schemas, which are ordered patterns that your child uses to understand his environment. These schemas become more complex over time, and your child uses them to help him think and react. For instance, early schemas for viewing or touching act independently—ultimately, however, your child merges them into particular schemas so that he can see an object as he is holding on to it.[69]

Piaget states that *adaptation* is the way your child receives new stimuli that is in opposition to his current knowledge. It requires her to follow two approaches:[70]

- *Assimilation*, which involves receiving new data and integrating it into current cognitive constructs.
- *Accommodation*, which requires transferring cognitive constructs to incorporate new information.

Piaget states that *equilibration* is the propensity to continually reach for balance, demonstrated by the ebb and flow of assimilation to accommodation. All systems within your child strive for equilibrium between herself and her world. However, if your child cannot cope with new and unexpected events within her current cognitive construct, then those structures reorder themselves, creating new mental patterns that merge the new events and thereby create equilibrium. As a result, when assimilation and accommodation integrate, they create equilibrium and cognitive development. All behavior transactions operate in this manner. For example, when your child moves from the breast to a bottle, she adjusts her sucking techniques to confront the new experience. In this way, she is using assimilation and accommodation to customize her original schema.[71]

A modification of Piaget's original idea is that a child's cognition is not a single advancement to formal thinking, but rather is influenced by particular content; in other words, what your child is thinking in relation to a specific problem, in conjunction with a cultural norm.[72]

Piaget believed that cognitive growth was a process regulated by both a child's maturation and the interactive relationship with his surroundings. He was the first psychologist to examine cognitive development, and he created an observational protocol, and a series of tests, to study children's cognitive growth. He wasn't interested in measuring how well children could add or subtract, spell, or problem-solve, but rather in the way children developed fundamental ideas about quantity, justice, causality, time, and so on. He challenged the idea that children were less capable than grownups, considering the idea that children's thought processes were significantly different from their adult counterparts'. Also, he was mainly concerned with focusing on children's mental growth, rather than learning. Therefore, his approach was void of memorization and learning techniques. What he discovered was that the critical stages of development could be identified by their qualitative characteristics, instead of an increased complexity of behaviors. He examined the specific mechanisms by which a baby, toddler, and child grows into a person who can think, first concretely, and then abstractly. According to Piaget, when a child grows cognitively, she readjusts her mental processes in relation to both her maturation and the interactions with her environment. She structures a view of her surroundings and is soon confronted by inconsistencies between what she thinks she knows and what she discovers.[73]

PIAGET'S FOUR STAGES OF COGNITIVE DEVELOPMENT

I. SENSORIMOTOR:

The sensorimotor stage is Piaget's first stage of cognitive growth, and it includes children from birth to two years of age. It is during the sensorimotor stage that your child learns about his world through his motor activity and developing senses. It is during this period that you first observe your child's metamorphosis from an infant who can only respond through reflex and random activity to a goal-driven toddler. Piaget's research indicated that the sensorimotor stage contains six sub-stages, which progress into one another as your baby's schemas become more complicated. In the first five sub-stages, your infant organizes intake and activity from his senses and environment. In the sixth sub-stage, your child begins to advance through hit and miss, learning how to use ideas and symbols to navigate obstacles successfully.[74]

SENSORIMOTOR SUB-STAGES:

Sub-stage 1: Birth to 1 month

In sub-stage 1, cognitive growth occurs in a "circular action." Here, your baby learns to reproduce pleasing and gratifying experiences that first happen by chance. Consequently, the chance discovery is integrated into a schema, one that is both new and novel. Also in the first sub-stage, your child will work and stretch her reflexes until she achieves a sense of control. Only then will she initiate activity, even though the original stimulation for that behavior is absent. Sucking is a perfect example, as your baby will suck whatever her mouth touches, ultimately focusing on her sucking in particular when she wants something to eat and is offered Mother's breast or a bottle. Soon, she will learn how to adjust and adapt her behavior, becoming more efficient at fulfilling her own wants and needs.[75]

Sub-stage 2: 1–4 months

During sub-stage 1, your child learns to replicate satisfying experiences that were originally discovered by accident. Piaget identified this as a "primary circular reaction." Now your child will be able to turn toward and follow sounds by organizing distinct and diverse sensory input, such as sights and sounds.[76]

Sub-stage 3: 4–8 months
Your child begins to learn about objects in her environment by touching and observing them. For the first time, she repeats her behavior to produce a desired outcome. Piaget called this deliberate behavior a "secondary circular reaction." For instance, your child may smile and babble just to get and keep your attention.[77]

Sub-stage 4: 8–12 months
Piaget called the fourth sub-stage the "coordination of secondary schemas." It is at this stage that your child creates new schemas scaffolded onto her old ones. Now she can connect and form associations, reaching back into her prior experiences for the answers to her current dilemmas. She becomes highly creative as she organizes and changes past schemas to problem-solve. Correspondingly, this stage is the beginning of your child's deliberate and intentional activity.[78]

Sub-stage 5: 12–18 months
By the fifth sub-stage, your child will begin to investigate his surroundings, experimenting with different modalities of reciprocal actions. This stage finds your child curiously trying out, adapting, and adjusting to new ways of behavior. A great liberator of this stage is walking. When your child is ambulatory, he is free to explore. This, stated Piaget, is a "tertiary circular reaction." Now your child begins to try different solutions to new problems, no longer simply repeating accidental behaviors.[79] Your child will thrill and delight you as he displays original thinking for the first time. Also for the first time, your child can successfully navigate problems. Through hit and miss, he experiments, figuring out the best way to reach his objective.[80]

Sub-stage 6: 18 months–2 years

In the sixth sub-stage, identified by Piaget as "mental combination," your child shifts and moves into the preoperational stage. Her mental range increases, and now she can symbolically and mentally represent items and behaviors. By employing symbols like numbers, your child finds herself liberated from the need for immediate experience, and she can access "deferred imitation" through memory. Imagination takes center stage as your child uses mental representation from her memory so that she can think about her behavior before acting it out. She finally comprehends that one thing can cause another. Now she no longer needs to go through the arduous task of testing out all of her assumptions to find solutions. This is what Piaget called "representational ability."[81]

	Key Developments of the Sensorimotor Stage[82]	
Concept or Skill	**Piaget's View**	**More Recent Findings**
Object permanence	Develops gradually between third and sixth sub-stage. Infants in fourth sub-stage (8–12 months) make A, not-B error.	Infants as young as 3½ months (second sub-stage) seem to show object knowledge, though interpretation of findings is in dispute. A, not-B error may persist into second year or longer.
Spatial knowledge	Development of object concept and spatial knowledge is linked to self-locomotion and coordination of visual and motor information.	Research supports Piaget's timetable and relationship of spatial judgments to decline of egocentrism. Link to motor development is less clear.
Causality	Develops slowly between 4–6 months and 1 year, based on infant's discovery, first of effects of own actions and then of effects of outside forces.	Some evidence suggests early awareness of specific causal events in the physical world, but general understanding of causality may be slower to develop.
Number	Depends on use of symbols, which begins in sixth sub-stage (18–24 months).	Infants as young as 3 months seem to recognize perceptual categories.
Categorization	Depends on representational thinking, which develops during sixth sub-stage (18–24 months).	Infants as young as 3 months seem to recognize perceptual categories.

Imitation	Invisible imitation develops around 9 months, deferred imitation after development of mental representations in sixth sub-stage (18–24 months).	Controversial studies have found invisible imitation of facial expressions in newborns and deferred imitation as early as 6 weeks. Deferred imitation of complex activities seems to exist as early as 6 months.

Piaget included six key developments in his sensorimotor model:

1. **Object permanence** appears gradually between eight and twelve months. It can be observed between the third and sixth sub-stages, and according to Piaget, it occurs when your child realizes that something exists, either an object or a person, even when out of sight. Moreover, your child recognizes that she exists separate from others, including both objects and people. Piaget described a process called A, not-B error, a situation in which an 8–12-month-old child will continue to look for a hidden item in the location where she originally saw it, even though she saw the object moved to a different place.[83]

   By integrating visual and motor input and observing the outcome of his own behavior, your child gains information about space and objects. As soon as he is ambulatory and can crawl or walk, he can reach objects nearest to him and contrast the size, shapes, and locations relative to other objects. When he adapts and adjusts, he gradually becomes more efficient at judging the distance and size of objects in his path. Having already achieved object concepts, for which he now understands that objects and people exist when out of view, he no longer feels insecure or fearful if Mom or Dad is out of sight. Now he recognizes that they still exist and have not abandoned him. The game of peekaboo is highly significant at this stage of development because peekaboo serves to help baby confront and overcome anxiety when his mother is out of sight. Further, peekaboo allows baby to think about the appearance, disappearance, and existence of people and objects beyond his view. Consequently, it helps baby learn how to take turns, which transfers to the protocol necessary for conversation. Finally, peekaboo gives your baby a chance to practice and rehearse active attention, which is a skill for focus, concentration, and learning. Piaget calls this development object permanence.

Peekaboo also encourages cognitive development, for the game requires baby to anticipate the facial expressions and voice modulations of each player. This places baby on high alert as he waits, anticipating what lies ahead. By the time your baby is one year of age, he is no longer a passive observer, but rather initiates peekaboo himself, using physical and vocal cues to encourage others to come and play.

When playing peekaboo with baby, it is essential to use a scaffolding approach as baby reaches cognitive competency gradually. As a result, you can stimulate baby's task mastery building up her skill a little at a time, always motivating and prompting her to a more advanced stage of competence, coaxing her to interact at her most advanced level.

All manner of toys can be used as participants in the game of peekaboo, as Mother decides how much and what kind of scaffolding to use to support baby. Though at first you may need to gain your baby's attention, he will quickly become a part of the game, modeling your behavior until he integrates it as his own. At twelve months of age, baby becomes more receptive to verbal commands, and it therefore becomes easier to instruct him on the rules of the game by reinforcing his excitement and pleasure at predicting future experiences. By the time baby is two, scaffolding is no longer necessary, as he can not only imitate peekaboo, but also add his own creativity to the game.[84]

2. **Spatial knowledge** is linked to your baby's self-locomotion, the integration of his motor knowledge and visual sense. Here, baby can make judgments spatially, which appears to develop just as egocentrism dissipates.[85]

3. **Causality** evolves gradually, from around four months to one year of age. As baby uncovers the mystery of his own behavior and its effects on his physical world, he discovers the concept of causality, or cause and effect. This development is slow and steady, proceeding in direct coordination to baby's general awareness of the effects of his actions on outside events. Once your baby is able to grasp items, he becomes aware of his impact on his environment. This is really how causality evolves, as baby becomes conscious of his own intent. As your baby gathers knowledge about how things act, he is able to transfer the idea of causality to other circumstances and conditions.[86]

4. **Number,** according to Piaget, requires the facility of symbols. Therefore, number appears in the sixth sub-stage, 18–24 months. Though babies as early as five months can identify and even use small digits, there doesn't seem to be a true understanding of what the number symbols represent.[87]

5. **Categorization** is the fifth development. At about 18–24 months, your baby will begin to think in a representational manner. This means that she'll be able to see visual distinction. In fact, your two-day-old baby can already see the difference between a curved line and a straight line, being more partial to the curved line. Furthermore, she can recognize simple and complex patterns, being more partial to complex patterns. At this age, your baby can even recognize the difference between a two-dimensional and a three-dimensional object, favoring the three-dimensional object. She can also identify the difference between a picture of a face, as opposed to a picture of a thing, and identify the difference between what is familiar and what is new.[88]

6. **Invisible imitation**, according to Piaget, appears at approximately nine months, when baby can imitate parts of her body that are invisible to her. A little before this is the onset of visible imitation, when baby can imitate with her body those things that she can see before her, such as fingers and toes. Then, at approximately eighteen months, your baby begins to defer imitation, now able to imitate a physical behavior she remembers from her past. Overall, Piaget's research asserts that immature cognition gradually moves to mature cognition.[89]

Now, your baby attends more to new and different stimuli, rather than familiar stimuli. According to Piaget, this is called a "novelty preference." By eighteen months, your baby can contrast and compare new information to old, creating mental representations. Current information suggests, contrary to Piaget, that your baby may even be able to demonstrate a novelty preference at birth. This is most evident in the area of sound, where baby can distinguish his own mother's voice at one day old. Piaget explains deferred imitation "as reproduction of an observed behavior after the passage of time by calling up a stored symbol of it." Now, your baby can copy behavior without seeing it.[90]

Piaget perceived that information processing was founded on the principle of habituation, in which your baby's knowledge of something lessens his response. Whereas in dis-habituation, there is an acceleration in responsiveness to a new or novel stimulation.[91]

Studies can measure the efficacy of your child's information processing by noting how rapidly she can habituate to something familiar, as well as how quickly her focus shifts when given a new stimulus, in conjunction with the time in between, paying attention to both new and old information. The proficiency of habituation in conjunction with the ability to process information is often used as a predictor of cognitive development, as well as IQ. However, "predictions based on information-processing measures alone, do not take into account the influence of environmental factors. For example, maternal responsiveness in early infancy seems to play a part in the link between early attentional abilities and cognitive abilities later in childhood and even at age 18."[92]

Also, Piaget, stated "that the senses are unconnected at birth and are only gradually integrated though experience. If so, this integration begins very early." For instance, a baby might look toward sound, indicating that she connects the idea of hearing with seeing. Correspondingly, Piaget defines this integration, as a cross-modal transfer, meaning that now your baby is able to take knowledge from one sense, to lead her toward others.[93]

WHAT TO LOOK FOR IN THE SENSORIMOTOR STAGE

At this stage, your child will obtain self-awareness, comprehension, and knowledge through her sensory and motor experiences. First, your baby begins to investigate her body and sensory impressions. Once ambulatory, she will examine and manipulate everything within her reach. Then, through a method of trial and error, new schemas form, which help her develop cognitively so that she can understand her environment.

The most important advance in the sensorimotor period is object permanence. At this stage, your child recognizes that something exists regardless of whether it is visible or concealed, and that capacity necessitates a mental representation of the unseen object.

WHAT YOU CAN DO TO POSITIVELY AFFECT THE SENSORIMOTOR STAGE:

1. The most central concern of the sensorimotor stage is that your child is free to explore in a learning rich environment that is safe, secure, stimulating, and, most important, loving.
2. Be sure to create a safe environment that is also rich in objects to manipulate, textures to touch, and exciting and interesting visuals to observe.

3. As your little scientist extends out into his world to explore and expand his range of influence, it is important for him to know that you are nearby, within his frame of reference, and that he can look back and see that you're there with him to support his journey.

4. Bonding at this stage is everything. Thus, your baby will be free to explore his surroundings when he can depend and rely not only on your love, but also on your presence. In this way, he can build the security needed for positive attachment, and it is that secure attachment that will translate into trust. If he trusts you, he will trust himself, and if he trusts himself, he can trust his environment. This security will further stimulate his cognitive development, as he extends out each day into the unknown.

II. PREOPERATIONAL:[94]

Piaget's next stage of cognitive development is the preoperational stage, 2–7 years of age. In this stage, your child becomes more knowledgeable about symbolic thinking. However, she is still unable to think logically. Piaget tells us that only in concrete operations will your child be able to use logic, and that won't occur until middle childhood. Because she thinks egocentrically, preoccupied with herself and her world, your preoperational child will find it nearly impossible to see another's perspective or point of view. Yet thinking symbolically allows her to represent one word or item for another, so that she can transfer the symbolic meaning of one thing to something else. It is in the preoperational period that your child gains a more sophisticated understanding of numbers, identities, causality, categories, time, and space. Some of this more sophisticated and symbolic thought has its beginnings in infancy. Advances in preoperational thought continue from early toddlerhood through middle childhood.

PIAGET'S STAGES OF COGNITIVE DEVELOPMENT IN EARLY CHILDHOOD:[95]

Symbolic function: By the time your child is four years old, she can desire something without needing a sensory cue. For example, she may want a slice of birthday cake by retrieving its image from her memory, rather than experiencing it through her senses. Therefore, she can now ask for birthday cake based on her memory of its sweetness, rather than from any current sensory input. Piaget calls this mental process the "symbolic function," which reflects your child's capacity to use mental representations wedded to a meaning, without the use of sensory or motor cues.[96] Here, symbols assist your child's memory and help her to think about things that are not in her presence. The use of the symbolic function can be seen in deferred imitation, for example in imaginative play. Even infants use deferred imitation as they remember and recall the mental image of something they've seen. Likewise, when your child makes one thing represent another, for instance a toy for a friend, she is also using a mental representation. You can see this all through childhood as your child participates in symbolic play, using her imagination to have one object represent another. Even language is part of the system of mental representation, as words are symbols used to speak.

Understanding of identities: Piaget discovered that the understanding of identities is intrinsic to your child's developing sense of self. It is now that your child can view the world in a more organized and predictable manner. For example, with a more developed understanding of identities, your child can recognize that objects and people are similar, though they may be altered in size or shape. This knowledge leads to the emergence of your child's self-image.[97]

Spatial thinking: By the age of three, children have a more developed capacity for representational thinking, which allows them to make better decisions about spatial relations. Before the age of three, your child will have difficulty accurately discerning the connection between a model or a picture and the space or object that they depict.[98]

In conjunction with spatial thinking is the concept of dual representation hypothesis, which is the idea that your child cannot understand spatial relationships, as it requires her to maintain several mental representations simultaneously. But after the age of three, your preschooler will be able to not only understand easy maps, but also to transfer her spatial comprehension to other models or objects reciprocally.[99]

Causality: Though Piaget realized that toddlers comprehended the relationship between reactions and actions, he didn't believe that they could think logically. Rather, he asserted that they connected or linked a myriad of experiences with or without understanding the logic of cause and effect. He called this system "transduction." Children using transductive reasoning are not reasoning logically, but rather generalizing from one experience to another, often seeing a cause that isn't there.[100]

Categorization: Your four-year-old can now classify objects, people, and things by comparing and contrasting what makes them similar and what makes them different. To do this, he has to be able to identify both qualities. Most four-year-olds can recognize approximately two such criteria. The process of categorizing allows your child to create order out of chaos and, in a very positive way, organize small parts of his life. For example, he may identify someone as good, someone as bad, and so on. Here, the capability to categorize demonstrates cognitive growth, as well as emotional and social development.[101]

Animism: Until the age of four, children think that inanimate objects are alive: the sun, the moon, the clouds, and so on. But at about four, your child will begin to understand that while people are alive, toys are not. As a result, animism is the propensity to assign life to inanimate objects. Correspondingly, your child's culture and customs can influence

211

his tendency toward animism. For example, certain cultures may attribute qualities of life to inanimate objects, as they do historically in Japan. It is customary for a traditional Japanese garden, for instance, to have particular arrangements of rocks and sand that are often seen as animated: not only living, but also having emotions.[102]

Number: Between three and four years of age, your child will develop vocabulary for comparing and contrasting things, qualities, and quantities. She will compare and contrast size, saying that one thing is smaller than another, or complain that one ice cream cone is larger than another. If she has a piece of candy and you give her another piece, she knows that they have more candy than she had before. If she gives some of her stash of candy to another child, she realizes she has less candy. Further, though qualitative and quantitative information appears in all cultures, it unfolds at various speeds based on the relevance and style of counting in each society.[103]

In the East, five-year-olds have the ability to count to twenty or higher and also understand the difference between size and number amounts. By the time your Western child is five, she can add and subtract using single-digit numbers. Five-year-olds also seem to have an inner knowing or intuition that allows them to create a method for adding and subtracting, by using items such as buttons, stones, fingers, or toes. Then there are those children who simply intuit an answer without knowing how they got there. Once again, a particular culture and its numeral system play a part in how soon children begin to count. In the United States, children begin to count from one to ten at approximately three; in China, it's quite similar. In the US, a four- or five-year-old can count to twenty, while children in China use a more sophisticated system based on tens and ones. Therefore, the Chinese child surpasses the American child in counting by the age of five.[104]

According to Paplia et al. in *Human Development*, your toddler begins to understand five fundamental concepts of counting:[105]

1. The 1-to-1 principle: say only one number-name for each item being counted ("One . . . two . . . three . . .").
2. The stable-order principle: say number-names in a set order ("One, two, three . . ." rather than "Three, one, two . . .").
3. The order-irrelevance principle: start counting with any item, and the total count will be the same.
4. The cardinality principle: the last number-name used is the total number of items being counted. (If there are five items, the last number-name will be "5.")
5. The abstraction principles above apply to any kind of object. (Seven buttons are equal in number to seven birds.)

IMMATURE PREOPERATIONAL THOUGHT:

According to Piaget, *centration* is a limited approach to preoperational thought in which your child concentrates on only one part of an event while ignoring others. That limitation of focus often creates an illogical thought process. Because your three-year-old is engaging in an immature aspect of preoperational thought, he has difficulty decentering, or focusing on more than one aspect of an event simultaneously. This is why centration inhibits your child's thought process in relation to social and physical interactions. Piaget asserted that your child decenters when he can think about more than one part of an event simultaneously. As a result, centration occurs when your child cannot decenter and thus can only concentrate on one part of an event, ignoring the rest.[106]

CONSERVATION

Piaget stated that conservation is the understanding that two equal amounts or items, based on a particular measure, continue to stay equal even though there is a change in perception, such as an alteration in shape. The only criterion is that nothing is either subtracted or added to the item. Piaget discovered that preschool children did not understand this concept, and that it was only in concrete operations that other types of conservation developed. Piaget's most well-known study of conservation is the water conservation method, in which water of equal amounts is put in two different sized glasses, one tall and one short. The children are asked if the glasses contain the same amount of water, and inevitably the preschoolers will identify the taller glass as containing more water. When the investigator shows the children that he is pouring the exact same amount of water into the tall glass and the short glass, the preschoolers still maintain the idea that the taller glass holds more water. This is an example of your three-year-old focusing on one part of a situation while ignoring others, therefore thinking illogically. In a sense, your child is unable to recognize that an activity can be carried out in more than one way. The definition of "irreversibility," according to Piaget, is the inability to comprehend that an activity can be completed in several possible ways. Finally, Piaget explained that your preoperational child focuses on "successive states," unable to discern the shift from state to state.[107]

EGOCENTRISM

Piaget tells us that egocentrism is an aspect of the preoperational stage. He defined egocentrism as a form of centration in which your child is unable to take another person's perspective into consideration. Even though an infant is more egocentric than a toddler, both feel as if the world revolves around them. Piaget believed that egocentrism was one of the reasons why your child might have difficulty distinguishing fact from fiction and have little grasp on cause and effect. A perfect example of egocentricity is when a three-year-old believes that he is responsible for his parents' divorce.[108]

Piaget used a format called the "three-mountain task" to study egocentricity. In this experiment, Piaget sat a child at one end of a table and a doll at the other, while on the table he placed three large mounds. Then he asked the child his opinion on how he believed the doll viewed the three mounds. Though preschoolers were unable to give the right answer, they talked about the "mountains" from their point of view. This example demonstrates that a preoperational child is unable to see another's perspective.[109]

EMPATHY

Piaget felt that egocentrism inhibited empathy, which is the capability to put yourself in another person's place and understand their feelings. Yet there seems to be a natural inclination toward empathy. If your ten-month-old baby sees another baby crying, she may try to comfort the other child or start crying herself. By fourteen months, your baby will exhibit comforting behaviors such as hugging or patting a crying baby. By a year and a half, your toddler may offer a crying child her own toy for comfort, or ask you to help if the child is injured. Empathy can be seen all through early childhood development, increasing as your child grows. Ironically, empathy is one of the few things that can be taught, and it is one of the most significant deficits of a bully. However, empathy appears early on in a child whose family of origin discusses emotions and the cause and effect of actions and reactions. My empathic process is a wonderful way to teach empathy to your child and will enhance her self-esteem and expand her ability to get along with others.[110]

PIAGET'S THEORY OF MIND

In 1929, Piaget researched the theory of mind, in which he noted that children aged three to six became self-aware of their own thinking, as well as the thinking of others. He concluded that once the theory of mind emerged, it continued to grow all through early childhood, at which time children begin to recognize that when someone succeeds in fulfilling their desire, they are satisfied and even joyful, whereas when they fail, they may be unhappy and even teary-eyed.[111]

UNDERSTANDING THINKING

From three to five, your child will understand that thought is an interior behavior taking place within his head. Not only that, but he comprehends the difference between reality and imagination, cognizant of the fact that he can hold the thought of one thing while observing another. At this age, your young child is already mindful that if he shuts his eyes and covers his ears with his hands, he is still able to engage in thought about objects, people, and places. He may also assume that if a person is quiet, they are most likely thinking, recognizing that thought is different from sight, speech, touch, or knowledge.[112]

It is not until middle childhood that your child will understand that his mind is constantly thinking, whereas your preschooler views the mind as something that turns on and off. In essence, your preschooler is unaware of the part that language plays in thinking, unable to comprehend that he and others think in language.[113]

THE DIFFERENCE BETWEEN FANTASY AND REALITY

From eighteen months until three years of age, your child can participate in imaginative play, communicating to those around him that what he is actually doing is pretending. Nevertheless, there is a thin veil between what is imaginary and what is real, and there are those times where that veil is pierced, blurring the distinctions. Somewhere between four and six years of age, your child will exhibit magical thinking in an effort to understand situations that are not clear or easily explained. Then, there is just the fun of imaginative play in which imaginary friends such as Peter Pan and Tinkerbell and others participate. Interestingly, your child at this stage does in fact understand that he is using his imagination in creating his fantasy play, though leaving the door open to the potential reality of his experience. Your three-year-old can appreciate the concept of a "false belief," but when he cannot, it is often because of his egocentricity and inability to be "aware of mental representations."[114] At this age and stage, it is sometimes difficult to determine if he is pretending or being sincere, so once again, it is important to know your child.

DECEPTION AND INCORRECT BELIEF SYSTEMS

Your three-year-old child, according to Piaget, is still unable to distinguish fantasy from reality, because she still is in egocentric thought. By four or five years of age, your child can recognize that she and others can have fantastical thoughts and ideas. The reason she is able to understand this is that she realizes that some children use mental representations that are incorrect. While your three-year-old can't accept or appreciate that another child or adult thinks differently from the way she does, with different wants and needs, your four-year-old can. On the other hand, because your four-year-old is less egocentric and has a better grasp of mental representations, she is able to recognize and accept the opinions and belief systems of others. Furthermore, by the time your child is six, she will understand that different people can view similar events differently. Research indicates that children who have high social skills are more capable of identifying false reasoning.[115]

Since "deception" is the idea of putting an untrue idea into another's mind, it asks your child to repress what she knows to be true. Nevertheless, between the ages of two and five, your child will be able to participate in deception. The determining factor is the particular kind of deceit that your child is asked to perform. If it is a simple deception, a young child is more likely to succeed. Piaget asserted that your younger child is unable to differentiate between a deception and an error, thus considering that every mistake is a lie. Nonetheless, your three- to six-year-old is better able to recognize the difference between a mistake and a lie, understanding the part that intention plays in falsehoods. By the time your child is five or six, she appreciates the difference between reality and appearances, and now she can see the distinction between what is real and what is not.[116]

WHAT YOU CAN DO TO POSITIVELY AFFECT THE PREOPERATIONAL STAGE:[117]

1. When your child is 2–7 years of age, in Piaget's preoperational stage, it is important to talk and read continually. All that talking and all that reading keeps building up that associative mass, creating more and more synapses and more and more cognitive connections from which your child can draw.

2. Remember that even though your child is getting older, he still needs lots and lots of bonding, TLC, touch, and affection. By cuddling and holding, praising and supporting, you can validate your child's sense of self by letting him know you value him, accept him, and love him unconditionally.

3. By fostering your child's sense of self, you are building his strong inner core. It is that resource that will inoculate him against peer pressure and self-doubt. Now he has the confidence to venture beyond his comfort zone, reaching for that next discovery. This is how he will learn to problem-solve. By teaching your child that he doesn't have to be afraid to make mistakes, you are freeing him up to be his best possible self.

4. In Piaget's preoperational stage, a child should engage in play that is simply imaginative and creative. His environment should be safe and secure, overflowing with color and objects to be manipulated and observed. Since your child is developing the ranges of his representational thinking, it is important to interact with him in games such as peekaboo, hide and seek, hide the doll, etc., always stimulating his perception of the symbolic function, which allows him to imagine and think about people, situations, and things that are not actually present. This is the place for pretend play.

5. As your child is now thinking logically, beginning to understand the idea of cause and effect, games that stimulate his understanding will encourage his development.

6. Your preoperational child can categorize and classify things both living and not. He is beginning to understand the concept of counting and quantity, while learning to make more succinct judgments about spatial relationships. He spends a lot of time in his imagination, playing along with his animism, which thrills and delights him. However, he still has the inability to decenter and doesn't understand conservation limited by

the idea of irreversibility. Introducing objects and games and interactions that enhance his understanding of conservation will further his development.

7. He is definitely in an egocentric place yet has the ability to be empathic. By using my empathic process at this stage, you can actually teach your child empathy. Model empathy for him in the course of your normal day. Also, tell stories and role-play situations that call for empathy. Finally, use my empathic process to invest your child in the real-life experience of empathy.

8. Between the ages of three and five, your child's theory of mind increases so that he becomes cognizant of his own thinking, separating himself from his oneness with Mother and capable of recognizing the difference between what is real and what is fantasy, what is false and what is true. It is at this stage that your child understands the difference between appearance and deception, so that imaginary games that encourage his fantastical play are joyfully received.

9. Discovery learning is most important at this stage. It involves guiding your child to actively explore and discover things for himself. Because discovery learning is not without structure, it is critical to fill your child's environment with those things of interest and stimulation that are necessary for his advancement. This is true individual learning. There should also be a focus at this time on play as it corresponds to learning. Learning by discovery, according to Piaget, unfolds naturally in accordance with your child's biological maturation. Once again, we see the importance of readiness, which includes appropriate stages, concepts, and information. For that reason, concentrate on the process of learning rather than the outcome. Create situations that confront your child with age-appropriate solvable problems. Organize collaborative as well as individual activities

that are age-appropriate so that your child can invite a friend
and they can stimulate, encourage, motivate, inspire, and learn
from each other. Finally, incorporate active methods, as they
involve the reconstruction and rediscovery of each problem's
solution.[118]

III. CONCRETE:[119]

Your seven-to-twelve-year-old child is in concrete operations. In this
stage, your child will be less egocentric, better able to think logically, and
have a better grasp on spatial relationships, recognizing cause and effect.
It is in this stage of concrete operations that your child will be able to categorize, make inferences, and display deductive and inductive reasoning.
She will also have an understanding of seriation, transitive inference, and
class inclusion. Only now can she use numbers efficiently and recognize
conservation; she is still, however, in concrete thinking, which creates a
horizontal décalage, leaving her logic, most obviously, in the present.
Piaget states that moral growth is connected in a very real way to cognitive maturation; this he says happens in two steps: morality of constraint,
which you can find in the preoperational stage, and morality of cooperation, which parallels concrete and formal operations. Furthermore, it
appears that your child's social interactions effect her rate of growth, in
concrete operations.

Here, though your child is thinking in symbols, he is still organized
around the construct of concrete thought and actions. Now, less egocentric, he can see another person's point of view. He is also more logical and
uses language more effectively, specifically to solve problems. For the first
time, reality and fantasy become distinct and autonomous. Accordingly,
reading opens your child to new ideas, thoughts, situations, and coping skills. By the time your child goes to school, he will be exposed to
new rules, and models for cooperation. Subsequently, he will establish
new relationships, friends, and cliques that begin at first with informal
rules and regulations but evolve into a hierarchy of more clearly defined

guidelines. As he gets older, this hierarchy gets tighter, and it influences music, clothing choices, behavior, and a sense of personal belonging. It is here that your child learns about matching his needs with those of others. And now you will see your child develop either a sense of industry and self-confidence or inferiority.

This concrete period is the turning point in your child's cognitive growth, for now she can think logically, with operational thought. She can problem-solve in her mind, and try things out in the physical world. More than that, now, she can conserve numbers, weight, and mass, while recognizing that quantity is identical though it changes appearance.

WHAT YOU CAN DO TO POSITIVELY AFFECT THE CONCRETE OPERATIONS STAGE:

1. First and foremost, your child needs a lot of bonding and encouragement during the ups and downs of concrete operations. By advocating your child, and letting him know that you are there for him no matter what, you will help him adjust to the changes of his physical, cognitive, and emotional world, which are all happening simultaneously.

2. You are his true North, the one person who can help him stabilize through this period of growth and change. At this stage, your child needs a lot of structure, scaffolding, support, and consistent discipline so that he can mature in a secure manner, adjusting to the day-to-day challenges with a positive sense of self.

3. The idea of readiness for learning is particularly important at this period, as it relates to what information should be taught, and when. Piaget tells us that your child should not be given particular learning constructs until he is learning ready and he has reached the appropriate age for each cognitive stage.

4. In a sense, your child is now an active learner, as he enters a period of discovery learning.

5. All learning at this point should be child centered, and discovery learning. Consequently, you become a facilitator, encouraging your child, helping him focus, discover, and construct ideas.

6. Your child can now learn both collaboratively and independently, so make learning fun by inviting other children for a play date and creating experiences that your child can master.

7. Construct events that contain problems that make your child think. By creating such disequilibrium, your child will seek balance and try to find a solution.

8. Observe your child so that you can know what stage he's in, so that you can create learning models that are age-, and stage-, appropriate.

IV. FORMAL:[120]

According to Piaget, your child enters formal operations at about 11 years of age and will stay in formal operations for the rest of his life. It is in this period that he will learn about abstract and critical thinking. Further, he will primarily test everyday hypothesis using logical concepts. Gradually, his grasp on abstract thought will increase and transfer to his understanding of morality, ethical principles, and justice. His firm grasp of logic allows him to think about rules and regulations. He can seek balance in problem-solving by using his facility of logic and reason and consequently develop a strong sense of self and a desire for independence. By 11 years of age, your child starts to experience self-reflection, thinking about who he is and his place in the world. His relationships shift in concert with his interests and social experiences; hence, now, he moves away from single-sex relationships and forms coed, as well as opposite-sex friendships.

WHAT YOU CAN DO TO POSITIVELY AFFECT THE FORMAL OPERATIONS STAGE:[121]

1. Education proceeds gradually and cumulatively, so it's important that you influence your child's learning by getting involved in her life. That requires you to participate in her schooling, encourage her advancement, and transfer positive reinforcement in conjunction with learning.

2. Become an active listener so that your child knows that you care about what she does. By paying attention and hearing what she has to say, you will validate her thoughts, and feelings.

3. When your teenager realizes that you care about her contributions, she will be more willing to share other information with you.

4. Your preadolescent and teenage child, above all else, needs your acceptance and love. She is particularly self-conscious and embarrasses easily. Thus, by expressing your respect for who she is, and what she does, you will encourage her to value and respect herself. Similar to the huge transition from 0 to 2, in which talking increased the synaptic connections, your preadolescent and teenage child also needs those open lines of communication. Thus, once again, you as a parent are called upon to talk, talk, talk. Freud called this period "Storm and Stress," and Aristotle, the age of insanity. We all can remember the highs and lows of hormonal changes that your child is experiencing, as she transforms from a child into an adult. Talk to your child about her changing biology and explain to her what is going on in her body, and why. By showing your teenager that you understand the biology and psychology of what she's going through, and that you respect her developing maturity, you will help her stabilize through her enormous physical, mental, and emotional changes.

No two children navigate Piaget's four cognitive stages at the same rate of speed, and that is because each child's biological maturation is unique unto himself. It is the combination of his biological maturation and his relationship with his environment that will foster his cognitive growth. And though the sequence of Piaget's four stages of cognitive development are similar for all children, each child still progresses at his own rate of speed.

PART TWO

6

TURN YOUR HOME INTO A LIVING LAB—EXERCISES AND MUSIC TO SUPPORT COGNITIVE AND EMOTIONAL GROWTH

Your child's brain is wired for discovery. A securely bonded child will explore his environment and test its limitations. To facilitate the most growth possible, you have to make sure that the environment will stimulate emotional and intellectual development. As you throw more children into the mix, it becomes increasingly important that you understand how to create an environment that caters to and fosters the right kind of growth for each child. From creating a print-rich environment to setting safe boundaries, I'll teach you how to create a home dynamic that allows your tiny explorer's natural curiosity and advances his higher-level cognitive and emotional development.

THE GIFT OF MEDITATION[1]

I began meditating not for any spiritual or religious reason, but rather to help my children become better students. I was a school teacher and therefore well aware that many very bright children were unable to get their act together and tap into the complete range of their abilities. One day after school, I came home to find a women's magazine that had been mailed to me as an advertising promotion. On the cover, in bold type, was a headline that stated that meditation increased concentration. I curiously began to

227

read. The article immediately grabbed my attention by stating that children could learn to focus and concentrate more effectively if they could just learn to meditate. I was hooked. I read the article from beginning to end and then followed the directions given for meditation. It was easy, and I learned it immediately. It was the most natural thing I ever did, because it focused on breathing, the one thing I knew how to do without instruction. As the days went by, I found that I looked forward to the few minutes each day when I entered a state of complete calm and quiet. Pretty soon, I noticed that I was receiving benefits just from those few minutes each day I spent in that peaceful space.

After putting my children to sleep at night, I would set my own alarm for twenty minutes, the time allotted in the magazine for each meditation session. By setting an alarm, I didn't think about the time and was freed up to just be. The article also gave a nonsense syllable to repeat as a mantra. The word they gave was *Nadam*. Though they described this word as a nonsense syllable, a word that was tonal and without meaning, I later learned that it was actually an early Hebrew name of God. Via the suggestion of the article, I played classical music, turned off the light, and sat down at the foot of my bed to meditate. I created my own practice, doing two twenty-minute segments each day, one in the early morning before I woke my children for school and the other after I put them to bed at night. Since I had no preconceived idea of what meditation could achieve, I just surrendered to the process, opening to the gentle flow of my breath with a beginner's mind. Soon, I noticed that I was not easily ruffled by outer events, and that fewer things seemed to bother me than ever before. What I didn't know was that my body and mind had entered into the alpha state of total relaxation, which caused my endorphins to elevate. This feeling of contentment spurred me on to continue meditating for twenty minutes twice a day.

What I later learned was that meditation can take you quickly into REM sleep, which is deep and renewing. Because half an hour of meditation equals approximately four hours of sleep, in only twenty minutes twice a day, I was gaining those residual benefits.

Soon, my mind and body worked so well together that friends and colleagues began to notice. Once, when I was competing in a tennis tournament, my competitor jumped the net and asked me if I was taking tranquilizers, which of course I was not. She just couldn't get over how calm and focused I was. I was never more than a B tennis player, but I did win that particular match. This natural state of ease continued for the rest of my life, often giving me the sense that I was walking through the day on a soft cloud. Though it seemed strange, I really did experience a state that is commonly referred to as being in the *tau*, or in the "the flow." No matter what I was doing—writing, reading, teaching, loving, parenting, or participating in sports—I felt cool, calm, and connected.

I continued my meditation practice for a month before I actually began teaching it to my children, recognizing that I needed to experience meditation before I could transfer the practice. One of my favorite stories about Gandhi illustrates this very idea:

There was once a poor woman in India whose son contracted diabetes. Though he was told that eating sugar was dangerous to his health, he continued to do so. And no matter what his mother did, she could not convince him to give up sweets. She had heard of the great master Gandhi, and wondered if he could help her child to stop eating sugar. Though she lived far from Gandhi, she used all of her money to travel for several weeks, until she finally arrived at Gandhi's door. Receiving an audience with the Mahatma, the woman immediately explained her fear that her diabetic child would die if he didn't give up sugar. Certain that Gandhi would help her, the woman asked if he would just command her son to stop. However, Gandhi looked in her eyes and in a commanding voice told her to return to him in three weeks. The woman couldn't believe it. She thought, "Three weeks, it took me almost that long to get here. I've used up all of my money, and my son is quite ill. Not only that, but he'll continue eating sweets until I return." She begged Gandhi to change his mind, but he did not. She followed his instructions to the letter, returning home with her son, only to repeat her trip three weeks later. Now, Gandhi looked at the boy in the eyes, and in a commanding voice said, "Stop eating sugar now!" The mother was shocked. "Stop eating sugar now? That's it?! That's what we had to make a three-week trip for, back, and forth, over land and sea, to have you say, 'Stop eating sugar now'?" And Gandhi replied, "Yes, madam, because when you were here three weeks ago, I was still eating sugar, so how could I tell your child to stop? But, in the three weeks that you were gone, I myself stopped eating sugar, and now I have the authority to tell him to stop."

This is one of my favorite stories, because it demonstrates what is central to parenting: be what you want to see. With that in mind, I felt I had to learn meditation before I could teach it.

Within a very short period of time, I was on the way to becoming a meditator, reinforced by the subtle and positive changes I experienced in myself. After several weeks, I decided that I knew enough to be able to teach my children, convinced that it could be a successful tool to help my young children focus, concentrate, and experience a natural love for learning.

First, we did a little stretching to help them settle down—before you can calm the mind, you have to quiet the body. Next, I put them both on the bed with me and just told them to feel their breath as they breathed through their noses, pointing out that the breath they breathed in was cool, and felt cool around their nostrils, while the breath they breathed out was warm, and felt warm around their nostrils. In this way, I engaged not only their rhythmic breathing, but also their senses of cool and warm. Pretty soon they were really into it, and each day, for just a few minutes a day, we sat on my bed breathing in and out, following an easy rhythm. This was all the more important because it was something we were doing together, something that they got to do with Mommy, and it was fun.

Once they were in the groove of focusing on their breath, I added a tonal mantra, which is basically a nonsense syllable that you can't attach any meaning to, so that it doesn't trouble the mind and can function as a benign point of focus. I gave them the same mantra I was using, *Nadam*, first saying it out loud, and then asking them to close their eyes and listen to it internally. I enlisted my older daughter, Dawn, who was seven at the time, to help her younger brother, Shawn, age four, to cut down on the giggling and silliness. By incorporating them into the process and giving them both a role to play, they became invested in the successful outcome of meditating. As a result, they rose to the occasion, especially because they were doing something so grown-up.

During the first month, we only meditated for five minutes. As their proficiency increased, I extended the time to ten minutes, twice a day. We would meditate at 4:00 p.m. when they came home from school, and at night after their prayers. That was our routine—and Shawn and Dawn loved it. When you teach anything new to a child, it is important to break it up into digestible bites, so when teaching meditation, pay attention to your child's ability to be still and concentrate, keeping in mind that all instruction must be age-appropriate. Only after your child has grasped the new concept can you extend the time accordingly.

The benefits of meditation were hard to miss. Not only did this mutual experience feel both bonding and intimate, it exposed my interest to my children, so that they felt that they were sharing in my life. Meditation by itself automatically slows you down—in fact, a meditator can always recognize another meditator by the calm and ease of his breath, conversation, and comportment. Yet people often resist the idea of quieting themselves so that they can experience what Aristotle called the inner journey. Perhaps because surrendering to the process of stillness can resurrect inner demons and insecurities. However, what is actually residing in your unconscious or inner psyche is the peaceful you. Thus, as you confront the demons at the gate, they dissipate, as all bullies do. And, for what seems like timeless time, you touch your inner resource, the you that you were meant to be. This is actually your destiny, to be able to quiet yourself so that you can hear your inner voice, the real you. And according to Carl Jung, that natural self is always better than the defended person you become when socialized.

From early childhood on, we begin to disown important parts of ourselves, and like an onion, we become layered by our defenses. But once you peel that onion, layer by layer through meditation, the individuated self comes forward, strengthened by the return of the creative energy that you've used up by suppressing your disowned material. Jung called this disowned material the shadow, stating that the shadow was neither evil nor bad, just unknown to you. It is in the shadow where all the fertility for your life resides. Therefore, once you recognize, integrate, and embrace it, you are complete, enlarged creatively, as your libido and vitality return.

In time, each of my children began to exhibit especially positive and empathic behavior. I remember in particular when Shawn was in the first grade and another child was being bullied because he was Jewish. Shawn stepped forward and protected the little boy, reminding the children that they were his friends, though he too was Jewish. Because Shawn was well liked, athletic, big for his age, and successful at school, he was able to influence the other children, causing them to feel empathy.

My favorite story about my daughter, Dawn, occurred when she was thirteen. Girls this age typically have a lot of birthday slumber parties, and Dawn's school chum was no exception. However, one of Dawn's other friends was left off the list. Dawn felt so sorry for her that she decided to stay home and invite her to a pizza sleepover at our house instead. I can remember this experience as if it were yesterday, because when Dawn gave up her place at her friend's birthday party, one invitation became available. Believe it or not, the girl that Dawn stayed home for accepted the invitation, leaving Dawn home alone. I said to Dawn, "I don't think this girl is really your friend, as she clearly doesn't share your values." Dawn quickly responded, "Mom, my friend has many nice qualities in her character, this is just one of the negative ones." Dawn was naturally empathetic, compassionate, and kind and always looked at the big picture, rather than getting caught up in the petty minutiae that teens and adults often experience in relationships.

Meditation had begun to play a larger part in my own life. I was very interested in the way it seemed to affect everything. I noticed that I was more optimistic than most and that the little things that seemed to bother my friends didn't faze me. Moreover, when I returned to school later in life, I not only learned material faster, but retained it better. Consequently, I began to examine the impact that meditation was having on my life, paying attention to the outer edges of my experiences.

Little by little, I realized that I was changing. Here I was, a working mother with a husband and two children, a condition that many today would consider stressful. Yet I seemed to navigate my life with ease. Having always had somewhat of a visual memory, my husband pointed out that my eidetic memory had increased. Somehow, I had stepped into a space where each day I felt self-contained, open, and happy. In the bath one evening, I cast a glance at my toes, bent out of shape from years of wearing high heels. As if seeing them for the first time, I felt moved with compassion and empathy for my poor little toes. I felt more loving with myself and others as I routinely and consciously quieted my inner critic. I realized that meditation had awakened me to my own inner resource and, by piercing the veil within, had released my inner light.

On my forty-second birthday, I went to Bangalore, India, to meet with the Dalai Lama. He was the keynote speaker at a mind-science summit there, titled "Science and Spirituality for the 21st Century," also attended by doctors, scientists, lamas, and monks. I had a private audience with the Dalai Lama on my birthday, but in fact it wasn't very private: there were many people there, and each of us filed in front of him for approximately one second. I felt that I couldn't get a chance to really talk to him and ask him the questions that I had prepared. The week that followed was filled with lectures and speeches on the power of meditation and its impact on science and medicine. I did have a second encounter with His Holiness the Dalai Lama at the end of the week, and when I returned to Houston, a friend asked if I would host the Dalai Lama's physician, who was coming to Houston to teach. He had been in seclusion in India for seven years, and this was his first reentry appearance. In his entourage were monks from Tibet, California, and Houston, one of whom became my teacher and was affectionately called Geshelah. During that visit, Geshelah asked if I would host the Dalai Lama when he came to Houston in 1991. Another synchronistic moment in which I fervently said *yes!* Soon after that, our daughter, Dawn, died at the age of twenty-four of cardiomyopathy with fibrosis. And on the one-year anniversary of her death, April 12, 1991, the Dalai Lama arrived in my home with twelve of his monks.

As he walked through my garden, the Dalai Lama told me about the death of his own brother from hepatitis. He said that even though he was the Dalai Lama, and knew there was no death, he missed his brother. We spent time meditating and talking, both sharing our stories. I experienced in a visceral way how meditation connects people in the soft space of understanding, a space that most people never allow themselves to feel. When you open to another's heart, pain, and suffering, you meet them at the edge of their feelings, and it takes you to a place of knowing. And, though I have studied with many teachers since, I still consider His Holiness the Dalai Lama as one of my primary teachers.

I hope that sharing my own personal meditation journey will alleviate some of the anxiety and resistance often accompanying new ideas. Reducing stress affects everything in your life, as you learn to walk more lightly through your world. In fact, I credit my ability to meditate with my being able to survive the death of my daughter, twenty-nine years ago. For it was there, in that open space, that I could find relief from the excruciating pain of loss. I often say that if I were on my deathbed, and a friend was nice enough to visit me, I would tell him or her that the only whisper of wisdom that I could leave as my legacy would be the word *meditation*. Even my late mother learned to meditate in her early nineties, which helped her adjust to the changes of her time of life.

Stress-reduction techniques, including massage and breathing exercises, are beneficial for your child at every age and stage of development. If you can help your child relax, he will perceive everything differently, his circulation will be better, and he'll think more clearly. When you teach your child how to release his stress, everything is better: the colors and light around him, the sights and sounds, all become more vivid and intense. Moreover, when your child is old enough to learn how to meditate, he will also learn self-discipline. For the very act of meditating requires your child to sit still and harness his mind, keeping it from wandering and bringing it back when it does through simple breathing techniques. This is the very process your child goes through as he matures, but now it's more pleasurable because it's self-directed. Therefore, when your child learns consciously how to put himself in a relaxed state, he will lower his cortisol and increase his endorphins. Not only is this a pleasurable experience, but it also teaches your child how to unlock his possibilities. Your child will be not only smarter, but also calmer.

All these relaxation techniques, including yoga, qigong, and creative visualization, can be learned at any time and in any circumstance. It is never too late, and whether you've meditated all of your life or for two months, the effects are the same. For example, a seven-year study at MIT indicated that people who had never meditated before but were taught meditation over a two-month period received the same benefits and abilities as the lamas and monks who had meditated since childhood.[2] And, as previously discussed and as noted in this study, Baroque music can also put the mind and body in a similar meditative state and as a result can accelerate learning. All of these behaviors build on themselves and over time can be used in combination to enhance focus and concentration as well as relaxation.

QIGONG[3]

A number of years ago, I completed a one-year pilot study in the Houston Independent School District, studying stress-reduction techniques and their effects on children's math, science, reading, bullying, and so forth. I created a video in which I taught children how to do qigong before we moved to meditation, followed by a guided conversation, so that children could unburden themselves from their problems before beginning to study. Choosing qigong was easy, as it is extremely powerful in its simplicity. In a sense, it is the root of all martial arts, including karate, tai chi, and so on. What is unique about qigong is its ability to unblock stress in the body by focusing on pressure points and meridians so that the practitioner relaxes almost immediately, opening more easily to meditation. Qigong is the teaching of carefully and skillfully unblocking the energy in the body, gathering it up for use in mental and physical health and healing. Qigong is an integrative practice of breathing, mental focus, and physical exercise.

Qigong can be used by all ages, primarily enhancing and storing energy. It is often used as a daily, or twice daily, technique, and it may be prescribed as a complementary approach to medicine. What is both exceptional and different about qigong is its adherence to the meridian structure.

Qigong is also set apart from other exercise methods by its physical properties, breathing techniques, and focused attention. Qigong is also essential for unblocking and circulating energy. This helps to lower stress, improving immunities, digestion, heart health, and the lymphatic system—accelerating recovery from illness by stimulating vitality. For those who practice qigong regularly, it increases a state of awareness and mindfulness, which consequently intensifies other states of consciousness. Finally, these mindfulness practices positively influence the properties of exercise while enhancing your total experience.

Qigong has the capacity not only to help emotional balance, but also to stimulate physical balance in children and senior citizens, in particular. Harmonizing the mind and the body by effectively balancing the meridians of both, qigong integrates the mind, body, and spirit. Qigong creates a positive atmosphere of wholeness and well-being, allowing you and your child to confront the negative self-talk that is so prevalent when these systems are unstable, or out of balance, by uniting or integrating your inner and outer life. This is wholeness.

There are many postures in qigong. Some supporting internal needs, and some external, all leading the practitioner to an ever more balanced, happy, and vital life.

I have practiced qigong for twenty-five years, and it is the approach that I use, in conjunction with meditation, as part of my daily practice.

YOGA[4]

Yoga can also be used as a prelude to meditation, and, as in qigong, young children can learn it rapidly. The word *yoga* comes from the Indian word for union, to yoke or to integrate, and the movements allow your child to redirect her frenetic energy. Soon your child will discover that the yoga postures demand focus and concentration, leading to a relaxed state of being. In fact, certain kinds of walking meditation fall under the spectrum of yoga. And when your child becomes more proficient at yoga, her poses will resemble meditation. Athletes call this state "being in the zone." When your child enters the zone on her own, she can learn anything with ease.

Three-fourths of the world practice some form of stress-reduction technique, and today yoga has become mainstream. Yoga uses not only postures and poses, but also breathing to balance the dual forces of mind and body. There are many forms of yoga, including Ashtanga (a high-energy, high-heat power yoga), Tantra (which include practices that awaken the kundalini life force within the body), and dozens more. Listed below you will find a primer for the various types of yoga, so that you can select the appropriate form for your child's age and stage.

Hatha yoga is the most popular in the United States because it includes all the positions. It is a general yoga that translated means "complementary forces"—or the balance between the sun and the moon. There are one thousand postures, called *asanas*, in hatha yoga, and many of these postures are based on the physical behaviors of jungle animals, especially from the cat species. Thus, hatha yoga is a favorite among children, and my personal favorite, as not only is it fun to imitate animal postures, but the results of relaxation and stress reduction are immediate. Most of the movements described in this book are taken from hatha yoga.

HOW YOGA BENEFITS THE MIND AND THE BODY[5]

The wonderful thing about yoga and its influence on both the mind and the body is that its benefits can be transferred to other areas of your child's life. For example, by simply controlling his breath, your child will have a feeling of peace and calm. Another advantage is that the postures themselves tone all the muscle groups while increasing strength and stamina. Beginning her day with yoga literally stretches your child's sense of well-being, affecting all of her interactions.

When the body and the mind work together in a harmonious fashion, your child's brain is used in concert. In a sense, as his body becomes limber, so does his mind. Though education in the West focuses on the mind in particular, the best possible approach is to integrate the mind and body. After all, your child's head is attached to his neck, and what affects one affects the other. Therefore, when the body and the mind are exercised together, he can concentrate his energy in a thoughtful and skillful way.

The first step in teaching yoga is the same as teaching all other relaxation techniques: the measured and focused attention to the breath. Because breathing is necessary and natural to our existence, we all know how to do that. If you lie on your back on the floor, you'll notice that you're not breathing from your chest, but rather from your diaphragm. This is the same way that your baby automatically breathes at birth. Asking your child to watch his tummy move up and down as he breathes in and out is the first concentrated effort at yoga. Asking him to feel the cool air as he breathes in and the warm air as he breathes out will direct your child's attention not only to his breathing, but also to the sense of the warmth and coolness against his nostrils.

Though breathing is taken for granted, by learning to control her breath in yoga, your child will soon realize that the rhythm and pace of her breathing will also affect her state of mind, her mood, her focus, and her health in general. In this way, your child gains control over something essential using the technique of breathing as a tool to help her manage her own stress and relax. Slowing down her breath, your child will train herself to deal with any difficult situation, including bullying. Moreover, by delaying reactive behavior through breath control, your child is also maturing. The more she practices controlling her breath in relation to the needs of her experiences, the more she will develop the strength of her own authority. Like the wise old turtle who carries the world upon his shell, keeping it steady and stable, your child will also be able to stay calm in the midst of chaos through the slow and balanced control of her breath.

Luckily, yoga is not a competitive sport, and anyone can follow it. In that respect, you don't even have to be flexible or well coordinated, for each person practices the postures in his own way and at his own pace. Yoga in particular discourages comparisons between children, asking them to take time in rather than time out. By calming the breath and learning how to use it to manage stress, your child will feel a confidence and a sense of knowing that will guide him toward more patience and less negative talk as he gains control over himself by confronting his inner critic. Then, yoga becomes the great collaboration between your child and himself.

YOGA'S POSITIVE EDUCATIONAL BENEFITS[6]

Yoga allows children to be in the present. It reinforces the idea of paying attention to the here and now. Whether in a classroom or any other educational setting, yoga teaches your child how to focus and concentrate. Consequently, he can learn not only with greater speed, but also naturally and with ease. The skill of yoga is that it teaches self-discipline, and self-discipline offers your child a feeling of self-control. Ultimately, that self-control transfers to an assured sense of self and positive self-regard. Anything learned in the early stages of life is integrated into the psyche and can be easily incorporated into your child's daily routine. In a sense, yoga learned early becomes second nature to your child. Then, as he spends time each day being, instead of doing, he automatically supports his own resource and intrinsic value. Now, your child will know how it feels to be self-satisfied and successful, listening to his own inner guide and finding his own truth.

Our culture is finally awakening to the ancient wisdom of stress-reducing techniques. Hence, there are now many schools across the United States that presently use yoga in their curriculum—it is a movement currently referred to as "om schooling"—and the academic results are impressive.

In 2001, *Time* magazine honored the Accelerated School, a public charter school in Los Angeles, with the School of the Year award. The Accelerated School incorporates yoga in its course curriculum, teaching yoga once a week to every child from kindergarten through high school. Further, the Accelerated School created an environment where children are self-aware, learning about health and wellness. As a result of practicing yoga as part of the school's culture, the children at the Accelerated School are calmer, face less bullying, and are more focused and prepared to learn. These children have been taught how to self-manage their stress, so that when confronted by bullying, they concentrate on their breath instead of hitting, taking time in rather than facing time out. The annual report from the Accelerated School indicates that "the students benefit from the positive effects of consistent yoga practice. And the results are visible in the classroom."[7]

Another school using yoga for kindergartners is Todd Elementary School in Briarcliff Manor, New York. Here, children as young as five practice yoga exercises in which they imitate the animal postures of lions, dogs, and house cats. At the end of their yoga routine, these children are asked to lie down on their backs on mats, placed evenly apart on a clean floor. Then they are asked to think about and visualize something that makes them happy, and to experience what it feels like to be in their body. This state of rest is really our natural state, and thus children respond to it much more easily than adults. According to Claudia Teicher, who taught yoga at Todd Elementary, children are often told to calm down without having the tools or skills to get there.[8] In a *New York Times* article, Teicher stated that yoga is the tool that has proven to help children reach a state of calm.

THE HEALTH AND WEALTH BENEFITS OF YOGA

The medical community is using yoga and other stress-reduction disciplines to not only help patients manage their stress and lower their blood pressure, but also to reduce the need for pain medication, accelerate recovery time, lower anxiety, and stimulate healing.[9]

According to a study by Dr. Dean Ornish, clinical professor of medicine at the University of California, San Francisco, patients who practice yoga for an hour each day, while following a low-fat diet and moderate exercise, reversed coronary blockages 82 percent of the time. Dr. Ornish proved that there was a direct correlation between practicing relaxation techniques, such as yoga, and the ability to create a state of calm, reducing stress, and hence reversing coronary blockages.

In another study, students who practiced yogic breathing for only ten days were able to increase their spatial memory 84 percent more than a similar population of students without any yoga instruction.

Research also indicates that women just beginning yoga increase their heart and lung capacity when regularly monitored on treadmill tests over the course of four weeks of yoga lessons.

Yoga is beneficial for everyone, whether they understand its philosophy or not. It's not a religion, though there are people who find spiritual solace from its practice. Moreover, though it tones the body and helps focus the mind, it is not a sport or exercise. According to Georg Feuerstein and Stephan Bodian, in their book *Living Yoga: A Comprehensive Guide for Daily Life*, yoga "infuses our whole being with vibrant energy, thus energized or enlivened, we can go about the business of our daily living in a harmonious manner. We become highly creative, establishing order where there is chaos, instilling life where there is a vacuum, causing comfort where there is distress, in other words, because we are full of joy and life, we become a healing presence in the world."[10]

In the following section, you will find particular yoga exercises specifically structured for your child's age and stage of development. But be careful—once your child practices yoga, he may really like it.

MEDITATION[11]

Meditation is neither a religious practice nor a philosophy, but rather a technique to focus on a single point by quieting your mind and concentrating on your breath. Though there are many variations on the theme of meditation, they all rely on this same approach. As you increase the range, intensity, and scope of your concentration, your body unwinds and your circulation improves, sending more blood to the prefrontal cortex and your executive function. This allows you to process information better, hold images longer, and use your mind more efficiently. Furthermore, meditation influences the default Mode network when the mind wanders, as negative thoughts find their way into an inner critic; but when focused on a single point such as in meditation, negative thoughts dissipate as positive thoughts override them. Therefore, meditation is one of the most preeminent forms of self-discipline. Through meditation, you connect to your sense of self, strengthening your inner core, so you can follow your own course and productively redirect the energy and power of your ego, better known as your function. Meditators will tell you that meditation can expand all aspects of your life, including your memory and your ability to learn.

HOW TO TEACH MEDITATION TO YOUNG CHILDREN[12]

Children as young as three can learn to meditate. After a short period of meditation, your child will feel alert, relaxed, and ready to learn. Because meditating feels so natural, your child will respond joyfully, soaking up anything that she encounters, like a blossom catching the sun.

When your child meditates, he learns how to alleviate his anxiety and tension and gain inner control over his mind and body. As soon as he grasps the basics of meditation, your child will immediately receive benefits. And when he gets older, you will find that he reaches for meditation independently, whenever needed, to self-manage his stress. Even something as simple as focused breathing can help him diffuse the intensity of a bullying child or a disgruntled adult.

Whether at home or at school, children who meditate can solve their problems internally. Thus, instead of needing "time out" to reestablish a sense of stability, your child can use "time in" as a tool to reset her inner state.

WHERE TO START

1. An easy way to introduce meditation is as part of rest, whether before naptime or before bedtime. Because children are curious, your child like most children, would rather not miss out on activity, whatever that may be. Since meditation is something to do, and is not sleep or taking your child away from where the action is, she will be more willing to participate and engage in something new and fun. Since meditation is relaxing, and when done correctly can put your child in a state similar to sleep, it offers your child all the benefits of feeling refreshed and revitalized without any angst or tears.

2. Especially with toddlers, it's important to keep meditation time short. Only a few minutes per sitting will do, definitely no more than five minutes. After your child has learned how to meditate, you can build on that timeline, slowly but surely increasing the five minutes a day to seven, ten, and so forth, until one day your little meditator is actually meditating twice a day, once in the morning and once in the late afternoon. For small children, ten minutes twice a day is sufficient.

3. Create a quiet space in your house without distractions. It is helpful at first to play Baroque music, in particular, in the background. Why Baroque music? Because it is in sync with your child's heartbeat, sixty beats per minute, and automatically relaxes her, preparing her to meditate. As your child's breathing slows down in time with your Baroque music selection, she will naturally relax.

4. Now, ask your child to lie down, flat on his back, with his arms at his sides. This can be done either on his bed or on a mat on the floor. The idea is to keep the spine straight, but not rigid. It's more difficult at this age to teach children to sit and meditate. But if they lie down, their little backs immediately straighten out, and they actually breathe correctly from their diaphragm. All children, no matter how young, breathe from their tummies when placed on their backs. They know instinctively the right way to breathe, and you're reminding your child of this when you ask him to lie down in a meditative pose.

5. Be sure to keep a blanket handy, because when the body relaxes, the body temperature lowers, and you want to keep your little meditator cozy and warm so that he can focus on his breath.

6. Use a progressive relaxation exercise (described in the following section) to isometrically relax all of the body's muscle groups, beginning at the feet and working up to the top of the head. This will put the body in a state of rest as your toddler prepares to meditate.

PROGRESSIVE RELAXATION TECHNIQUES[13]

Progressive relaxation is a simple isometric exercise in which you tense and relax all your muscle groups from head to toe, relaxing the body by releasing muscle tension. It's a good idea to begin meditation with a little progressive relaxation routine to help your child settle down and pay attention to his body. This technique can be used anywhere, at any time, standing up, sitting, or lying down. In fact, your child can learn, when faced with a difficult task or test, to simply give a total body squeeze to relax all of his muscles at once, isometrically. Progressive relaxation is even a great tool to use at night, helping your child self-soothe and fall asleep.

You can use progressive relaxation as a part of almost any activity. Similar to a basic vegetable or chicken stock recipe, progressive relaxation forms the foundation for a variety of other meditation routines.

Progressive relaxation actually takes less time to practice than it does to describe. The more your child practices this technique, the more rapidly she will tune into her body, learning how to relax those few muscle groups that remain tense. Soon, she will be able to command her muscle groups one by one to relax. Eventually, she will be able to go through the entire progressive relaxation routine and achieve a full-body tension release in a few short minutes. It is one of the most important techniques you can teach your child, one that can be used again and again—at every stage in your child's development. It is the basic prescription for relaxation that people of all ages can follow.

LET'S BEGIN:

First, ask your child to lie down flat on his back with his hands a few inches away from his thighs. Then, tell him to close his eyes while asking him to think about how his body feels without commenting on it. This sets the stage for guiding your toddler to quiet down.

Direct your child to squeeze his toes while thinking, "squeeze, squeeze, squeeze." This allows him to tense and release his toe muscles three times. Next, tell him to let go and tell his toes to relax.

Then, ask your child to squeeze his calf or leg muscles three times, while repeating to himself the words "squeeze, squeeze, squeeze" three times. Now, tell him to let go and command his leg muscles to relax.

Following the path of muscle groups, ask your child to isometrically squeeze his thigh muscles three times, while saying to himself, "squeeze, squeeze, squeeze." Now tell him to let go and tell his thigh muscles to relax.

Now, ask your toddler to squeeze his buttocks three times, while repeating to himself, "squeeze, squeeze, squeeze." And letting go, silently repeat the word *relax*.

Then, ask your child to put both of his hands on his stomach, asking him to breathe in, filling it with air like a balloon. Then ask him to hold his breath, repeating the words "hold it, hold it, hold it," three times. Then ask him to blow out the air from his tummy while repeating to himself, "blow out, blow out, blow out," feeling his tummy recede. Now, tell your child to tell his tummy to relax. Remember to use age-appropriate language and information matching your child's age and stage of development. Thus, for older children, you'll use more complicated and accurate words, such as calling the "tummy" a diaphragm or abdomen and using words such as *exhale* and *inhale* instead of "blow, blow, blow" or "breathe in." Nevertheless, it is still important to tell your child of any age to continue to hold his breath until he blows or releases it out on the exhale, saying to himself, "blow, blow, blow," or "exhale" three times. This will remind him that not only is he breathing in and out, but deeply and slowly.

Next, ask your child to place both of her hands on her ribs, filling her chest up as she inhales. Once again, tell your child to place her arms gently by her sides, asking her to breathe in while repeating to herself three times, "slowly in, slowly in, slowly in," and then breathing out, repeating to herself three times, "slowly out, slowly out, slowly out." Finally, ask her to silently repeat the word *relax*.

Next, with his hands down at his sides, ask your child to stretch out his fingers as far as they'll go while repeating three times to himself, "stretch, stretch, stretch." Then let go and silently repeat the word *relax*.

Then, ask your child to make a fist, squeezing his fingers while repeating three times to himself, "squeeze, squeeze, squeeze"; and letting go, silently repeat the word *relax*.

Moving up to your child's arms or biceps, ask her to squeeze her arms while repeating to herself three times, "squeeze, squeeze, squeeze"; and letting go, silently repeat the word *relax*.

Ask your child to shrug her shoulders so that the top of her shoulders can almost touch the bottoms of her ears while repeating to herself three times, "squeeze, squeeze, squeeze"; and letting go, silently repeat the word *relax*.

Ask your child to gently move her head from side to side three times in each direction. Then, ask her to bring her head back to center while silently repeating to herself the word *relax*.

Then, ask your child to stretch her mouth open as wide as she can while repeating to herself three times, "hold, hold, hold"; and then letting go, silently repeating the word *relax*.

Next, ask your child to make a funny face by scrunching up her nose. Once again, ask her to repeat silently three times, "hold, hold, hold"; and then letting go, silently repeating the word *relax*.

Now ask your child to squeeze her eyes tightly shut, making a funny prune face while silently repeating to herself three times, "squeeze, squeeze, squeeze"; and then letting go, silently repeating the word *relax*.

Next, ask your child to scrunch up her forehead while repeating to herself three times the word "squeeze, squeeze, squeeze"; and then letting go, silently repeating the word *relax*.

Finally, ask your child to remain at ease and feel what it is to be in her body. This peaceful state is the real her. Then, ask her to check in with her body and say to her toes, "Toes, are you relaxed?" To her legs say, "Legs, are you relaxed?" Then to her thighs, "Thighs, are you relaxed?" And then to her buttocks, "Buttocks, are you relaxed?" Then to her tummy, "Tummy, are you relaxed?" And then to her ribs, "Ribs, are you relaxed?" Then to her chest, "Chest, are you relaxed?" Then to her fingers, "Fingers, are you relaxed?" Then to her arms, "Arms, are you relaxed?" Then to her shoulders, "Shoulders, are you relaxed?" And then to her head, "Head, are you relaxed?" And to her mouth, "Mouth, are relaxed?" Then to her nose, "Nose, are you relaxed?" And to her eyes, "Eyes, are you relaxed?" To her forehead, "Forehead, are you relaxed?" By checking for tension, your child becomes aware that she is a partner with her body and that she can affect the tension in all of her muscles groups by simply tensing and releasing each one. If any one group is still holding tension, she can return to that muscle group and attend to it again. Then, with one mighty squeeze, ask your child to squeeze and release her entire body while telling her whole body to relax.

THE BREATH IS NEXT[14]

As soon as your toddler learns the progressive relaxation exercises, he is ready to approach meditation. And the easiest way to teach your child meditation is by asking him to follow his breath. By deeply focusing on his breath, your toddler is becoming familiar with his own body processes and how to control them.

LET'S BEGIN:

Ask your child to pay attention to his breath, focusing on breathing in and breathing out. Then, ask him to notice that when he breathes in the air feels cool around his nose, and when he breathes out it feels warm.

Now, ask your child to continue concentrating on his breath while repeating a nonsense syllable both on the in breath and out breath. Allow your child to pick any nonsense syllable he wishes. As he continues breathing, your child should repeat the nonsense syllable, paying attention only to its sound. It is important for his word to be a nonsense syllable and tonal so that he can't associate it with any image—only then will he stay focused. Otherwise, he can easily be distracted by the meaning of his word. In meditation, we call this situation "monkey mind." Once your child has picked his nonsense syllable, it is a good time to explain to him that if any other distractions enter his mind, like the sound of a car or truck passing by, or music, he should just say "hi" to that distracting sound and invite it, whatever it is, into his meditation. In this way, he can easily return to his nonsense syllable or mantra, repeating it again and again, with each in breath and out breath. Pretty soon, not only will his nonsense syllable fall away, but his focus on his breathing will fall away, as he relaxes deeply into the peaceful state of meditation.

Once again, ask your child to check in with his body, asking each body part if it's relaxed. If there's any tension anywhere, he can attend to it himself by telling that particular muscle group to relax.

After your child has checked in with his body a second time and is satisfied that he is relaxed, he will return to his breath and the nonsense syllable of his choice. Little by little, he will synchronize the pace of his breathing with the repetition of his sound, keeping his mind focused.

When your child is ready, ask him to slowly open his eyes. Then, add a positive affirmation similar to "now you are ready to begin a wonderful day." Next, ask your child to move slowly and carefully as he returns to a standing position, reminding him how peaceful and quiet his body feels. Finally, give your child a few moments to acclimate before beginning his next activity. In this way, he will savor and remember this peaceful feeling that he can return to anytime he wishes throughout his day.

It is important to recognize that meditation is an active experience, rather than sleep. At the end of his meditation session, your child will feel wide awake, alert, and restored.

MEDITATION TIPS FOR YOUR OLDER CHILD[15]

When your older child (five years or older) begins to meditate, set an alarm clock for five minutes. In that way, she won't worry or lose her concentration, wondering when five minutes is up. Increase her meditation little by little, building on the ease at which she settles into practice. Your older child will find that meditating twice a day for fifteen-minute increments will serve her best. If she meditates before school, she will begin her day refreshed and alert, and if her second meditation session begins directly after school, she will once again restore her concentration and focus so that she can approach her homework revitalized and ready to go.

As time moves on, your older child will deepen her meditation. She will be able to quiet herself and enter a meditative state more easily. Soon, her feelings of well-being will support and scaffold her feelings of calm, increasing her focus and stimulating her desire to meditate. After even a short session of meditation, your child will find herself wanting more.

To begin with, ask your older child to lie down on the floor, or if she prefers, to sit comfortably on a cushion or chair. The only prerequisite is a straight back, so lying down on a mat will also get the job done. Be careful here—while you want your child's back to be straight, you don't want her to overdo it and make it rigid or tense. So use words such as "soft" or "elongated" when describing the posture. If she's sitting, tell her to think of a string attached to her head, stretching her straight up. If she's lying down, tell her to imagine a string tied to her toes and moving straight up to the top of her head. Now, tell her to relax while opening her chest and softening her breathing. Next, ask your child to check in with her body, making sure it's relaxed, reminding her that meditation requires her to keep her mind quiet and concentrated on one single point.

Some older children meditate with their eyes open, though this can be somewhat unsettling and distracting. Other children prefer to meditate looking at a lighted candle or a blank wall. Regardless of your child's choice, it is important that it not be distracting. If she closes her eyes, she should keep her inner focus on the space between her eyebrows, often called the "third eye." With her eyes closed but tilted slightly up, ask your child to direct her attention inward.

Now, ask your child to focus on her breath, breathing in deeply, as slowly and rhythmically as possible. Direct your child's attention to how cool the air feels against her nostrils on her in breaths, and how warm it feels as she breathes out. Remind your child that by paying attention to her breath and using all of her senses, disquieting thoughts dissipate, as slow and steady breathing relaxes her body and calms her mind.

Your child may find that if she listens quietly and attentively to her breathing, she may hear an inner hum or tone. This first experience with both focus and concentration is fun for your child, as she receives the added benefit of being in sync with her body. For the first time, her body is responding to her efforts in a new and exciting way.

Most children find it easier to use a mantra in concert with their breathing, giving them a concrete distraction from their distractions. By choosing something tonal, such as the word *om, ah,* or *one,* your child will be able to concentrate on a word that is free of association, and hence free of thought. Here is where she begins her journey to mindfulness, the idea of paying attention to her thoughts and feelings.

At first, you will ask your child to say her chosen mantra out loud. Soon, she will progress to saying it to herself, hearing it only in her mind. Listening to her interior mantra, she will quiet herself, making it possible to hear her own inner hum or tone. By drawing her attention inward, your child will soon not only hear, but feel the pulsing sound of energy coursing through her veins.

Earlier in this chapter, we discussed the idea of the "monkey mind," in which the mind is thinking, thinking, thinking, constantly connecting thoughts but never at rest. As your mind flips from thought to thought, it resembles a monkey climbing from tree to tree. If your child experiences "monkey mind" while meditating and finds that her mind is wandering, instruct her to simply invite the unwanted guest of distraction into her meditation. What resists persists, so by not resisting random thoughts, they dissipate, and your child can easily bring her mind back to following her breath. This technique will help your child deepen and focus her concentration while capturing her "monkey mind."

If you teach your child to maintain her calm, even when bombarded by uninvited thoughts, she will easily grasp the notion that those outside thoughts are not her problem. Thus, uninvited, they leave.

Otherwise, if your child resists outside interruptions and interferences, they will gain importance and disturb her meditation. I typically say to the uninvited guests in my meditation, "Welcome, come join my meditation." By surrendering to what is, all tension goes away. Most important, your child's focus will not be diverted. This is how to meditate.

CREATIVE VISUALIZATION (OR CREATIVE IMAGINATION)[16]

There are a number of ways to describe creative visualization: visual imagery, visualization, creative imagination, and so forth. However, regardless of the name, the process is the same, one of imagining specific images, feelings, senses, and scenes focusing the mind on a particular task. Concentration and memory are used together as your child imagines himself achieving a desired goal. By engaging all of his senses and feelings, your child can actually experience the steps needed to successfully complete his objective. So by seeing and feeling himself practice and rehearse the moment-by-moment steps required, your child will be on his way to successfully reaching his target. Whether your child is learning to tie his shoe, or your grown-up child is competing in the Olympics, the approach is the same. The process works.

In the past, educators taught children that if they were positive thinkers, they could will themselves to achieve success. Unfortunately, this attitude, though uplifting and goal-oriented, seldom works. That is because success is much more than simply the "power of positive thinking." It is the integration of both imagination and willpower. Here is how your child can use creative visualization to help her achieve her goals throughout her life. When your child combines her left-brain activity—logic, language, and will—with her right-brain activity—creativity, visual images, dreams—she will have the full thrust of her brain's capacity. She'll be able to process information better, hold images longer, and store memories deliberately. This last piece is the key to creative visualization, because when your child stores a memory it's always attached to emotion, the emotion she felt when the experience occurred. Therefore, when she uses a creative visualization technique, she is deliberately storing an imaginary memory of her successfully achieving a desired goal. Your child's brain cannot recognize whether the imagined experience is real or not—when it stores that memory, it stores it as real. When your child engages all of her senses while imagining an experience, her body reacts to the event as if it were real, including changes in her bodily functions such as blood pressure, heart rate, and breathing. Creative visualization is no different from what you experience in a movie theater, when your imagination places you within the story. Even though you know what you're watching is fiction, you still respond physically. If it's a scary movie, for instance, you may hear yourself scream.

MAKING CREATIVE VISUALIZATION WORK[17]

There are two important parts to creative visualization: the first is for your child to relax while imagining accomplishing her goals. The idea is similar to watching a movie and uses your child's creative function to visualize the specific steps needed for success. It could be as simple as asking your child to imagine that she is buttoning her coat, and practicing and rehearsing in her mind's eye the exact steps needed. Older children might visualize winning a competition such as a spelling bee, acing a test, or winning a sports match.

Creative visualization will be a lot of fun for your child. Mastering the art of summoning her imagination, while using it successfully to achieve a particular goal, can be thrilling. Now she can practice this technique anytime she wishes. In time, your child will learn that not only can creative visualization be used to relax, but also to enhance memory, increase learning, reduce pain, and lessen anxiety.

Because creative visualization is so effective in relieving pain, controlling blood pressure, and changing behavior, it is highly regarded as a treatment protocol in many medical contexts. For example, heart patients have been known to improve their clogged arteries, lower heart rate, stabilize blood pressure, and reduce stress. Cancer patients have been known to use creative visualization to imagine that their white cells are aggressively fighting off their cancer cells, using familiar formats similar to video game scenarios or movies to create the appropriate backdrop or environment for the theme of their imagination. One of my professors who was undergoing chemotherapy told me that he imagined a war similar to a Pac-Man video game in which his cancer cells were overwhelmed and killed by his protective white cells. He also engaged his other senses in the battle, heightening his experience by playing the soundtrack from the movie *Alexander the Great*. This all served to engage all of his senses, and reinforce his memory, while adding to the reality of his imagination. His doctors were truly amazed at the results of his chemotherapy, telling him that never before had they witnessed such a rapid reduction in the size of a cancerous tumor. Today, there are many such anecdotal accounts of the successful use of creative visualization in conjunction with cancer treatments. Thus, a treatment protocol that was once considered out of the norm has now become mainstream. Rallying a patient to use his own resources through imagination and creative visualization to confront his illness restores a sense of control that is lost when faced with the reality of a serious disease.

A number of years ago, I read an article in the *New York Times* Sunday magazine section reporting on research from Johns Hopkins on the impact of the mind on the body. This research revealed that when cancer patients were given placebo chemotherapy, they exhibited the same side effects as those patients who had received the real drug—losing their hair, becoming nauseated, and experiencing exhaustion, similar to their counterparts who were treated with the real drug. A further study indicated that patients who were taught how to utilize creative visualization and self-manage their own stress were able to vividly imagine their chemotherapy as an ally. By not resisting their treatment, but rather supporting it, they were able to substantially reduce the historically difficult side effects of chemotherapy.

Neuroscience in the twenty-first century teaches us that the mind affects the body, and that the body can be commissioned to affect the mind. Inasmuch as the body is a metaphor for the mind, both can be called upon to operate as a unit. For instance, even when you hug yourself, your mind translates the hug as personal, oblivious to the identity of the person doing the hugging . . . and the benefits are the same. Regardless of who gives you a hug, your psyche feels the connection, intimacy, love, pleasure, and warmth. Similarly, when you smile, your brain receives that smile with all the positive feelings that it invokes, whether you are truly happy or not. Regardless of your genuine feelings or present situation, the practice of creative visualization can have a powerful effect on your emotional and physical outcome.

CREATIVE VISUALIZATION BASICS FOR YOUR CHILD[18]

It bears repeating that before you harness the power of the mind to work in harmony with the body, you must relax both. Begin by guiding your child through a progressive relaxation exercise, so that he can take the physical edge off before he engages his mind. Then, add a visual technique by asking your child to imagine stepping on an escalator and, while breathing deeply, seeing himself moving down to the next floor. Another visual relaxation technique incorporates color with that escalator ride, following the rainbow spectrum down to the next floor. This incorporates more of your child's senses as he feels the warmth of the color and relaxes into a joyful state. You can direct your child to first see an ultraviolet color on the seventh floor, riding down color by color, purple on the sixth floor, blue on the fifth floor, green on the fourth floor, yellow on the third floor, orange on the second floor, and red on the first floor. Not only will your child feel relaxed, but he will also access his creative function to gain control over his stress.

Now ask your child to think of something or somewhere that makes her feel especially happy and peaceful. It might be lying in a bath of warm water, on a sandy beach, on a float in the ocean, or in a favorite spot in her garden. Some children need a little nudge to think of such an imaginary place, in which case you can offer them some of your favorite spots, or just suggest things such as balloons rising in the air or sleeping in a tent or a cave. A creative way to help your child find her place of peace and calm is to tell her a story that takes your child along on a journey. I use this technique with my grandchildren, walking them through a meadow so that they use more of their senses, feeling the wet grass under their feet, hearing the babbling brook to their left, and seeing a mountain in front of them, with different color terraces that move up, instead of down, to a state of relaxation.

All of these ideas have one central focus in mind: to help your child relax. Once you and your child have found a favorite spot, ask your child to close her eyes and describe to you, in detail, what she sees. Children love this practice because they love to hold your attention by telling you a story. Your child will soon become adept at clearly defining her peaceful place. Soon, without any prompting, she will be able to go there by herself. Practice active listening while your child recounts visual, auditory, physical, and sensory details of her story. She may include the chirping of birds, nature sounds, smells, and so forth as she tells you what it feels and looks like to walk up the terraces on the side of the mountain. Help her emphasize, and elicit all the descriptors along the way, so that she can recall them in detail through positive association. For example, how the warm air feels calming, or how the water ripples, cool against her toes. With each detail, your child will find herself more authentically a part of her creative experience.

Although this particular autogenic exercise takes a little extra time at first, the more clearly your child can visualize her peaceful spot, the more quickly she will relax, until soon she can go there at any time she wishes, in no time at all. So, what originally may have required twenty minutes' practice can now be effective in five minutes or less. What's wonderful about this approach is that your child can use it independently, whenever she is under stress or anxious, as well as to heighten her performance.

In summary, the first step in using creative visualization to help your child reach his goal is to guide him toward his peaceful place so that he can relax and experience a state of calm and quiet. The second step, however, is to show your child how to use autogenic training to set his goals so that he can use creative visualization as a tool to accomplish them.

HOW TO TEACH YOUR CHILD TO SET GOALS

Regardless of which relaxation technique you use, the most important step is helping your child discover the goals she wishes to achieve. Setting goals is not as easy as it seems, because speaking isn't doing. It won't work to just say "I want to button my jacket" or "I want to tie my shoe," because to achieve her goals, your child has to integrate her thoughts with her actions. If not, she will be doomed to create and repeat ineffective patterns of behavior.

Your child has the best chance to achieve his goals if he envisions them succinctly. Each detail should be identified and built into the image he holds in his imagination. The more complete and realistic he can be, the better he will be able to visualize his target. Short-term goals are more effective at first, as your child can see an immediate result, which only serves to reinforce this new technique. In this way, success builds on success, and your child learns that his long-term desire, whatever it may be, whether tying his shoe or learning to button his coat, is just a series of small visualizations, built on themselves, until his goal is attained.

GOALS AND HOW TO ACHIEVE THEM

Your child's goal should be meaningful to her, for only then will she concentrate her energy toward accomplishing it; and the more she values her goal, the more attention she will focus on her imagination.

At this time, it is important to invest your child in the process, completely, by asking her what she thinks it will take to achieve her goal. Then, ask her to describe the necessary steps to reach her objective. Now, together you can investigate what actions promote success. By helping your child find clarity, you can work out, together, a definite timeline to master her task. An extra bonus of working with your child is that you become a team, and an intimacy develops as you pay attention to her progress, helping her make the needed refinements and adjustments to her plan. Soon, you will both be aware of the right time to adapt and move on to the next step.

You and your child have become collaborators, working together to reach a common goal. And because it is her goal, she recognizes that she can depend on you to be her support and guide her through her creative visualization process. By teaching her to make a detailed description of her objective, you are actually giving her the tools for self-mastery . . . to harness the power of her own desires. By showing her the efficacy of being flexible and adjusting her aim when needed, your child will experience the confidence that leads to competence and success.

THE END: NOW IT'S TIME TO VISUALIZE GOALS

At this point, it is time to guide your child to practice and rehearse the specific steps leading to his target. Until now, he has been using logical, left-brain processes. Now he will engage the creative right brain to achieve his endeavor. Here your child learns to use his whole brain like a symphony, tapping into all of his inner creative resources to attain his objective.

Remember to first ask your child to practice his progressive relaxation techniques until he feels that he is in a relaxed and peaceful state. Once relaxed, he is ready to focus on the projected image of his goal. Since he has already prepared his plan of action, he can easily construct a detailed paradigm of his aim.

Rehearse and practice your child by reviewing the particular steps needed to master his goal, always paying attention to his level of success as you move him toward self-mastery. To begin with, ask him to relax, closing his eyes while he guides his mind toward imagining his aspirations. Then, direct him to take the appropriate actions to accomplish each part of his plan. For example, if your child wants to learn how to tie his shoes, break down that objective into small, doable increments. Next, tell your child to imagine going through the exact motions of tying his shoe in his mind's eye. Direct him to envision himself putting on his shoe while imagining what it feels like to touch the coolness and the texture of his laces. As his fingers move to perform the steps necessary to accomplish his task, instruct him to think of how he feels emotionally as he succeeds in completing his effort with ease.

Finally, the more you guide your child to visualize and review the steps needed to achieve her goal, the more able she will be to summon those images on demand. Because the creative visualization experience takes place within your child's mind, it can be practiced and rehearsed anywhere and at any time, including naptime or bedtime. Returning to these images again and again will help your child stay focused on her objective, while the creative imagery will infuse your child with the positive reinforcement that is essential for success.

MUSIC FOR LEARNING

It is impossible to overstate the importance of music. As the poet William Congreve (1670–1729) stated in his play *The Mourning Bride*, "Music hath charms to soothe the savage breast."[19] And though many remember this iconic quote incorrectly, often stating that music has charms to sooth the savage beast, if we had actually used music to learn this quote, you might have remembered it correctly. Regardless of this quote, I think that you can agree that music affects us deeply, in ways we don't understand.

Science has long recognized the unique qualities that music has to affect us emotionally. Music has also been shown to influence the body's healing abilities, as well as certain types of learning. Baroque music in particular has the capacity to optimize and accelerate learning in general.

So you might say that music has an almost magical quality to affect our lives. Advances in neuroscience show that music can enhance your memory and activate each part of the brain, allowing you to learn and recall information more efficiently. For instance, think of how you learned the ABCs. Probably your mother sang the letters to you with a now-familiar song that all children know, a song that matches the alphabet to the musical scale, teaching children a particular note for a particular letter. No matter how old you become, you can still sing that alphabet song, especially when looking up material in a library or dictionary. Then there is the Jiminy Cricket tune by which we all learned to spell *E-N-C-Y-C-L-O-P-E-D-I-A*.

Whether it's a nursery rhyme or a bedtime story, whatever material you learn accompanied by music is more easily remembered. And you remember the words to the songs you learned as a child throughout your entire life.

Why does music impact our memory? Neuroscience researchers can now qualitatively measure how listening and playing music enhances not only the function of your brain, but also its form. Brain scans indicate, for example, that music bridges the right and left hemispheres of the brain. That's why stroke victims who have lost their ability to speak can often sing the words needed to communicate. The right hemisphere of the brain can learn the melody while the left can learn the words. As a result, many stroke patients can still speak if phrases are sung to music.

When you listen to music, it activates both hemispheres. The entire brain is activated, opening to more modes of thinking and processing information. And listening to Baroque music expands the brain, making you happier, healthier, and more able to perform at a peak mental capacity.

Music has been an important part of every human endeavor and affects people all around the world in a universal way. Thus, you can easily see how music can be deliberately used in our modern world to affect specific outcomes. When you shop in a grocery store or shopping mall, the music selection piped into the store is upbeat, encouraging you to shop. If you go the doctor's office, the music selection is often meditative or calming, and if you go to a gym, the music there is often fast-paced and stimulating, encouraging you to exercise.

Music that accelerates learning should be relaxing, because relaxing music follows a rhythm and beat that's in sync with your heartbeat, approximately sixty beats per minute. When you listen to relaxing music, it puts you into a meditative state, sending more blood to the prefrontal cortex, the seat of your executive function, and improving circulation in general. As you relax, your focus can turn inward, which is the perfect condition for accelerated learning.

Not all music however, evokes the same response. Most music listened to throughout the day falls under the category of entertainment and is designed to lift our spirits and stimulate excitement. This type of music is more intense with a faster tempo. Faster music accelerates your heartbeat, which is fun and exciting, but not peaceful or calming.

But music that is in sync your heartbeat will put you in the optimal state to learn. While it calms you down, it increases your ability to concentrate and focus. As restful music quiets you naturally, it regulates your heartbeat to a deeply relaxed state in which your brain waves change from their beta frequency of 13–39 cycles per second (cps) to an alpha range, about 8 cps. The Earth has a particular harmonic resonance or electrical magnetic field, which also pulses at approximately 8 cps. By quieting your body and your mind to its natural state of relaxation, your mind becomes more alert and receptive to learning.

In particular, it is the slow "largo" or "adagio" movements of Baroque music, written by Vivaldi and Bach in the eighteenth century, that are in sync with the normal rhythm of your heart. Accordantly stringed instruments, such as the harp or violin used to play Baroque music, offer the most benefit for improving health, memory, and focus. That's why you often see a harpist playing in spaces orchestrated for healing modalities, including the lobbies of hospitals and senior citizen facilities.

Music in general has an almost magical ability to inspire and stimulate learning. A University of Kansas music therapist, Janalea Hoffman, used Baroque music as background while giving a homogeneous number of nursing students a test. Using an experimental model for her research, Hoffman did not administer the music treatment to the control group. The outcome of her study demonstrated that the nurses who received the music treatment had higher test results and lower heart rates than those in the control group. Hoffman verified her preliminary finding that slow music, approximately sixty beats per minute, reduces stress, lowers blood pressure, and reduces pain, all important protocols to accelerate healing while protecting the body against illness.[20]

At St. Luke's Hospital in Cleveland, doctors used music as a protocol during surgery, discovering that their patients needed less sedation and less pain medication. Some of their music choices were Baroque, including works by Vivaldi and Brahms. Furthermore, Dr. Raymond Bahr, once head of the coronary care unit at St. Agnes Hospital in Baltimore, noted that thirty minutes of Baroque music in the andante movement had the same impact as 10 milligrams of Valium.

Music has been used to enhance mnemonic memory training for years. In fact, foreign-language schools often employ the Tomatis Method, which relies upon music in conjunction with a mnemonic memory approach for language acquisition. Though the Tomatis Method has been successfully used in Europe, it is still not as accepted in the United States.

Baroque music in and of itself is meditative and thus relaxes the body, increases circulation to the prefrontal cortex, and helps the mind focus. If you did nothing else but listen to Baroque music while completing a task, you would benefit greatly. I was determined to use classical music as background in my own children's lives. When I became a grandmother, I encouraged my children to load their iPods with Baroque music in particular, to be played around the clock in their baby's nursery. To this day, a selection of Baroque music can be heard in my grandchildren's rooms when they study or play. Since music improves both physical health and brain health, it can also make your child smarter, happier, and healthier. So why not put on Baroque music? Such an easy step to positively affect your child's ability to learn.

When using music as a teaching tool, perhaps teaching your child a nursery rhyme, lullaby, or ABCs, try "chunking," or breaking up into small chunks, the task to be learned. The small chunks should be able to be stated or read in less than four seconds. Then pause for a few seconds to let the new information find a home. Then add the next chunk of information, once again stated or read in four-second intervals. Remember to pause for about four seconds between chunks, giving the new information time to sink in, all the while having Baroque music playing in the background.

Chunking information into small units has been used successfully, for years, as a memory tool. Further, neuroscience reveals that the brain also learns new material more efficiently when it is chunked. Because chunking breaks up new material into small bites, it creates a singsong rhythm, helping you to remember new knowledge effectively. This approach is similar to remembering a telephone number, address, or zip code by chunking a long number into smaller segments of two, three, four, or five.

When teaching your child anything new, it is important to elicit different styles of learning—auditory, visual, and kinesthetic. In this way, the two sides of your child's brain will be better at communicating with each other. By maximizing the use of both sides of your child's brain, you will encourage brain plasticity, increasing blood flow to both hemispheres, reinforcing the brain's capacity to change and grow. When your child uses his brain like an orchestra, he will increase brain synapses, which can enhance learning.

When a child's brain is relaxed, it is uniquely receptive to outside stimuli and performs optimally, in concert. In order to perform at its best, each section of the orchestra must be focused, waiting for its turn to contribute to the music. A small amount of good stress helps the musicians be on high alert, waiting for their turn to perform. However, too much stress, rather than keeping them on their toes, can cause them to play poorly or even shut down. Without a coordinated effort, each musician playing his part, the show may not go on. The same is true for the brain.

CREATE YOUR OWN ACCELERATED LEARNING PLAYLIST

It is the slow movement of Baroque music that enhances learning. I've compiled a personal playlist of the selections that I prefer from classical Baroque recordings, but you can find your own Baroque music that best encompasses your taste, tempo, and style. While gathering recordings of Baroque music, you may find that you prefer more modern composers such as Stephen Halpern, whose music carries a similar tempo and rhythm.

RECOMMENDED BAROQUE CLASSICS

- **Telemann:** Largo from Double Fantasia in G Major for Harpsichord
- **Vivaldi:** Largo from "Winter" from *The Four Seasons*; Largo from Concerto in D Major for Guitar and Strings; Largo from Concerto in C Major for Mandolin, Strings, and Harpsichord
- **Bach:** "Jesu, Joy of Man's Desiring"; Largo from Harpsichord Concerto in F Minor, BWV 1056; Air for the G string; Largo from Harpsichord Concerto in C Major, BWV 975; Lute Suite in E; "Sheep May Safely Graze"
- **Corelli:** Largo from Concerto No. 10 in F Major from Twelve Concerti Grossi, Op. 5
- **Caudioso:** Largo from Concerto for Mandolin and Strings
- **Albinoni:** Adagio in G Minor for Strings
- **Handel:** *Messiah*

- **Purcell:** *The Fairy Queen*
- **Monteverdi:** *Vespers*
- **Schütz:** *Musicalische Exequien*
- **Scarlatti:** Sonata
- **Rameau:** Overtures
- **Johann Pachelbel:** Canon in D major

At this level, your child's music experience is not only enjoyable, soothing, and fun, but also educational. Studies indicate that children who play the piano experience educational gains. According to neuroscientist Gordon Shaw,[6] children ages three to five who participated in six months of piano lessons showed significant gains in spatial-temporal reasoning, which is the very aptitude needed in engineering, math, and chess. Not only that, but when compared with children who received singing and computer lessons, or no lessons at all, the children taking piano lessons still performed at a higher rate of success—and the older the child, the more significant the improvement of spatial-temporal reasoning. For instance, when second graders from a poor district in California took piano lessons twice a week for a year, they not only improved their math scores, but they performed on par with fourth graders from a neighboring affluent school system.

ADDITIONAL RELAXATION EXERCISES

The following exercises will help your child focus and relax:

EYE RELAXATION EXERCISE

Relaxation exercises can relax and strengthen the eyes.

1. Ask your child to look up at the ceiling without moving his head.
2. Then, ask your child to look right, toward the right wall.
3. Now, ask your child to look down toward the floor.
4. Next, ask your child to look left, toward the left wall.

5. Now, ask your child to look around in a circle two times, then ask him to make a circle by moving his eyes in the opposite direction, for two more rotations.

6. Then, ask your child to reach his hands out in front of his eyes and stare down at his hands for seven seconds.

7. Now, ask your child to look across the room and stare at the opposing wall for seven seconds.

8. Finally, tell your child to rub his hands together, back and forth, as if he were rubbing two sticks together to make a fire. Then, tell him, when his hands feel warm, to put each palm over one of his eyes, feeling the warmth bathe his eyes for several minutes.

BREATHING RELAXATION EXERCISES

Your baby automatically breathes correctly, lying on her back while breathing from her diaphragm. But by the age of five, she starts to breathe more shallowly from her chest, and shallow breathing is not relaxing. The following relaxation techniques will help bring your child back to a healthier, deeper style of breathing. If at any time your child feels dizzy or lightheaded, just direct her back to her more familiar shallow breathing.

BLOWING BUBBLES

Teaching your child how to blow bubbles in a clear glass of water is the easiest way to help her direct her attention to her breathing in and out. Ask your child to make her blowing action steady and smooth, and if using a bubble loop, encourage her to blow out evenly and deeply. Another fun approach to blowing bubbles is to use Baroque music as your background while using a bubble loop. You can find a simple bubble loop in any toy store or online.

MEASURED BREATHING

Ask your child to lie down with her hands resting quietly at her sides. Then, ask her to notice whether her breathing is fast or slow. Now, ask your child to try and slow her breathing down. Next, ask her how slowly she can breathe without holding her breath, by simply and evenly breathing out and breathing in.

BREATHE IN WARM AND BREATHE OUT COOL

Now, ask your child to notice how cool the air feels against his nostrils as he breathes in, and how warm the air feels against his nostrils when breathing out. Ask him to take several slow deep breaths, as he continues to notice that his in breath feels cool, and his out breath feels warm. By becoming aware of the change in temperature from cool to warm, your child is also focusing on his breath, which will automatically relax him and place him in a meditative state.

TUNE INTO YOUR TUMMY

Now, ask your child to place his hands on his tummy. Then, ask him to fill his tummy up with air like a balloon, by breathing in as much as he can. Next, ask him to push the air out of his tummy by breathing out. Soon, he will notice that when his tummy fills up with air, it expands, and when he breathes out, it goes down. Then, ask him to fill his tummy with air one more time while holding his breath for thirty seconds, repeat "hold, hold, hold," and then tell him to breathe out, letting his tummy return to normal.

MEDITATION FOR TOTS

Meditation gives your child an opportunity to tune into herself, practicing time in rather than timeout. Through meditation, your child will learn how to focus, concentrate, and process information effectively. It is these very skills that will serve her well throughout her life, helping her to unite the hemispheres of her brain for optimum results.

INSTRUCTIONS BEFORE YOU BEGIN:

1. Explain to your child that she may get cold during meditation, so you will place a blanket at her side if she needs it.

2. Next, tell her that she can either lie down or sit up on a floor mat, though lying down is more comfortable.

3. Then, explain that you will dim the lights and put on Baroque music in the background to help her relax.

4. Then, introduce the idea of focusing on a sound such as *om*, or *ahh*. Explain that she can pick her own sound, but that the sound should not hold any meaning, so that it is free of associations, which can distract her during her meditation.

NOW YOU ARE READY TO BEGIN:

1. Help your child get comfortable. Ask her to sit or lie down on a mat. If she lies down, ask her to place her hands gently at her sides, an arm's length away from her body, palms up.

2. Place a light blanket to the side of her mat, reminding her that she can use it anytime she wishes.

3. Turn the lights down low.

4. Now, ask your child to tell you her sound. She will love this part of her meditation preparation, as she will get to tell you her choice of a sound and why she likes it. You can tell her now that her sound is called a mantra, and that all meditators, including Mommy, have one. If she is stumped for a sound, tell her that she can use the mantra *om*, which is a universal tone that is used worldwide and can be found in words such as the Arabic word Assalam Alaykom or the Hebrew word Shalom. Whatever word she chooses is fine—the idea is to repeat her special word over and over again, quietly to herself, by using her inner voice.

5. Then, instruct your child to repeat her mantra slowly, out loud, ten times. She will delight in the fun of hearing her voice speak her special sound. Next, direct her to try and match her chosen sound with her breathing. Then, ask your child to close

her eyes, hearing and feeling her sound as it resonates with her breathing. Next, ask her if she can hear the sound of her breathing. Now, ask her to bring the sound of her word inside so that she can hear it with her inner voice. By making her word silent, but audible in her mind, she is preparing herself for future silent reading. And by matching the sound of her word to her heartbeat, your child is crossing the threshold into meditation and relaxation.

6. This first meditation practice should be done for five minutes each day. Then, slowly, you can increase your child's meditation time. Ultimately, you can build up small increments of time until your child is meditating for ten minutes once a day. Of course time should be flexible, as meditation should be experienced as fun, playful, and useful, not as an obligation to be resisted. The benefits of meditation are so evident and so immediate that soon your little meditator may want to meditate twice a day.

PRESCHOOLERS AND YOGA

Your preschooler is unbelievably flexible. If you've ever watched your child dance to music, you know what I mean. When you introduce her to yoga at this age, it is amazing to watch the feats she can perform. Your little yoga master may even outperform you—as the animal poses so excite her imagination, she might get lost in the sheer revelry of doing full-fledged yoga poses. Each animal position is constructed to build on your child's sensory awareness, ability to follow instructions, growing coordination, and sense of self. My grandchildren used to love going to the park with their mom to practice yoga, and when I visited, I was met with a complete demonstration.

THE TURTLE EXERCISE

Show your child a picture of a turtle. Then, ask him if he has ever seen a turtle. Now, ask him to make believe that he is a turtle, while showing him the following turtle movements, which will help him relax.

1. Tell your child to let his head reach gently toward his chest. Tell him to feel the weight of his head as he leans forward.
2. Ask your child to raise his shoulders up toward his ears, then to raise his head. Now, ask your child to lower his shoulders and raise his chin toward the ceiling.
3. Ask your child to move his shoulders in a circle, while keeping his hands at his sides. Now, ask your child to reverse this action, forming a circle moving his shoulders in the opposite direction. Before you begin step number four, make sure your child knows his right side from his left side; if not, this can be a wonderful teaching moment.
4. Ask your child to look over his shoulder, first to the left side, as far as he can see. Then, ask him to do the same on the right. Then, go through the turtle exercises one more time, so that your child will relax.

THE ELEPHANT POSE

This pose helps to increase lung capacity while energizing your little yogi.

1. Ask your child to stand straight with her feet apart, clasping her hands together while allowing her arms to drop in front of her like an elephant's trunk.
2. Next, tell your child to breath in through her nose and, like an elephant, swing her arms up and over her head, being certain to arch her back while widening the expanse of her chest.
3. Now, ask your child to blow air out of her mouth, while swinging her imaginary trunk with clasped hands gently

from side to side, and then down through the center of her widespread legs.

4. Finally, direct your child to breathe in again, repeating the entire movement by first breathing in and then breathing out with each complete set.

THE LIGHTED CANDLE

This yoga pose helps your child relax her body while focusing her mind.

1. Tell your child to sit on her knees with her hips resting lightly on her heels.
2. Then, ask her to inhale deeply while stretching her torso.
3. Now, with your gentle touch, help your child hold the stretch in her spine on her out breath.
4. Next, direct your child to roll her shoulders back, allowing them to fall on her down movement.
5. Then, ask her to stretch open her chest as wide as she comfortably can.
6. Now, direct her to drop her chin, relaxing her face and neck.
7. Then, ask her to clasp her hands together in front, imagining that she is a candle with her hands as flames.
8. Tell her next to close her eyes gently and relax with her eyes closed for ten seconds.
9. Now, ask her to breathe naturally and feel what it feels like to be a candle.
10. After one minute, tell your child to slowly, slowly open her eyes, look around quietly, and smile, paying attention to how good she feels.

THE ROCK POSE

The rock pose is wonderful for recharging and restoring your child's energy level.

1. Once again, ask your child to sit back gently on his knees, with his hips resting lightly on his heels.
2. Then, help your child drop his body forward until it rests on his thighs. Now, let his forehead fall forward until he can gently place it on the mat in front of him, just beyond his knees.
3. Now, ask him to put his hands at her sides close to his body with his palms facing up.
4. Next, ask your child to check in with his body while telling his face to relax.
5. Next, ask him to be very quiet as he listens to his breathing, feeling the cool of his in breath and the warmth of his out breath.
6. Then, with one final movement, tell your child to feel what it feels like to be in his body, asking him to try and connect with the earth or floor beneath him . . . and be still.

BE A CAT

This yoga pose helps your child practice quieting her mind and body.

1. Ask your child to think of what a cat looks like as she lazily stretches.
2. Then, ask your child if she can tell you something about a cat, for example, what a cat does. She will probably answer that a cat purrs, meows, and stretches.
3. Now, ask her if she can show you how a cat stretches and meows.
4. Then, direct your child to get down on her hands and knees as she imitates a cat, placing her hands right underneath her shoulders, and her knees directly under her hips.
5. Then, while still on all fours, direct your child to spread out all fingers as far as she can, while pointing them straight ahead.
6. Then, with straight arms, ask your child to press down on her hands and breathe out while rounding her back up toward the ceiling as high as she can . . . just like a cat.

7. Next, ask your child to breathe in while looking at the ceiling and arching her back, placing one leg behind her, like a cat stretching.
8. Have your child repeat this sequence, first rounding her back when breathing out, and then arching her back when breathing in, but this time stretching the opposite leg behind her, like a cat stretching all the way down his back to his tail.
9. This pose can be repeated as often as comfortable. Remember, however, to keep arms straight and movements slow and smooth.

THE DOG

Ask your child to imagine herself as a gentle little puppy while she practices each puppy pose.

1. First, ask your child to get down on the floor on her hands and knees, placing her hands right under her shoulders and her knees directly under her hips.
2. Ask your child to open her hands wide, spreading her fingers while pointing them forward.
3. Next, ask your child to curl her toes and press her hands and feet into the ground while pushing her hips up to the ceiling.
4. Then, let your child's head drop forward, as far as she comfortably can, so that she can look through her legs.
5. Now, ask your child to stretch her back while straightening her legs and arms, pressing her heels through the floor.
6. Next, ask your child to open her mouth wide as she imitates the way a dog yawns.
7. Finally, ask your little yogi to hold this yoga pose for five breaths before lowering herself back down to her knees and hands.

THE SQUIRREL

Ask your child to think of a squirrel. Then ask him to try to imagine that he's a little squirrel.

1. Ask your child to sit on his knees with his hands on his thighs.
2. Ask your child to come up to a kneeling posture, bringing both hands out in front of his face.
3. Then, ask your child to stretch each arm up, one at a time, as high as he can while making believe that he is looking for a nut.
4. Next, ask your child to gather up the nuts and place them on his chest while taking turns reaching for another nut with his other arm.
5. Finally, ask your child to return to the rock pose, happy that he was able to store his nuts for the winter.

THE WHITE CLOUD

This creative visualization is designed to help your child relax by teaching him to quiet his mind and focus his attention. When your child visualizes himself as a little white cloud, he will feel relaxed and able to engage in any activity, prepared to learn.

1. First, go outdoors with your child and ask him to lie down on his back on a mat, either on the ground or on the grass.
2. Then, ask him to look up at the clouds, imagining that he is one of the clouds in the sky, and feel how relaxing it is to just float on by.
3. Now, return to the house and ask your child to lie down on a mat on the floor while doing one minute of breathing exercises to quiet his mind.
4. Then, ask him to imagine that he is outside on a warm, sunny day looking at a blue sky.

5. Next, tell him to ask his body to relax while doing one complete body isometric squeeze to relieve any body tension.

6. Then, ask him to imagine that he is relaxed and happy, looking up into the clear-blue sky.

7. Now, tell him to imagine what it feels like to be calm and peaceful as he sees a tiny fluffy cloud floating by.

8. Ask him to watch the cloud and feel how happy it makes him when it stops right above his head.

9. Tell him to continue watching the cloud, imagining that he is now the fluffy white cloud.

10. Then, ask your child to make believe that he's that little fluffy white cloud floating by in the sky, feeling joyful and relaxed.

11. After this exercise, your child will take that feeling of well-being and relaxation with him wherever he goes throughout the day.

EXERCISES FOR INTELLECTUAL DEVELOPMENT

When introducing these exercises and games to your child to enhance intellectual development, be careful never to impose any exercise on your child. If she is resistant, move on to something else. Let her guide you toward her interests. If she isn't stimulated, interested, or excited, she won't participate.

When your child is ready, her own inner teacher will encourage her to explore. At this stage, her task mastery is its own intrinsic reward. By mastering the object of her attention, your child will experience a feeling of success, which will motivate her to move on to the next stage of development. Now, she will learn even more, and this feeling of confidence will guide her to a strong sense of self and self-confidence. By reacting to outside challenges with only an intrinsic reward, rather than responding to the opinions of others, your child is demonstrating the beginning of her own maturation.

If at this stage your child is having fun, let her. When your child's interest is focused and she is concentrating on a project—let her be. This focused activity is what your child thinks of as her work, and it is this focus and concentration that she will transfer to the art of learning.

THE GAME OF MEMORY

In this game, your child will be encouraged to notice things in her environment. The idea behind the game is that the more objects you recognize in your surroundings, the more you learn. Repeat this exercise over and over again. Each time your child plays the memory game, she will be able to notice more details. Soon, she will point out objects from her environment throughout her day, all the while building up her memory.

Ask your child to lie down quietly, close her eyes, and practice a short breathing technique until she feels relaxed. This should not take more than two minutes. After one minute, ask your child if she is feeling relaxed yet. She will tell you how she honestly feels and if she needs more time. Now, you are collaborating and working together . . . having so much fun!

Next, with your child's eyes still closed, ask her to imagine her surroundings here and now. Direct her to picture, in her mind, what objects are immediately in front of her. Then ask her what she remembers. Now, ask her what colors she can remember from her surroundings. Finally, with her eyes still closed, ask your child what she can see in her mind as she looks to her right and left side.

Then, allow your child several minutes to simply use her imagination. Ask her what she imagines is around her. Next, ask your child to open her eyes and take a second look. Then, ask your child if she imagined most of the things or only some of them. Be sure to tell her that this is only a game. We are only having fun. Point out to your child that today her answer might be one way and tomorrow another. But little by little, each day, ask her to notice what she observes in her surroundings.

Your child will love playing this game with you if you keep it light and let her tell you everything that she remembers, answering questions such as:

What color dress did you wear yesterday? What color shirt did your friend wear today? or What did you eat at lunchtime? Always remind your child that the more she notices and remembers, the more she will know about her environment.

STIMULATING OBJECTS TO MANIPULATE, FEEL, OBSERVE, AND SORT

At this age and stage, one of the more significant intellectual activities your child is compelled to engage in involves any object that she can classify, sort, number, or order. Your child can participate in any of the following games using common household objects, as long as they can be classified, sorted, numbered, or ordered. There are a variety of categories that can be used in these activities. For example, objects can be sorted by size, texture, color, or shape.

Thus, it is a good idea to keep a large stash of interesting and brightly colored items for counting, sorting, manipulating, and classifying. Some easy candidates are pots, pans, plastic lids, plastic bowls, different textured fabrics, and the proverbial large button. Fruits and vegetables are also great for sorting, numbering, ordering, and classifying by a variety of categories, such as color, texture, size, shape, and smell.

ASKING YOUR CHILD TO SORT THROUGH HER SENSE OF TOUCH

Ask your child to categorize the different textures he feels while identifying them. For example, soft, silky, smooth, rough, bumpy, and so on. Help your child separate out the objects in each category that are the same and put them all together.

ASK YOUR CHILD TO LINE UP OBJECTS BY THEIR SIZE

Direct your child to make a line of any particular category. For instance, large buttons, toy cars, baby dolls, and so on. Now, ask him to separate out, from each category, specific sizes such as small cars and large cars or large buttons and small buttons. Ask your child to hand you the smallest object in each category. Then ask him to hand you a bigger object from each category. Finally, ask him to hand you the biggest item from each category.

HELP YOUR CHILD SORT BY SEVERAL DIFFERENT CLASSIFICATIONS

This sorting game teaches a concept called multiplicative classification. Here, your child will learn that there are sub-classes of items and objects. For example, under the larger class of wooden beads, there may be various colored wooden beads, such as blue and red. Here your child learns by observing, manipulating, touching, and feeling interesting and unique items. Even before she can verbally describe the relationships between objects, she is beginning to understand them.

First, spread out piles of buttons that are different in size, shape, and color on a low child-sized table or on the floor. Then, ask your child to join you in sorting them, using one category at a time. For example, color. Here you can say to your child, "Let's take all the blue buttons and put them into one pile."

Now, ask your child to join you in sorting the buttons using two classifications. For example, size and color. Ask your child to join you in putting all the large green buttons in one pile. Ultimately, you will want to increase the properties for sorting, adding one new classification at a time. For three properties you may classify texture, size, and shape.

WHAT YOUR CHILD CAN LEARN BY EMPTYING THE DISHWASHER

Invite your child to help you in emptying out the dishwasher, by putting dishes, glasses, forks, knives, spoons, pots, and pans away. You are giving your child an excellent object lesson in sorting by category. For example, say to your child, "The dishes go here in the dishwasher and now the dishes go here in the cupboard." Item by item, object by object, you can use this exercise to classify and sort by category.

Moreover, you are giving your child work, which he is naturally pre-disposed to desire. Children love to participate in household chores. As he works by your side, he will feel a great sense of accomplishment as he models grown-up behavior. Partnering with your child during household work makes him feel part of the team, and it is an amazing bonding experience. This small window of opportunity is yours to enjoy—while chores can still be perceived as fun.

ASK YOUR CHILD TO HELP YOU SORT THE LAUNDRY

Similar to emptying the dishwasher, your child will love sorting laundry. This task provides a great lesson in sorting by category. When sorting laundry, you automatically put like objects with like objects, such as all dark socks go together, which can be further categorized by black, blue, and brown socks (good luck finding all your matching pairs of socks!).

ASK YOUR CHILD TO PLAY THE COUNTING GAME WITH YOU

Here is another creative, fun experience that your little explorer will love. Now he can learn the physical correspondence of items on a one-to-one basis, such as numbers and objects.

TEACH YOUR CHILD COUNTING SONGS: "THIS LITTLE PIGGY"; "THE ROLLOVER SONG"; "TEN BOTTLES OF OJ ON THE WALL"; OR ANY OTHER COUNTING NURSERY RHYMES

Your child will love to count. And when she is ready, she will count everything. So when you recite nursery rhymes to her, for example, "This Little Piggy," be sure to touch each of her little toes as you count them. Touch in connection with language and mathematics creates a physical cue that stimulates memory. Then nursery rhymes, by themselves, add a creative visualization to the art of counting, as she visualizes each particular nursery rhyme. This is when your children start to comprehend that numbers are symbols, though at this stage, they don't completely understand why.

HELP YOUR CHILD POUR WATER INTO DIFFERENT-SIZED GLASSES

Though this exercise is somewhat complex and abstract, your child will begin to master it by the age of six or seven. Nevertheless, you can begin to expose her to it earlier. This exercise is what Piaget called "conservation." The concept is that if you pour the same amount of water into different shapes, it is still the same amount of water. However, children in the preoperational stage, before the age of six or seven, think that because the shapes of the glasses are different, some tall and some short, the taller shapes must contain more fluid. This is an important concept to grasp and leads to mastering more complicated math skills in the future.[21]

1. First, place several cylinders of different sizes and shapes on a small child's table. Point out that you have one measuring cup. Next, fill the cup with water and show your child what you are doing, pointing out that one measuring cup is filled with water. Then, ask your child to pour the measuring cup of water into the tall cylinder. Now, have your child pour the water from the tall cylinder into the short cylinder. Next, ask your child which cylinder holds the most water.

2. Then, place short and tall glasses on a small child's table. Once again, point to the measuring cup of water, telling your child that it contains one cup of water. Now, ask your child to pour one measuring cup of water into each of the two glasses. Finally, let your child see and compare how each measuring cup of water looks different in each glass, while the amount is exactly the same.

14 BUTTONS ARE 14 BUTTONS

Here is a variation on the conservation theme.

1. Ask your child to count out 14 large buttons and put them in a pile.

2. Ask him to count out another 14 buttons.

3. Next, direct your child to divide the second group of 14 large buttons into smaller groups, such as 7 and 7, 10 and 4, 8 and 6, and so on, telling him to count the large buttons in each group.

4. Now, ask him to count out all of the large buttons in the first group. Soon, he will see that regardless of how you group the buttons, the quantity 14 will always remain the same.

5. Finally, invite your child to join you as you try this game with other objects: toy cars, blocks, etc. In that way, he can see that the same approach works with all items.

SPATIAL RELATIONSHIPS SUCH AS BEHIND, INSIDE, FRONT, BACK, LEFT, RIGHT

Since your child, at this stage, is still egocentric (lost in a state called egocentrism), it is still difficult for him to appreciate another person's perspective. Therefore, he will still struggle with spatial concepts and relationships that depend on the viewpoint of others.

1. Teach your child to help you set the table, which requires complex concepts including right, left, and mirror images.

2. Show your child how to put a place mat on the table.

3. Help her hold a dish with two hands as she places it in the center of the mat.

4. Next, show your child that the napkin goes on the left side of the plate, while the water glass goes on the right.

5. Now, show her how to set the table with the knife on the right side of the plate and the spoon to its right, followed by the fork to the left of the plate. While teaching this important concept to my own children, I added a story, telling them that the fork was a princess who was being protected by the knife, who was a knight. So, that is why the knife is always turning in, with

the sharp edge toward the plate. I added that the spoon was the princess's and knight's baby. By making a family, including a princess, a knight, and a baby, setting the table caught the attention of both my son and my daughter, who immediately added their own versions to the tale.

6. After your child has learned to set the table, turn the place mat in all different directions, placing it on one side of the table and then the other. Now, your child can see, in concrete terms, that no matter which way you turn the place setting, the relationship of the fork on the left side of the plate and the knife and spoon on the right stays the same.

GAMES THAT TEACH MIRROR IMAGING

Children at this stage often have difficulty understanding the concepts of mirror images, as well as left and right. Therefore, games such as the Hokey-Pokey, which uses these concepts, help make these concepts less confusing, as well as fun. This kinesthetic way of learning teaches your child to use his whole body by connecting his sensory movement with his logic. This helps him have a clear understanding of not only mirror images, but also the concept of right and left. Remember that the Hokey-Pokey incorporates both singing and dancing.

1. First, make a little circle with your child by holding hands while singing the Hokey-Pokey.
2. Ask your child to repeat after you, as you sing, "you put your right hand in" and instruct him to put his right hand into your circle along with you and any other participants.
3. Next, sing "you take your right hand out" and tell your child to follow you as you take your right hand out of your circle.
4. Continue singing the Hokey-Pokey as you teach your child the game. He will be thrilled to play along with you as he learns all about spatial concepts.

5. Complete the song, following all of the Hokey-Pokey instructions with your child. You will have a ball as you see his little face light up with glee each time he gets it right. Let the song lead you as you incorporate each particular body part.

BUILD A 3D ACTION-PACKED HOUSE

This is my favorite game, as it is filled with happy memories of my own childhood play.

1. First, help your child build a house out of blocks.
2. Next, add a small car, boy or girl doll, soldier, knight, etc.
3. Then, ask your child where he would like to put the doll, the car, etc. For example, should the toy car go on the top of the house or in front of the house?
4. Now, ask your child to help you to make up a story. Perhaps with a giant bird or dragon hiding in the backyard or behind the house.
5. Ask your child to tell you where he would like to put all of the participants in the house.
6. Now, ask your child to tell you the story. Then ask him what to do, so that you can follow his sense of play.
7. Let your child's story be created by him, including which actions should take place.
8. Finally, let the action of the story be directed by your child's imagination.

CONSTRUCT A SUNDIAL

Comprehending time helps the brain to think in a logical sequence by recognizing special concepts that help to develop logical thinking. Time, in and of itself, is difficult to grasp without a visual aid. The sundial is such an aid, and it is simpler to make than you might think.

1. The first step is watching the sun's shadow as time moves through the day.
2. Help your child draw a circle on a piece of cardboard or construction paper and draw a clock face on the circle, with lines designating each hour of the day.
3. Then, lay your clock face on the ground outside, while pushing a pencil through the middle of the dial.
4. Next, return during specific time segments throughout the day, so that you and your child can see how the pencil's shadow moves around the circle.
5. This will give you and your child a look at abstract thought by using a concrete method.
6. Now, you and your child can congratulate yourself that you made a sundial.

BAKING COOKIES

Another fun exercise is baking cookies so that children can measure time. Not only that, but you will teach her important mathematical concepts. Baking cookies engages all of the senses. More than that, your child will learn how to delay gratification while waiting for her cookies to bake, an important step in maturation. The smell of the baking cookies and their delicious taste will help to focus your child's attention on her work.

1. As you and child prepare your recipe for cookies, your child will concentrate on measuring the necessary ingredients, a beginning lesson in conservation and mathematics. By paying attention to how long the cookies must bake, you are also teaching your child to measure the passage of time.
2. Read the instructions in the recipe so that your child knows exactly how long the cookies are required to bake in the oven.

Point the time out to your child on the clock. Invite her to watch the clock as it measures off the allotted time for baking.

3. Before the cookies are finished, ask your child if she knows how much longer they need to bake. Here, she may guess based on an inner knowing or sense of time. Whether her answer is right or wrong, redirect her attention to the clock, praising her for such a good answer.

GROW CARROT TOPS

Help your child grow carrot tops so that she can measure time.

1. First, cut off the top of the carrot and place it in a glass of water.
2. Next, take a calendar and show your child the corresponding days of the month, marking off each day, so that she can calculate mentally as well as visually how fast the carrot root has grown.
3. As you and your child monitor the growth of the carrot top, you can point out to her how much the carrot top has grown within a particular period of time.
4. In this way, your child will not only have the pleasure of watching something grow, but she will also have the ability to gauge the passage of time.

TIME FOR CHORES!

Teach your child how to help you with chores, so that he can estimate time.

1. Show your child your watch and point out the time.
2. Now, ask your child which chore he would like to do first. Then ask him how long the chore will take.
3. Now, work together with your child to complete the chore.
4. Finally, check your watch again so that you can point out how close his estimate came.

LANGUAGE DEVELOPMENT CAN BE STIMULATED THROUGH THE ART OF STORYTELLING

Your child first learns language in the womb at approximately four months gestation. After birth, language can be stimulated by talking, talking, talking to your child. Complex language can increase IQ development. At this stage, girls often move ahead; however, language evens out by preschool. The best way to engage your child is to stop, look, and listen to her.

1. First, tell your child a story.
2. Now, ask your child to tell you what the story was about.
3. Ask your child to tell you a story.
4. Now, you tell your child what her story was about.
5. Finally, create a story together with your child, using characters from each of your prior stories.

WRITE YOUR CHILD'S STORY

Help your child create a storybook or storyboard to expand his imagination and bring his story to life.

1. Tell your child to tell you a story, while you write it down on paper.
2. Then, make the story into a little book.
3. Sew the pages together with brightly colored yarn.
4. Ask your child if he would like to draw some pictures in his book.
5. When the book is finished, read it together all over again.
6. This same process can be used by writing your child's story on a large piece of construction paper and taping it to the wall, where he can color and draw on it to enrich his story.

ORGANIZE AND STRUCTURE A PRINT-RICH ENVIRONMENT FOR YOUR CHILD

1. Buy some construction paper and label familiar objects in your house with large block letters. For example: BED, BATHROOM, DOOR, WINDOW, and REFRIGERATOR. Use brightly colored crayons to color each block letter. Next, tape the labels to each object, using masking tape so it doesn't cause any damage. Soon, your child will connect the word with the object and begin to remember and identify which word belongs to which object. Though you are not teaching reading or spelling, your child is becoming familiar with both. By creating a print-rich environment, you will improve his intellectual environment.

2. You can also create a print-rich environment by naming the things in it. For example, if you are reading a book, you can point out the name of the book; if you go into the kitchen, you can point out the name REFRIGERATOR that is on your refrigerator door; if you open your refrigerator, you can point out the name MILK on the carton of milk; and you can point out the name EGG on the carton of eggs, etc.

3. Words are all around your child. By showing your child which word belongs to which item, you are enriching his environment with print.

BEDTIME AND STORYTIME

By reading a story to your child, every night at bedtime, she will get into the habit of reading. If you allow her to read along with you, while looking at the words on the page, she will mimic you and try to read. When she makes mistakes, don't correct her, just listen to her read you her story. In time, your child will become a reader as she begins to recognize the words on the page and memorize their meaning. This is a deeply bonding activity that will serve her well for the rest of her life, while teaching her good language skills.

SOCIAL AND EMOTIONAL DEVELOPMENT EXERCISES

Talking gives your child the chance to express herself in a welcoming environment, which leads to feelings of value, validation, and self-actualization. Passing through the stages of each exercise will support good language skills and good self-esteem.

SIMON SAYS TO TEACH SPATIAL RELATIONSHIP CONCEPTS AND RULES

1. By playing Simon Says, your child will explore spatial relationships, including placing your hand on top of your head, over, under, and so on.
2. It also teaches children about rules and that they have to know the rules, so that they can follow them.
3. The game of Simon Says also exposes children to the idea of taking turns. For example: Simon Says tells your child he should do something . . . and he must listen and follow, so that he can play.

WHEN YOU PLAY WITH YOUR CHILD, TALK, TALK, TALK

Your child loves to talk and can't wait to tell you all the things that have happened to him, whether at home with his family or in his own little nest. Take advantage of your child's natural proclivity to enhance his language, expressiveness, and communication skills playfully, but do not make it a teaching moment or lesson. According to Singer and Singer,[22] children who scored high as imaginative during play on physiological tests also had better language skills.

For your best outcome, combine physical activity with conversation, such as putting on plays, puppet shows, baking, singing, and so on. The dinner table is the best place to talk, and families that eat together do better in all things, including school. In my own home, I used to play a game with my children and husband called serendipity. Each person around the table took turns sharing one good thing that happened to them during the day. Everyone in my family loved this game, and what's more, it sparked all kinds of ideas and conversations that enriched our dinnertime. In my family, as I am sure in yours, each child loved having the floor and capturing everyone's complete attention.

7

YOUR 3- TO 5-YEAR-OLD'S EMERGING SENSE OF SELF

Children as young as three begin to separate in play based on gender. This behavior seems to be universal and present in most known societies. Yet, by middle childhood, gender influences manifest more prominently. Thus, by three, you see a difference in the way most children play. Boys and girls in general play dissimilarly, neither gender appreciating the other's style.[1] At first, boys play more aggressively in greater numbers, while girls are more into relationships and often prefer one-on-one play. Regardless of the toy, and regardless of how exceptional the toy, children still seem to prefer to play with their own sex.

At age four, boys often match up with each other, and by age six, they participate in coordinated and competitive play.[2] Girls pick up approximately six social cues, including tone of voice and facial expressions, while boys, on the other hand, pick up one or two. Girls make eye contact, boys do not—something deep and biological in the male feels that looking another boy in the eye is a challenge for dominance. The boy wonders if he can beat the other boy in competition; the girl will give you her favorite doll if you'll be her friend. Why is this?

From a purely biological perspective, these gender influences on play appear in societies as children begin to grow up and master the conduct necessary for survival. The aggressive play engaged in by boys prepares them to mate; while the relationship play, engaged in by girls, prepares them to birth the next generation. Actually, these are the very same gender characteristics practiced by all other primates, the evolutionary necessity for reproduction, endurance, and the continuity of existence.

As most boys mature, their gender affects their dramatic play. Their stories represent danger and crisis, stories of war and battles. Whereas girls, for the most part, are concerned with establishing relationships such as building a home and family.[3]

HOW BOYS AND GIRLS LEARN DIFFERENTLY

When talking about parenting strategies, it is helpful to note that boys and girls learn differently. Men are from Mars, women are from Venus . . . or are they? Are the differences between boys and girls really that great? Or is our biological determinism more of a self-fulfilled prophecy? Neuroscience tells us that yes, boys and girls *are* different. Boys' brains are larger, but girls' brains grow faster, and typically their interests and learning styles vary somewhat. But are these differences as significant as we once thought?

New studies tell us that it is the environment we create for our children that has the greatest impact on the way they learn and what they learn. We can go back through history and point out notable men and women who have gone against gender stereotypes. We can talk about Wolfgang Mozart, Leonardo da Vinci, and Michelangelo—men who had fine motor dexterity, could sit for long periods of time, had beautiful handwriting, and who were interested in arts, literature, music, and writing.

We can talk about women such as tennis legend Billie Jean King, astronaut Sally Ride, civil engineer Marilyn Jorgenson Reece, aviator Jacqueline Cochran, doctor and researcher Elizabeth Blackburn, and so on—women in history who were interested in athletics, math, engineering, and science.

In today's world, the outliers are more the rule than the exception, and parents have the greatest impact on both the suppression and enhancement of our children's genetic makeup.

ALL GENERALIZATIONS ARE FALSE, INCLUDING THIS ONE

It is true that many boys pick up fewer social cues than their female counterparts, and that girls make more serotonin and oxytocin, so they are calmer and more interested in emotional connection. Boys mature more slowly than girls, and girls have more of their cerebral cortex defined for verbal function. Girls have a larger corpus callous, which correlates to their superior verbal fluency. Boys, on the other hand, have more of their cerebral cortex defined for spatial relationships. As a result, they learn easily through movement and visual experience. Also, because girls have more serotonin and oxytocin, they can sit for longer periods of time more easily than boys, who may need movement to feel comfortable.

However, there is very little gap between what girls and boys can learn, and herein lies the rub. The differences are most pronounced in young children, and as they grow older, their home environment, their interests, and their peers have the greatest influence over their behavior. By the time children are in the twelfth grade, the differences between boys and girls are subtle. Understanding these subtle differences can help educators guide their students in a positive way, meeting them and their needs where they are.

When little boys don't want to make eye contact and fidget in their seats, and little girls are caught talking and sending notes, a savvy teacher will organize her classroom, taking into consideration that little boys need to move around and little girls need to express themselves verbally, and interpreting this as part of biology rather than misbehavior. A smart teacher will also create playtime opportunities during the day for both boys and girls to unwind and express themselves in a creative way. In fact, allowing children, especially little boys, to start school a little later, perhaps even by a year, gives them an edge, as a more mature child can handle school material much more affectively.

In my years as a researcher and educator, I've found it to be true that boys and girls perceive their school problems in different ways. Girls tend to take their problems and failures personally and are much more self-critical. Boys, on the other hand, see their problems in more focused ways and will assign their failure to a particular area of study rather than overgeneralize and consider themselves as lacking. Ironically, girls tend to do better in school than boys and are more likely to stay in school and graduate.

So what can we do to help boys *and* girls have a happy, fulfilling, well-rounded, and successful school career?

1. Be certain that your child's school has a recess program that includes unstructured playtime.
2. Be careful not to label children, especially with labels such as ADD or ADHD, unless they are diagnosed by a health-care professional. Many boys and some girls are just on the outer edge of active and are being mislabeled.
3. Encourage girls to play with toys and activities that allow them to use their spatial relationship and manipulation skills.
4. Encourage boys to take study breaks and allow them to be active during those study breaks.
5. Help your daughter talk through her feelings about schoolwork and school problems. Because girls may focus on communication, relationships, and attention for approval, they can easily get caught up in intense emotional experiences. Often, a girl will subvert her own feelings and needs to get the approval of others, and this causes self-esteem issues.
6. Engage your daughter in sports to help her build confidence.
7. Help your son creatively with literacy skills, including reading, writing, journaling, drawing, fantasy, humor, war, and mythology. Boys are action-oriented, often competitive and impulsive risk-takers, so giving them an opportunity to express themselves creatively and explore their interests is very important. This will help connect their words to their feelings and validate both.

8. Offer your daughter the opportunity to experience STEM (Science, Technology, Engineering, Mathematics), using everyday examples. By having access to a computer, girls can build, design, and explore anything from architecture, medicine, and engineering to culinary experiences. You can also enroll your daughter in one of the many STEM programs around the country.

9. Make sure teachers understand the different learning styles of boys and girls so that they are able to create learning environments that meet the needs of both by teaching different modalities capturing girls' needs for spatial learning practice, including geometry, and boys' needs for enrichment projects.

YOUNG CHILDREN AND GENDER

Children first realize that they are either a boy or a girl between the ages of eighteen and thirty months. In fact, it's their first attempt at categorizing using terms such as "he" and "she" to distinguish between boys and girls. Further, children get a lot of sexual cues as infants from their parents. When parents interact with boys and girls, they are also expressing their own idea of sexuality in the different ways in which they speak to their male and female children, the different ways in which they cuddle them, and the different ways they play and socially interact with them.

Social learning and role-modeling are a big part of gender develop-ment, not to be confused with sexuality. As in all other things, parents and primary caretakers are their children's first teachers. Young children learn about trust, gender, and sexuality by observing and interacting with parents, family, and other children. Media, daycare, and elementary school teachers can also affect the way in which children perceive them-selves in relation to others. Children role-play in early stages of gender development by imitating their same-sex parent. They are also learning to understand the value of relationships by observing and experiencing the social interactions of the meaningful people in their lives. This social behavior broadens the context of the building blocks needed for sexual development.

Young children between three and six start understanding gender differences as they recognize and notice, perhaps for the first time, that boys and girls have different genitalia. Girls may think boys look fancier; boys think girls have something missing. These external observations lead to gender constancy, where children start acting congruently with their gender, while also realizing that if a girl wears pants, and a boy wears a dress, it doesn't in any way affect their gender.

Then there is the cultural impact of the way we perceive the roles of boys and girls within society. Here is where stereotyping can create a narrow idea of what boys and girls should be. This can be a problem, since stereotypes are limited and, in many cases, incorrect. For example, in our own culture, we see men who cook and are chefs, and women who become lawyers and congresswomen. So, as children move along in their gender development, it is helpful to broaden their horizons and scope by the types of experiences we create for them. If we expose them to all kinds of toys, for example building blocks, mechanical games, things generally considered male, as well as crafts and dolls, toys often considered female, then we have the opportunity to allow our children to find their passions and tap into their full capacity. In fact, mechanical toys and building blocks may help a girl do better in math and science, which may lead to a career in medicine or engineering. Boys allowed to play with pots, pans, and cooking utensils as well as paints, dolls, etc., may become great chefs, designers, or artists.

The important thing to remember is that gender develops from infancy to puberty and is different from sexuality. It has more to do with what we expect from boys and girls rather than what is related to their sexual anatomy, including biology and DNA. Children's understanding of their own gender helps frame the way they perceive their body image and feelings of self-worth. Television, movies, and computer games have changed the way we perceive gender identity in our culture. We have women such as Captain Marvel and Wonder Woman demonstrating very physical and masculine machismo, while, conversely, you have males as single parents cooking and raising their children, exhibiting what was once considered stereotypical feminine behavior.

There is a condition called Gender Identity Disorder. This is rare, but if it occurs, parents need to understand what it means and how it affects the relationship with their child. Studies show that this occurs more in boys than girls and needs to be diagnosed by a health-care professional so that parents know how to help their children find their place in the world. Children's development, whether gender identity or gender stability, has an ebb and flow throughout childhood. However, once gender identity is stabilized, a parent has a great opportunity to help their child become a well-rounded and well-adjusted person.

CULTURE DOES AFFECT PLAY FROM AGES 3-5

The importance of play can be seen around the world in all cultures. The repetitiveness and forms of play are unique to the cultural and cognitive structure of each specific society. These aspects of play mirror, in essence, each culture's morals, ethics, and values. The most important thing is to let your child play. Give her the time and space needed, in a safe, secure, and rich environment, with age-appropriate objects to manipulate, touch, observe, and experience so that she can play creatively.

GIVE YOUR CHILDREN AN INDEPENDENT ZONE SO THAT THEY CAN SAFELY TEST THEMSELVES AGAINST THEIR ENVIRONMENT

Three-to-five-year-olds are very active; they progress quickly in both gross motor and fine motor skills as well as eye-hand coordination. It is at this point that they begin to gradually gain control over their eye-hand coordination and develop increasingly complicated systems of activity. Though they are not as practiced in using their fine motor skills, they are quickly discovering how to master the use of their fingers and hands. Though they may appear somewhat clumsy at first while trying to tie their shoes, button their clothes, use a spoon or fork, or hold a glass of milk, nevertheless they show rapid improvement daily. Therefore, when spills and accidents happen, it is important to stay calm, reminding your child that though mishaps occur, you can always solve the problem together. Now you've enlisted your child to be your partner in creating a solution without any residue, conflict, or guilt. At this time, your three-to-five-year-old can benefit greatly from a safe and age-appropriate space that he can call his own, one in which he can try things out by himself. It is now that he needs opportunities to play creatively, move around, and explore his surroundings, either independently or with others, without generating any conflict with parents and siblings. What your child needs at this level of development is an independent zone where he can try things out, pushing against his boundaries, as he prepares for independence.

Your three-to-five-year-old seems to be running on extra, somewhat like the little Energizer Bunny that keeps on going. In fact, according to Emily Glover, there have been studies where top athletes follow three-to-five-year-olds around for a day, and by lunchtime, the athlete has reached the end of his endurance, while the toddler is just getting started. As you watch your child play, run, hop, skip, dance, and so on, to the absolute outer limits of her capacity, it becomes clear that you have to institute a time for rest. By establishing a consistent nap period at a regular time each day, so that she isn't surprised and knows what to expect, you will cue your child into her own body awareness, teaching her that there is a time to play and a time to rest and restore.[4]

These are the days when you will hear the echo of "Mommy, I want to do it myself" again and again. Yet there will be times when your three-to-five-year-old is still having difficulty controlling his fine motor skills. Things that require eye-hand coordination such as tying a shoe, picking up small items, and buttoning a shirt can all be challenging. Nonetheless, advances are made rapidly as your child develops a more complex system of action.

By giving your child opportunities to practice and rehearse eye-hand coordination through games and objects that he can touch, manipulate, hold, and observe, he will soon master the art of feeding himself, dressing himself, and picking up small things, as well as drawing, coloring, and using plastic scissors. Be patient as your child refines his gross and fine motor skills as you encourage him toward new levels of independence.

By age three, the dominance of one brain hemisphere or the other becomes evident in the handedness of your child; this, of course, will affect her coordination. Another aspect of brain growth can be seen in your child's interests in expressing herself artistically. Now, she scribbles everywhere, on everything, as she creates and designs shapes, objects, and pictures. Never, under any circumstances, change your child's handedness—it can have devastating effects, both physically and emotionally. You want your child to develop naturally without any obstruction or resistance.

Piaget's preoperational level of cognitive growth extends from ages two to seven, and you can observe your child's progress in almost every domain of cognitive growth.[5] For the first time, he will actually understand the world in which he lives, not simply through his senses, but by thinking. He will understand that symbols represent items, people, and events that are not actually there. Here, he can transfer his thinking from symbols to objects. It is at this point that your preoperational child becomes efficient at using language and drawings to describe his feelings, family, and friends. In a sense, your child is beginning to think logically, and he has the ability to put things into categories, like living and non-living. He can conserve, decenter, count, and classify, and he can judge between fantasy and reality.

At the beginning of this stage, your child is still egocentric, believing that the universe revolves around her. Therefore, your child may appear selfish but in reality is unable to perceive another's perspective. Soon, however, she will begin to detach from egocentricity, appreciating another's point of view and recognizing that not everyone sees the world as she does. When logical thinking and empathy begin to influence your child's thinking, she will learn to interact with others and play more collaboratively. Then, she will develop a theory of mind, which exposes her to an understanding of her own thinking process. Now, she will be better able to separate reality from fantasy, make more precise judgments concerning spatial relationships, and recognize deception.

LANGUAGE EXPLOSION

One of the greatest cognitive leaps your child takes between three and five is language acquisition. As soon as language takes off, your child talks and babbles to herself in a constant monologue of sounds, rhythms, and stories. An example of egocentricity, your child is quite comfortable carrying on a lengthy conversation with herself in what is commonly called private speech. It is thought that private speech helps move your child toward self-regulation, a behavior that dissipates at approximately ten years of age. Between three and five, your child's vocabulary explodes through fast mapping, as grammar and syntax become refined. Also, your child will become ever more efficient in pragmatics as she gradually increases her social conversation. Though the reasons for delayed speech are still not clearly understood, it is important to recognize it early so that it can be treated without creating serious consequences cognitively, emotionally, and socially. Eventually, your child socializing with adults leads to the social speech needed for the advancement of emergent literacy.

Remember the Art Linkletter program *Kids Say the Darndest Things*? Well, keep in mind—they do. Once your child gains even a little command of the English language, he will repeat anything he hears with sheer abandon, taking pleasure in talking like a grown-up. So be warned: any phrase you don't want to hear repeated, don't speak in front of your child. Some of the most embarrassing moments between families and friends have been initiated by a tiny person repeating a wicked remark overheard in private. In our own family, I can remember distinctly when my four-year-old son went over to a cousin at a family wedding and asked him if he was the cousin they called "meathead." (He was.)

BE YOUR CHILD'S TV MONITOR

It is important to limit television viewing. In fact, you have to be your child's TV monitor. TV is not interactive, but rather hypnotic. It creates passive experiences, thereby thwarting imagination and creative play. Not only that, but studies show that TV can cause a malaise similar to depression, even in very young children. If the educational shows your child is watching flash numbers and letters at him, while his brain is in hyperdevelopment before the age of two, it can create learning problems similar to ADD and ADHD, where your child's growing brain reacts to patterns of flashing stimulation, putting him on high alert.[6] After the age of two, however, shows from the past such as *Sesame Street* and *Mister Rogers' Neighborhood* not only can support confidence, but can also promote self-esteem. In families without fathers, shows such as *Mister Rogers' Neighborhood* offered children a parental substitute for a kind, loving, and accepting dad. A positive male role model is critical, as children thirst for that missing parent, while having no idea what that parent should be like. Therefore, exposing them to a positive male model gives them the opportunity to emotionally interact and gain the necessary psychological input that is so needed from a loving father and is missing in a single-parent home. Studies indicate that boys without a father to emulate are at a higher risk for delayed maturity, as they are forever seeking the confirmation and bonding from a missing dad.

Only allow your child age-appropriate screen time and be certain to control any violent programming at home. There is so much to say about the effects of violence on a growing brain, and you will find more on the subject in Chapter 2. If an adult watches one hour of violence a week, his brain stores that visual memory as abuse—thus, consider your child's developing brain creating memories from TV violence that she experiences personally. Because your child's imagination places her in the story, watching violent images creates violent memories that can generate false memories of abuse. It is important to screen your child's TV and online video viewing, supervising all of it, making certain to protect your child from violence, just as you would from a violent stranger.

Be your child's home companion. By watching television together, you will be available to explain and discuss what your child is seeing, asking and answering any questions that may arise. In that way, you can confront opinions that don't support your value system. Then, you can generate an active conversation, talking about the subjects and characters in each show. If you want your child to benefit from television programming, he must be actively engaged. Additionally, communicate your thoughts and feelings about each program, expanding your child's judgment to discern fact from fiction. By pointing to the difference between a program and a commercial, fantasy from fact, you are teaching your child to become a discriminating and intelligent viewing audience.

DEVELOP AUTONOMY, HOW INDEPENDENCE INSPIRES SECURITY

In early childhood, your three-to-five-year-old begins to conceive of herself as separate from others. She shifts from a single representation of herself to representational mappings of herself in relation to others. Before this, she cannot distinguish her real self from her ideal self, but by experiencing her feelings and recognizing the emotions that point to herself, she begins to understand the simultaneous feelings that emerge in early childhood. Now, as her self-concept evolves, she begins to understand her feelings. Erikson tells us that this crisis stage is initiative versus guilt.[7] If this developmental stage is successfully navigated, your child will reach a sense of virtue of purpose. This successful resolution endorses a state of self-esteem and is experienced globally, relying on parental approval. But because early childhood self-esteem can be based on achievement or accomplishment, it holds an inferior pattern of helplessness, infecting the way your child thinks and interacts with others.

We've already discussed the importance of play, but we haven't discussed the kinds of play that demonstrate your child's cognitive and social development. Both Piaget and Sara Smilansky discuss play as parallel to functional, constructive, pretend, and formal stages of development.[8] Remember that once your child engages in formal play, he will also progress to knowing the rules and following them. Pretend play is most important, though you'll see a lot of physical play appear in early childhood.

Further, Mildred B. Parten reminds us that play becomes very social at this stage of development, gradually increasing as children grow older.[9] At this age, children begin to buddy off by gender, and your child will have one or two best friends. Because of the increased sociability, children may change friends often, open and flexible to making new friends. There also seems to be a more strident preference for gender-specific toys, as boys and girls imitate parental role models. Gender preferences with toys and activities emerge by kindergarten. Three-to-five-year-olds gravitate to other children who are like them, echoing their future choice of friendships based on common interests. Children who are more social are more popular than those children who bully and assert themselves aggressively.[10]

Once your child enters into the pact of friendship, she will experience both positive and negative behaviors with those friends she holds most dear. You can help your child develop her social skills and teach her how to make friends. Wanting to be liked and accepted, while feeling less popular than others, is the real emotional crisis of early childhood. In fact, your three-to-five-year-old will tell you just how she feels, expressing her emotions openly, vulnerable to heartbreaking tears of rejection, along with angry outbursts. Likewise, jealousy is common in early childhood, as children compete for the attention and affection from their friends and family.

Your three-to-five-year-old is still egocentric, believing that everyone she knows thinks and feels the way she does. She is just beginning to recognize that some people have wants and needs that are different. At this point, she's developing a conscience and a moral structure. Not only that, but she's beginning to know the rules, understanding that there's a right and wrong way to do things. As her spatial relationship develops, so does her judgment, and as a result, she senses that her actions will be assessed in relation to those rules. However, it will take some time before she really comprehends the reason for those rules and why they must be followed. Gradually, her thinking will evolve so that she will even question whether those rules can be changed.

HOW TO HELP YOUR CHILD MAKE FRIENDS

Learning to make friends is one of the most important skills your child can learn that will benefit him throughout his entire life. Having close friends has been known to help people live longer, happier lives, as well as become more successful at school and work.

Not all children are innately socially adept; some children who may be shy or have behavioral disorders such as ADHD may need additional assistance in learning age-appropriate social skills. However, all children can benefit from their parents guiding them in the friendship department.

THERE ARE SOME KEY TECHNIQUES YOU CAN USE WITH YOUR CHILDREN TO HELP THEM MAKE FRIENDS, EVEN FROM A VERY YOUNG AGE:

- **Teach simple, daily social greetings.** If you have a toddler or preschooler, you can teach your child about kindness by practicing simple daily interactions. You can ask your toddler to practice saying hello and good-bye, with a smile, to others, as you are out and about at the grocery store or at the park.
- **One-on-one playdates are important.** Invite one of the neighborhood kids over to your house for an afternoon of arts and crafts, playing dolls, or playing in the backyard. Take a trip to the library or museum with your child and invite a mom friend and her child of a similar age to join you. One-on-one playdates are the best opportunities for bonding and shared experiences that your child can build on when he goes to school.
- **Teach your child how to have conversations that lead to connections.** When my children were young, I would give them

icebreakers before we would enter social situations. They learned to ask questions such as "What's your favorite color?" or "What type of books do you like to read?" This helped them, from a young age, to make connections with others through shared interests and experiences. It also taught them the importance of being a good listener.

- **Help your child find interesting group activities.** Does your child like to sing or paint? Is your child really into sports? Help her by engaging her in clubs and activities with others who share her interests. Children like "sameness," and while you don't need to teach them to be followers, you can help them feel comfortable by leading them to situations where they have the opportunity to interact with other children who have similar likes and dislikes.

- **If you have a particularly anxious child, always listen and observe him carefully.** Give this child more time to rehearse and practice what he might say in social situations. Practicing and rehearsing social skills in a safe and warm environment, such as home, will support your child by teaching him social cues, as well as age-appropriate social skills and practices. Also, impulse control and empathy can be taught to your child. These strategies can help your child relate to his peers in a positive way.

- **Be what you want to see.** Modeling good social behavior yourself, of course, is one of the best ways to teach by example. Show your child how you warmly greet friends, how you empathize with them when they are dealing with a difficult situation, how you ask questions and listen carefully to their answers. Emphasize the importance these friends have in your life.

- **Keep in mind that your child will make mistakes socially because she is still immature and doesn't understand.** There's nothing wrong with your child; she just needs to be taught social skills and problem-solving on a regular basis until she can fully understand.

You have to know how to *be* a friend in order to *have* a friend. As a parent, you can help your child understand what it is to be a friend. It is your job to teach her about the importance of relationships rather than keeping her isolated, so that she can learn to build meaningful friendships throughout her lifetime.

One consistent conflict that parents grapple with in this area is the idea that children should share. There have been many diverse opinions on this subject. We discuss it briefly in Chapter 4. In my own family, I chose not to make my children share their personal things. My feeling is that when you force an action that involves someone else's belongings, whether it's a toy, clothes, or food, you diminish your child's sense of self, rendering her own control impotent. This behavior can cause your child to feel helpless and hopeless, believing that even her belongings don't belong to her. Your child has to have some sphere of influence, where she can learn independence and gain self-control. But if you make her share, you violate her tender and growing autonomy from which her own authority evolves. Yet there are consequences for not sharing, and these consequences are governed by your child's own choices. Now, you are teaching her about cause and effect, empowering her to make and trust her own decisions. This is how you build her sense of self, her security and self-esteem. As always, any lesson taught must be a lesson followed, so be what you want to see. The best way to teach about sharing is to share. Nonetheless, whether your child shares or not, it is imperative for you to honor her decisions. By honoring her choices, you are in essence validating your child, and the payoff here is that she will feel respected and valued. Similarly, the consequences of not sharing must also be accepted, and your child should know that if she doesn't share her whatever, with whomever, they don't have to share with her, either. These experiences are teaching moments, because if you are present and a problem arises, you can point out that the current situation might be the result of not sharing. Speak to your child in a nonthreatening, calm tone, explaining the natural consequence of not sharing. Over time, your child will share on her own, once she realizes that she doesn't have to defend herself against sharing. Ultimately, left to her own devices and peer-group socialization, your child will begin to share automatically. When she is ready to share on her own, she will.

HOW TO EFFECTIVELY DISCIPLINE YOUR CHILD WITH COMPASSION; THERE CAN BE NO FREEDOM WITHOUT LIMITS

You are well aware that your child needs structure to thrive. But structure for structure's sake misses the real objective: your routines must foster trust between you and your child. Letting your child "cry it out" in sleep training or resorting to corporal punishment floods your baby's brain with stress hormones that inhibit his growth in areas critical to higher-level thinking. You may have trained your baby to sleep—but you've seriously undercut his future.

There can be no freedom without discipline, and when two parents come together in one household, each bringing a different discipline style from their family of origin, it is important to mutually decide upon a discipline plan that works for your new family. Whatever it is, your plan must be consistent, fair, age-appropriate, equitable, and loving. The hard work occurs in the beginning, when you establish the rules and consequences for your child's behavior. My empathic process is a wonderful model for your family to all be invested in the process of discipline. When children are invested, even toddlers, in their own discipline, they are more likely to obey the rules that they helped craft. There are certain things, however, that are important in any discipline plan. For example, if you positively reinforce your child's good behavior consistently, he will perform consistently for your approval, as praise is one of the most effective reinforcing tools. On the other hand, if your child misbehaves, it is imperative to correct the behavior on the spot, without criticizing your child. For example, you could tell him that "he's a good boy, but that he did a naughty thing." By explaining to him that it was his behavior that was wrong, but that he is still a good boy, you inspire him, giving him the space to do better in the future. Always reiterate, no matter what the transgression, that you love him . . . though you don't like his bad behavior. An insecure child is more likely to act out, so what you want to do is consistently reassure your child that he is loved and valued. It is easier to reinforce good behavior than to remediate bad behavior.

Another important point is that in all intimate relationships, between parent and child or significant partners, the other must know that no matter what, whether she is right or wrong, she can count on you to be her advocate, because you love her. You want to build this in your child from the beginning, instilling in her that she can trust you, and that you will be there for her unconditionally. Trust is based on experience: if your child learns to trust you, she will develop self-trust. Moreover, by showing your child from the beginning that you can be counted on to be there for her, no matter what, she will feel he can call on you when she is in trouble. The most succinct letter I ever read was written by a therapist who worked with children involved with drugs and alcohol. As her son Johnny reached his teens, she wrote a public letter to him, which was published in the newspaper, telling him that though she hoped he wouldn't use drugs or alcohol, reminding him that such underage behavior was illegal, nevertheless, he could count on her to come and get him if he was inebriated . . . without any recriminations. This therapist was an advocate for her child, showing him that she could be depended on, while modeling for him what it is to be a reliable parent. Her essential message was clear and concise: she wanted him to trust her, and she wanted him to live. For her, what was most important was that he not have an accident and hurt himself or others.

ONE FINAL WORD ON DISCIPLINE

When creating your discipline plan, be certain to take your child's temperament into account. Each child's personality is unique unto himself. Some children just need a nod or a disapproving look to correct, adapt, or adjust their behavior, while other children may need a firmer approach. So, know your child, and you will save a lot of time and wasted energy by allowing his temperament to guide the discipline you employ.

Remember that young children dislike change, and some children have difficulty transferring from one activity to another, one place to another, or one event to another. In such cases, it is helpful to practice and prepare your child for change, so that he can transition smoothly, giving him enough time to adjust by telling him what to expect. Other children may still be more narcissistic, and therefore demanding. In those cases, it is helpful to create incentives and rewards, as well as positive reinforcement.

When talking about discipline, the question of spanking always comes up. And, as discussed in Chapter 2, research indicates[11] that children who are spanked are more likely to hit and display aggressive behavior. The American Academy of Pediatrics suggests[12] that corporal punishment is of "limited effectiveness with potentially deleterious side effects." Spanking found a home in past generations under the auspices of "spare the rod, spoil the child." But today, there are always alternative approaches that are more successful than spanking, without any negative side effects. Refer to Chapter 2 for more information on spanking.

MORALITY AND EMPATHY CAN BE TAUGHT

We first begin to see moral behavior at age three. It is at this stage that your child starts to think about her separateness, her place in the world, and her conscience. One of the few things that can actually be taught is empathy, and, ironically, what we notice about bullies and overly aggressive children is that they tend to have low empathy. Therefore, take advantage of this window of opportunity to teach your child the difference between right and wrong. Guide her to understand the consequences for her behavior and its effect on those around her. If your child is emotionally deprived in infancy, not touched enough, cuddled enough, talked to enough, she may not be able to experience either compassion or empathy for others, including the recipient of her behavior. Technology shows us that children so deprived in infancy don't fully develop cognitively and in some cases lack the appropriate connections for intimacy and close relationships.[13]

By raising your child to be empathetic and morally grounded, you inoculate him against the peer pressure that so often sabotages academic achievement. Even though children can't cognitively understand empathy until age eight or nine, your child will start modeling your emotional responses, reactions, and interactions as early as six months old. By using my empathic process, you can set the foundation for your child's sense of self-bonding, self-esteem, and a lifetime of meaningful relationships.

Teaching empathy to your child during this most important stage of social development will give you a full understanding of how empathy is passed on through environment, genetics, and epigenetics. In doing so, you'll remove social and emotional stumbling blocks throughout your child's entire life.

As a primate, you are a social learner, and according to Albert Bandura, you learn through imitation. As a parent, you can't help but notice that your child imitates everything you do and everything you say, whether you like it or not. So if you show empathy to your family and friends, your child will copy that. Knowing how social learning works, you can see how being polite, showing good manners, and having consideration will positively influence your child's social interactions. If you use words such as *please* and *thank you*, your child will do the same. If you make a point of setting a good example, your child will keep you on your toes, pointing out to you if you slip. It's a kinder, gentler approach than aggressive singular commands—it builds better language skills, a larger associative mass, and is a style that your child will be more inclined to respond to.[14]

FOSTERING BETTER CHILD BEHAVIOR

Your child is acting out, and you're feeling at your wit's end. You feel overwhelmed and frustrated and don't know what else to do. If you're a mom or a dad, you likely have—at one time or another—felt this way while parenting your child. While every situation is different, when a pattern of bad behavior emerges, there are a few elements that research has found to be consistent in fostering better behavior among children.

SIX STEPS TO A BETTER-BEHAVED CHILD

1. **Bonding.** Above and beyond anything is bonding with your child. If your child is well bonded, she feels secure and therefore may do better in all things. The secure child will be able to problem-solve better, stick to a task longer, and has better cognitive and social development. It is important, while bonding with your child, not to burden her with your problems. This can create anxiety and take her childhood away.

2. **Communication.** Active listening is the key to good communication between you and your child. In fact, active listening is the essential ingredient to family communication. It involves a safe environment in which confidences are kept. Trust based on experience is developed, eye contact is held, and full attention is given. Furthermore, it is important not to defend positions and to maintain empathy for all family members, including parents.

3. **Environment.** A safe space should be created in which you and your child sit together while communicating. This environment should not be anyone's power place such as an office, study, or bedroom, but rather a mutual place, such as the kitchen table, the heart of the house where alchemy happens. The empathic process should occur at least once a week at a set time—consistently.

4. **The Empathic Process.** My empathic process teaches empathy and mutuality by investing your child in family problem-solving, such as conflict resolution. Such participation in family

business empowers your child to feel that she has respect and responsibility, and therefore a choice in what happens to her, which establishes a win-win outcome for all.

5. **Consistent Follow-Through.** Following through in all things is imperative. If you are reliable and your child discovers that he can count on you to advocate for him—right or wrong—then he will value and trust himself. If your child values and trusts himself, he will transfer that trust to the world at large. This is how we make self-actualized children who are secure and proactive rather than reactive.

6. **Be What You Want to See.** Your child takes her cue from you. You are your child's first teacher, and as your child grows, she will look at you with a more critical eye. The best inoculation against behavioral problems with your child is to be a positive role model by having good nurturing skills, meeting her needs in a responsible way, and being reliable. Then your child will behave appropriately and choose to be responsible, with empathy and reliability.

When your child is invested in the process of creating the rewards and consequences for her behavior, she is more likely to behave. The empathic process has rules of engagement, which are flexible in relation to your particular family style. But in general, your child speaks for a prescribed amount of time while you listen intently, making eye contact. Then you, the parent, speak, giving your opinion without defending your position for the same amount of time. Then the entire family participates in the brainstorming period, which allows your child to be invested in the options for conflict resolution.

This is a successful problem-solving strategy, with positive regard for all. This approach works well for the assignment of chores, as well as their rotation, and allows you to keep a connection with your children, checking in on how they are doing in their social, emotional, and academic lives.

TEACH YOUR TODDLER EMPATHY

In our society, empathy is a critical component to helping us connect with others and interact with compassion and understanding. Being able to recognize another person's emotions and place yourself in their shoes, however, is a more complex skill than most people realize. It is not something you either have or don't have; we can each possess different degrees of empathy, and we can also continue to enhance our capacity for empathy throughout our lives.

Even though children don't have the cognitive skills to understand empathy fully until the age of eight or nine, parents can begin teaching empathy to their children early on. Even at six months old, babies look to parents to see how they react to strangers. However, the important developmental age is 18–24 months. This is when a toddler first realizes that other people have feelings that may be different from his own and begins to recognize himself as a separate person. At this stage, toddlers are able to soak up the social cues taught by their parents and build a foundation of strong social interaction that can help them grow into secure, compassionate adults.

TIPS TO HELP TEACH TODDLERS EMPATHY:

1. **Be what you want to see.** When parents model strong social interactions with others, children watch, learn, and mimic that behavior. When you show empathy to your friends, family, and strangers, your children learn that is how they should respond and interact with others.
2. **Involve children in charitable activities.** Even toddlers learn from accompanying you to donate used blankets and clothing to the local homeless shelter.
3. **Ask your child to think of others and role-play.** For example, if your child shares that his friend is moving away, ask your child not only how he feels about it, but also ask him to try to imagine what his friend feels about moving away. Empathy takes practice, and the more you talk with your child and ask

him to think about how others may be feeling, the more your child will begin to empathize with others on his own.

4. **Validate your child's feelings.** When your child is angry or upset, ask him to verbalize what he is feeling. Help your child learn to recognize and cope with these feelings, not push them aside. By learning how to be aware of his own feelings, he will be better equipped to know how to relate to others who are experiencing difficult emotions, as well.

5. **Praise your child when he shows empathy toward others.** Even though she may not realize what she is doing at the time, by pointing out that you saw her reach out and give a hug to that little boy who was hurt on the playground, you are reinforcing the importance and goodness of being compassionate toward others.

6. **Play a nonverbal guessing game.** When you're at the park, ask your child to guess how the child on the swings is feeling: "If she's laughing and her eyes are wide open, do you think she's happy and excited to be on the swings? What do you think?" or, "See that boy sitting by himself with his arms crossed, looking only at the ground? How do you think he is feeling?"

7. **As children get older, you can begin to engage them on a regular basis in my empathic process.** Each person gets equal time to talk without interruption, and without defense. Here, each child is invested in ideas and solutions. Everyone's feelings are considered. This process helps reinforce your basic social interaction modeling and teachings within your own family dynamic.

Teaching children empathy from a young age has many benefits, from helping them build a strong core to deflect peer pressure and bullying, to helping them grow into secure adults with the capacity for healthy relationships with others. Remember to have patience with your children; empathy is a complex skill that takes time to learn and understand.

Moral intelligence, like empathy, can be taught. There are many creative ways to help your child learn how to do unto others as she would have them do onto her. For example, games such as patty-cake and peekaboo reinforce the ideas of waiting your turn, give-and-take, and the necessity for reciprocity. And, your child will delight in actively participating in storytelling, where there is a moral to the story. Such morality tales can be the genesis for plays, games, active listening, the sharing of similar tales, and role-modeling, all fun activities, without once having to preach or lecture.

By the time your child is a toddler, she will have already recognized that certain games require certain rules, and she will respond appropriately. Though these rules are organized around games such as peekaboo, hide the cat, and so on, they are still laying the groundwork for moral reasoning. As your child participates in games with rules, she learns what is good and what is bad, what is right and what is wrong, and when she receives smiles and giggles, applause and approval for playing the game correctly, she is positively reinforced to follow the rules. It is only when your child understands the concept of rules that she can transfer that knowledge to a more developed sense of moral reasoning.

HOW TO MANAGE SIBLING RIVALRY

Ah, siblings. Your sisters and brothers may be your first friends . . . and your first enemies. Sibling rivalry is so powerful that it may even affect the roles that we take in a family, and the careers we choose for ourselves in the adult world. For example, due to competition with our siblings, what we pick for our life's passion may be in direct opposition to our brothers' and sisters' choices.

Strategies for preventing toddler sibling rivalry have the greatest opportunity for success, as they get the entire family off to a good start.

- Prepare your child for the birth of the new baby. Remember that your toddler didn't ask for a new brother or sister—in fact, he had no choice in the matter. The best thing that you can do to affect your child's security is to make him an ally. Include him in all preparations, such as shopping for the new baby, asking his opinion in the selection process. With a wink and a nod, this child can help you shop, choose toys, and even help select special foods for your new baby. If you bring your older child into the process, he or she will be more likely to participate with goodwill.

Furthermore, tell him the sex of the newborn ahead of time if you know it; involve him in the selection of the new baby's name, as well as all other planning activities, so that he feels in the loop. This invests your toddler in the process and will make him feel a part of things, so that he is more likely to feel secure and accepting of the new baby.

- Bring a gift for your toddler from the new baby when your new baby arrives home. This makes him feel special and connected to the baby and a part of the family unit.

- Never leave your toddler alone with your newborn. This is a prescription for trouble. Toddlers have no understanding of abstractions, and she can easily take her frustration out on the newborn without understanding the consequences.

- Reassure your child that he is loved and that there is a place for him in the family. Displacement is a common feeling for siblings and can be avoided by one-on-one time with Mom and Dad.

- Don't make your toddler give up his room for the new baby. No matter how you explain it, he will feel less then, and rightfully so. Moreover, do not make one sibling share his toys with the other. This takes away the newly found sense of control that children experience as they strike out toward self-mastery and independence. I can hear the oohs and ahhhs out there, but what belongs to your child is his possession, and only if it is his choice to share should it be brought into a common area.

- Remind your child of her place in the family. Show her family pictures that include her, as well as notes and cards saved from her birth. Children love to hear the story of their lives and bedtime is a perfect time for a cuddle and a real-life bedtime story.
- Reward your toddler for being the big brother by extending his bedtime ten minutes. This and other added privileges give a sibling the feeling that it is good to grow up, and that there are concrete benefits to doing so.
- Don't give the older child any added responsibilities associated with the new baby. This baby was not his idea and should not in any way become his burden. And that means to never make one child a babysitter for the other. Your child will learn to quickly resent the newborn if he is made to feel responsible for the baby.
- Space your children, if possible. Three years is good spacing, as one child is ready to get off your knee just when your newborn goes on.
- Be fair. Your child will look at you with a critical eye and already suspecting that you might love the new baby more. As a result, it is important that you be evenhanded in all things, including not always putting the baby's wants and needs ahead of his older sibling. Your toddler's feelings are very tender in this period of adjustment, and it is the wise parent who stays connected to his sensitivities and never compares one child with another.
- No competition, ever. No family games where one can win and one can lose. This is a family, not a sports arena, and children should be raised in collaboration, not competition. Never tell one child you love that child better than the other because she is behaving better. This is a form of splitting that can turn one child against the other forever.
- **Parents must parent.** This means to step into your adult, even overriding exhaustion to give each child some private time with Mom and Dad.

- **Never discount, demean, or embarrass your older children.** Never tell them to be a big girl or boy, to act grown-up, or to be understanding. They are children and they have feelings too. Instead, confirm their feelings with sentences such as "of course you feel this way, I understand completely." Your empathy goes a long way toward cooperation.
- **Never tell one child to do things the same way the other one does.**
- **Never discuss one child with the other.** You don't like it when someone talks behind your back; follow the same courteous behavior with your children.
- **Don't manipulate.** Manipulation is humiliation and makes your child feel undervalued, and he will not trust you, himself, or others if you diminish his self-esteem.
- **Practice and rehearse communication through listening.** Let your children tell you how they feel. If you listen with empathy, they will tell you everything, and together you can find ways to problem-solve. Invest your children in the process.
- **Finally, be prepared**. When holidays, birthdays, and family gatherings occur, think ahead and find ways as a family to come up with some rules, a plan that can help nip sibling rivalry in the bud.

Create a time and a quiet place to have a family conversation at least once a week where you can all take turns as a family talking about your feelings in an empathic way. This will help you to check in on your toddler and see how he is doing . . . and, most important, how he is feeling.

This empathic process should take place in a neutral space, such as a kitchen. It requires that each family member listen intently to the others without defense or discounting feelings, while investing one another in the options for problem-solving. This is how we make a family that is collaborative, not competitive—and whole, rather than split.

WHEN PARENTS FOSTER SIBLING RIVALRY

Remember when your mom asked, "Why can't you be as nice as your sister?" or "Your brother used to get A's in calculus, why are you barely getting B's?"

If you are a parent, have you found yourself making similar types of remarks to your own child? Sibling rivalries can be initiated by seemingly benign comments such as these. However, they can often escalate and plant the seeds for unhealthy sibling dynamics that can continue into adulthood. As a parent, you may be inadvertently fostering rivalry between your children; as a child, you may unwittingly be the pawn in your mother's or father's attempts at splitting and/or manipulating.

Parents who engage in this kind of conduct may, in some cases, actually be projecting their issues of low self-esteem, narcissism, lack of control, and insecurity onto their child. It's possible they were compared to their siblings and are now projecting their past experiences onto their own children. A form of splitting and/or manipulating occurs when parents compare and contrast their adult children in an effort to control them or make them jealous.

What's really happening is that parents use splitting and manipulating as a way of asserting their control. They play one child against the other or play favorites, implying that one child is preferred. But children are sensitive and perceptive and pick up on the nuances when it comes to matters of the heart. And when it comes to demonstrations of parental love and affection, they can detect favoritism and rejection immediately. If sustained over a long period of time, this parental splitting and manipulating can have lasting consequences.

All parents love their children; however, it is undeniable that for some parents, child-rearing is informed by their own problems. Ultimately, parents hold the power, and if they act in the best interests of their children, then they can leave a legacy of a happy, healthy family. In spite of their controlling and manipulating behavior, most parents do want their children to be close and not burdened with childhood jealousies.

WHAT CAN PARENTS DO?

1. Recognize and acknowledge your behavior. Ask yourself: "Am I creating hostility between my children in order to gain love, attention, control?"
2. Recognize that your children are separate individuals, and it is important not to compare them.
3. Step back and let your children individuate.
4. Seek counseling when needed.

Your first child receives 100 percent of what you have to give, and in the best of all possible worlds, that means a lot of love and attention. Therefore, your child has the best chance for bonding, nurturing, and having her needs met. Then, suddenly, without any choice, knowledge, or options, a stranger—the new sibling—is introduced into her world. Not only does this new person require a lot of time and attention, but also has seemingly replaced her as the center of Mom and Dad's universe.

At first, the new baby on board is a novelty, and your older child may even enjoy some of the busy activities going on, especially if she is included. But soon enough, your older child may begin to tire of the novelty and will want her place back as the sole recipient of Mom and Dad's attention. However, that is not going to happen. Not only that, but your child soon realizes that her place is gone . . . forever.

A nagging thought sits on the edge of the older child's consciousness: that maybe this new baby is loved the best. This is where things begin to heat up and the first sibling, out of frustration, may become duplicitous, as she tries to sabotage and even injure your new baby. A pinch or slap when no one is looking, hiding your younger child's toys, or even overt expressions of anger, such as "I don't want or like this new baby and I want you to send it back," are only a few examples of how difficult it can get.

The first sibling may become aggressive in general, even when your new baby is not around, or may regress into more childish and needy behavior, all in an effort to reclaim his rightful and now-lost place. This competition, if left without remediation, has the potential to generate a lifetime of negative patterns. Then, if another child is born into your family, the resources of Mom and Dad's time and attention are divided again.

And so it goes, until by the time your last child is born, the competition for goods and services is very scarce indeed. To further complicate things, your young child is thinking in concrete terms, meaning he is both egocentric and unable to process his emotions critically. Therefore, when he is emotionally upset, he strikes out reactively instead of thinking about things and choosing the best course of action.

His understanding of the here-and-now is concrete, and he doesn't really understand the difference between a city, a state, a universe . . . or life and death. He is magical in his thinking and believes that what is killed today will rise up tomorrow. Since the brain is still forming, your child might develop patterns based on these early frustrations that could stay with him for a lifetime, influencing the way he thinks and feels not only about his brother or sister but also about other significant relationships.

HOW TO HELP YOUR TODDLER THROUGH YOUR DIVORCE

Toddlers are still in need of bonding and attachment. Thus, divorce may create regressive, needy behavior in toddlers as a reaction to feelings of abandonment. When a parent leaves the home for good, it can be very disturbing, and visitation can cause both clinging and aggressive behavior. Parents can minimize the negative impact by working together as a team.

1. Engage in age-appropriate conversations with your toddler. You must support your toddler by explaining that there will be a divorce and that one parent will not be living at home. This conversation should happen *before* the divorce occurs.

2. Assure your toddler that she is not to blame for the separation.

3. Reassure your toddler that though you and your soon-to-be ex-spouse no longer wish to live together, you both love her.

4. Don't burden your child with your own emotional problems.

5. Never criticize the other parent or fight in front of your toddler.

6. Don't put your toddler in a loyalty bind. That will only backfire on your toddler, causing tension, stress, and emotional problems.

7. Stabilize your toddler as quickly as possible by sticking to routine and being consistent with your discipline.

8. Keep a structured schedule for your home routine and for parental visits. This will give your toddler a routine that she can count on—that alone can help reestablish security.

9. Talk with your toddler about her concerns and allow her to grieve and talk to others about her feelings. Secrets are suppressed feelings that can cause emotional problems.

Above all, shower your toddler with love. You can never love your child too much, and a divorce is a time when she will need your love and security the most.

HOW TO MANAGE SIBLINGS FROM BLENDED FAMILIES

Not too long ago, I was at dinner with some friends and they were all talking about their children. One of our friends made a most interesting remark when he said he was raising his wife's son and somebody else was raising his.

This made me think about all of the different family structures we have today, and how siblings from these different arrangements can find their way to one another in relationship. There is no longer any one face called family, but rather family types made up of full siblings, half-siblings, and stepsiblings.

Here are some steps you can take to ensure that your children be given the best chance for peace and harmony within their immediate and extended families, to secure a healthy and vital life together:

1. **Communicate.** Sit down with your mate and, using my empathic process, discuss what your different styles of discipline, traditions, and family expectations are. Ask what you can do together to build a new structure that fits your new family. By creating a "new normal," you and your spouse will allow children to let go of the past and be cocreators, forming something new that works for your family.

   Consider also that you, as well as your children, are in a transition period. Thus, to transform your relationship into a family, it may be necessary in the beginning to spend a little alone time with your biological children, so that they know their place is secure in your heart. Remember that this is the first time your children will have to share you with someone else's children—siblings that they neither asked for nor necessarily wanted. Because children of blended families have no options about new siblings, they may feel out of control. Helping them assert feelings of stability and security may require more parental time.

2. **Know the rules.** Using my empathic process, sit down with all siblings contained in your new family and actively listen to your children's feelings and thoughts about their new family. Ask them what they think the appropriate rules should be within your family unit. Divide time for discussion equally between parents and siblings, giving each child ample time to express his or her feelings without defense. Finally, bring the conversation together, so that each member of the family is invested in both the rules and the consequences for family management and discipline. This is how you proactively build

a new family model, with new ground rules including routine, structure, boundaries, and mutual respect.

3. **Create a family identity.** By creating a new family identity, you connect each member of the family to a future together. Let siblings share chores so that they have to depend on one another to accomplish them. Take family trips together, where games, outings, and activities—such as boating, camping, biking, and hiking—depend on cooperation and collaboration. Participate as a family in all sibling activities. Go as a unit to ball games, recitals, and school plays. Build your home team and create new memories, filled with family times spent together. This is how siblings become part of a family identity and feel that they belong.

4. **Ask for help when needed.** It is important to recognize when it is necessary to get outside guidance. Each parent knows his child the best. You know his history and how that history influences his behavior.

   Therefore, it is important to look for signs of distress such as behavior problems at home and in preschool or kindergarten, changes in sleep habits, weight gain or loss, threats of suicide, changes in friendships, regressive behavior such as bed-wetting, nail-biting or hair-pulling, sadness or depression. Consulting a professional can go a long way toward restoring your family's health and well-being. In the end, remember that your family is transforming, so move from your heart, with compassion and empathy.

WHY KIDS BRAG AND WHAT PARENTS CAN DO ABOUT IT

"I am the best reader in the whole class!"

"I am so much smarter than all of my friends."

Sound familiar? There are several reasons why children brag. They are still learning how to navigate socially in this world, and it is our job as parents to help guide them with love and compassion.

Reasons your child may be bragging:

1. If your child is bragging, it may indicate that he has low self-esteem, lacks self-confidence, or is immature. Therefore, bragging helps your child feel better by making him larger and more inflated than he really is. By enhancing his experiences and accomplishments, he pivots himself onto a higher plane than his peers. For example, if your child has something more than his friend or something better, and he feels insecure, then inflated achievements can make others appear less while elevating his status.

2. Your child may be bragging to establish her position in the family and the outer world. For example, a middle child who feels lost in her parents' attention may brag to find a space in which to feel special. All children want to be accepted and loved, and sometimes bragging is their effort to accomplish it.

3. Your child may be bragging to feel important and gain attention. Because your child doesn't have the social or coping skills that adults do, bragging becomes a technique to find and create friendships. Meanwhile, he is unaware that bragging can make others move away from him and even dislike him. Since bragging is an antisocial behavior, it can actually heighten your child's sensitivity, causing insecurity and loneliness.

4. Your bragging child may be modeling or imitating Mom or Dad, brother or sister. We are social animals, and we learn through social modeling. Children often copy what they see around them and what seems to work for others.

So what can you do if your child brags?

To curb bragging, it is important for parents to help develop a child's feelings of self-confidence and good self-esteem.

1. You can follow my empathic process. Discuss with your child, in a nondefensive and nonthreatening way, how others feel about bragging and why it's not working for him.

2. Teach your child better social skills and cues. Practice and rehearse those social skills at home until they become second nature to your child. Through role-modeling and creating new and healthier habits for social interactions, you will teach your child how to make friendships with both confidence and competence.

3. Help your child understand that others dislike bragging and avoid people who brag. You might ask how he feels when his friends brag, and what he thinks of friends who brag.

4. Teach your child that she is valued and loved unconditionally. In doing so, you will open the door for successful friendship experiences that will grow along with your child.

5. Remember to know your child and listen to your child. Then, you can offer praise when it is earned and love unconditionally.

6. Finally, be what you want to see. Your children will mimic your behavior. Don't brag yourself, or you will find that you are fostering this behavior within your own family.

By making sure your child knows how important and loved she is, she will not need to make herself larger in the eyes of others. Remember that your child is vulnerable; she needs to be noticed and seen to feel that you are proud of her and that you appreciate and love her for who she is. Then, she doesn't have to brag to feel good about herself or to feel as if she belongs. This will help her find her place within your family and her social circle.

WHO IS THE GIFTED CHILD? CHARACTERISTICS, SPECIAL NEEDS, AND APPROPRIATE INSTRUCTIONAL TECHNIQUES FOR THE GIFTED CHILD

Gifted children are, by definition, "children who give evidence of high performance capability in areas such as intellectual, creative, artistic, leadership capacity, or specific academic fields, and who require services or activities not ordinarily provided by the school in order to fully develop such capabilities."[15]

According to a study by Thompson, Berger, and Berry[16] there is a biological difference between the gifted child and the typical child. The gifted child seems to have an increased cell production, which also increases synaptic activity. This all adds up to an increased thought process. The neurons in the brain of the gifted child seem to be biochemically more abundant, and, as a result, the brain patterns that develop are able to process more complex thought. There seems to be more prefrontal cortex activity in the brain, which leads to insightful and intuitive thinking.[17] Gifted children have more alpha wave activity in the brain. They not only get more alpha wave activity faster than the typical child, but they also sustain it longer. This allows for more relaxed and focused learning with greater retention and integration.[18] The brain rhythms of the gifted child occur more often, and this allows for concentration, attention, investigation, and inquiry.

The characteristics of the gifted child, according to Barbara Clark, the author of *Growing Up Gifted*, include self-disciplined, independent, often antiauthoritarian; zany sense of humor; able to resist group pressure, a strategy developed early; more adaptable; more adventurous; greater tolerance for ambiguity and discomfort; little tolerance for boredom; preference for complexity, asymmetry, open-endedness; high in divergent thinking ability; high in memory, good attention to detail; broad knowledge background; needs think periods; needs a supportive climate, sensitive to environment; needs recognition, opportunity to share; high aesthetic values, good aesthetic judgment; freer in developing sex role integration; lack of stereotypical male or female identification.

However, the characteristics of the gifted child do differ on the basis of sex.[19] The characteristics of the female gifted child include liking school, especially courses in sciences, music, and art; liking their teachers; regularly read news, magazines, and other nonrequired reading and special reports; active in dramatics and musical productions; do not go out on dates as often; are daydreamers.

The characteristics of the male gifted child include disliking school; disliking their teachers and thinking they are uninteresting; doing little homework; dislike physical education and seldom engage in team sports; are regarded as radical or unconventional; and often want to be alone to pursue their own thoughts and interests.

The gifted child also appears to have his share of emotional stresses. Studies indicate that the gifted child, in fact, may have lower self-esteem than the average child. There seems to be a direct correlation between the high expectations that the gifted child has for himself and the unrealistic goals for which he strives. This situation tends to cause anxiety, as the gifted child pushes himself unrealistically. Another factor in the gifted child's often low self-concept seems to be that parents feel obliged, on occasion, to push this child, feeling that having such a child creates the extra responsibility to oversee his educational progress. Teachers and parents alike can help the gifted child with problems of self-esteem if they first recognize that the problem exists and then help establish more realistic goals for them, more appropriate behavioral responses. As a result of the pressure placed on the gifted child by himself and his adult community, he becomes frustrated, developing compulsive behaviors such as perfectionism. Not only can this child establish unrealistic standards for himself, but he all too often develops high expectations of others. This creates a strain in his interpersonal relationships, as he becomes unaccepting of more typical behavior. Parents and teachers can alleviate this situation by helping the gifted child understand the dynamics of his behavior, teaching him more appropriate responses.

Another issue that arises with the emotional interplay of the gifted child and his community of peers is the feeling of self-doubt. Because the gifted child is usually heterogeneously grouped, he can usually participate in class without the same preparation needed by his peers. As a result, he may find himself becoming a lazy student who has developed poor learning habits. The gifted child is often so verbally skilled that a little bit of bluff goes a long way. Unfortunately, all of these behaviors tend to create an environment in which the brain function of the gifted child slows down. Because he doesn't need to develop his learning skills and integrate them with his abilities, he risks the potential for loss. This child's high intellectual ability is often accompanied by a high anxiety level, for he is in a sense bright enough to be extrasensitive to himself. When asked to perform academically in an area for which he is not prepared, the gifted child will become very upset, feel helpless and lost, and begin the process of blocking. Couple this with the fact that parents and teachers often withhold praise from the gifted child, saving it as a behavioral modification technique, causing him to become confused and discouraged. He can lose his sense of reality in relation to his abilities, for without appropriate appreciation for quality work, this child has no parameters by which to judge himself. His contributions lose their relevance, and the gifted child can develop negative feelings about his own self-worth. As a result, the gifted child may decide to copy the behavior around him, the behavior that seems to be getting all the rewards. While imitating others for acceptance and approval, the gifted child often misplaces himself. For an older child, this behavior can present itself by underperforming academically, showing off, and acting silly. Seeking conformity and peer acceptance, the gifted child will adapt to whatever it takes to make him feel good—and as bright as he is, his adaptability is quite strong. In a culture that doesn't really reward intellectual precocity (Torrance, 1969), the gifted child may, in fact, lose his gift simply because he is not being nurtured and understood.[20]

This raises the issue of just how much a role the environment plays in the life of a gifted child. There seems to be a direct relationship between the level of gene activity and cell development (Krech, 1969; Rosenzweig, 1966), and, furthermore, this activity directly influences learning. Differential experience can change not only the anatomical picture of the brain, but also its chemical composition. In a study that appeared in the *Journal of Comparative Neurology* involving two groups of rats from the same genetic strain, it was concluded that environments could, in fact, alter the brain's capacity to learn. One group of rats was raised in a nonstimulating environment, each one living alone in a small, dimly lit cage. The control group was allowed to have a mesh wire cage from which they were allowed to venture for thirty minutes a day. This group was also given toys to play with and experienced the general interaction that was present in the laboratory environment. Both groups were given identical food and standard health care. The rats that lived in the stimulated environment, upon examination, had significantly larger brain cortexes that were also thicker and fatter than the deprived group. And the glial cells, which are directly connected to the nutrition received by the neurons of the brain, affecting the learning potential of the brain, were increased in size and number. There was also evidence that the diameter of the blood cells that supply the cortex were larger, and there was a chemical change in these brains. They had more acetylcholinesterase, which is the enzyme present in the Tran synaptic conduction of neural impulses, and cholinesterase, another enzyme that is found in glial cells. Further studies indicated that there is a reduction of these enzymes with age and, hence, the loss of both memory and brain function so prevalent in the elderly. When the rats that lived in the stimulated environment were placed into a deprived environment, their brains went back to their normal size. However, the chemical changes remained stationary. Additionally, the rats from the enriched environment with enlarged cortexes and chemical changes were, in fact, smarter. Another experiment quite similar to this was undertaken with blind and seeing rats. In this study, the blind rats were placed in the stimulated environment. As a result, the blind rats, though handicapped, were better learners.

In conjunction with these studies and others like them, educators and researchers are beginning to feel that early intervention in education and stimulation in the gifted child's environment is imperative. Even traumatic stimulation was shown to be preferable to no stimulation. Another study demonstrated that stimulated animals were more emotionally stable, more curious, and more able to learn to concentrate and have appropriate coping responses.[21]

The needs of the gifted population, therefore, are very important. The gifted child needs, first and foremost, a teacher who is trained to teach gifted children—one who is not intimidated, threatened, or irritated by the gifted child. Then this "gifted teacher" needs both home and school cooperation so that he or she can hand-tailor a curriculum that is individualized for the gifted child. The gifted child needs to be appreciated, respected, and rewarded appropriately for quality work and quality behavior. Furthermore, this special child's sensitivities need to be understood, for the gifted child can learn negatives with the same fervor and accelerated ability that she can positives. She is the leader of tomorrow, and therefore it is our responsibility to train her so that her best assets can be used in service to the community.

Clearly, one of the most significant steps in educating and guiding the gifted child is an individualized curriculum created for his needs. Torrance suggests that educators create a curriculum that encompasses a cooperative learning environment. Several appropriate instructional techniques include individualized teaching, homogenous grouping for certain subjects, small cluster grouping, and an environment that fosters the freedom to continue learning at one's own rate of speed. The teacher must become the facilitator. Educators must include in their curriculum the concepts of differentiating characteristics, related needs, organizational patterns, and classroom strategies. In the final analysis, the variable for all people is love and understanding. Thus, with a nurturing environment, the gifted child will obtain his best opportunity for growth.[22]

WHO IS THE UNDERACHIEVER? CHARACTERISTICS, SPECIAL NEEDS, AND APPROPRIATE INSTRUCTIONAL TECHNIQUES FOR GIFTED UNDERACHIEVERS

Gifted underachievers have personal characteristics that are quite different from their gifted counterparts, and the environment plays a significant role. According to Torman and Oden, the characteristics of the gifted under-achievers are that their academic performance does not equate to their measured IQ cognitive ability or intellectual aptitude; their behavior fits an explainable pattern of insecurity and low self-esteem; lack of self-confidence; the inability to persevere; lack of integration to goals; the presence of inferiority feelings; and a narrow range of interests as psychological energy is drained from repressing negative feelings. The cost of expending all that negative energy eliminates that energy from creative and productive behavior, leading the gifted child to blame others for his failures.[23]

A significant factor in the underachieving gifted child is his relationship with his nuclear family. Pierce and Bowman state that the father is a factor of potential influence to this child. In a study that they conducted with both high achievers and underachievers, they reached the following conclusions:[24]

1. High achievers felt that their father was the most important influence in their lives.
2. Underachievers named males other than their father; for example, a teacher, an uncle, or a priest.
3. The underachievers had inadequate relationships with their fathers and were unable to express their negative feelings.

From this information, both Pierce and Bowman demonstrate that the underachieving gifted child, in effect, has lost his parental role model in relation to family values and standards. Also, it appears that the more reject-ing and punitive the father, the more this child suffers from low self-es-teem.[25] In another study conducted by Karnes, McCoy, Zehrbach, Studley, and Wright, the fathers of underachievers were more hostile than the fathers of students who achieved to their fullest potential. This study also indicated that gifted underachievers are not bored, which is a popular myth, but rather undercreating and having trouble in their social relationships. The underachiever from these studies scored lower, for example, on fluency, flexibility, and originality and had lower ratings in peer relationships.[26]

Finally, the pupil who feels unhappy in an unaccepting home environment develops defense mechanisms for coping. The very mechanisms that she uses to maintain an equilibration at home create an unaccepting view of the world at large. This child has, in fact, learned through experience and imitation and therefore reflects back to the world what she has learned from her family's interaction.

The mother's role in the family unit seems to have less influence in relation to the underachiever. The most dramatic influence that mothers can have is one of a laissez-faire attitude. As discussed in his book *Family Interaction, Values, and Achievement,* Strodtbeck studied family and cultural relationships and concluded that when the power structure was equal between parents, children had the best opportunity to achieve to their fullest potential.[27] However, if the power balance in the family unit was tilted strongly in the direction of the punitive father, the pupil was more likely to underachieve. He further concluded that a strong, dominant mother could offset a rigid and authoritarian father. And if the mother and father were both rigid authoritarians, then the same situation would occur. Also discussed in Strodtbeck's book, in a study that he conducted on the emotional issues of the underachieving gifted student (which appeared in the book *Family Interaction Values and Achievement*), Pierce found that a significant problem that arose from a strong and unaccepting father was the child's failure to identify with the values of his dominant parent. If the child happened to be the same sex as his father, then he had the further problem of not being able to introject or take into himself the standards and values of his parent. Because the pupil rejects the role-modeling from his family, he turns to his peer group for parenting. Unfortunately, he gravitates to peers who are similar in ideology to himself.

Therefore, this gifted underachiever often relates to an underachieving social clique. A study conducted by Walsh indicated that because underachieving boys felt less accepted by their families, they were more constricted in their actions and more negativistic and defensive to their outside community.[28] Therefore, since their families displayed unfriendly attitudes toward them, they were hesitant to accept the values of that family or society. They harbored feelings of hostility as a result and expended a lot of energy both controlling and disguising that hostility. This expenditure of energy is so great that these children often have little left for creative outside interests. The investment of preserving some semblance of balance causes them to shift the blame for their failures onto others. An interesting characteristic of these children is that they block their feelings of insecurity and fail to realize that they have the capability to help themselves. These children become very magic-oriented and hope that fate or luck will intervene on their behalf.

The distinguishable behavioral patterns of underachieving gifted children manifest early in their lives. Studies have been done in which the records of adult underachievers were tracked back into elementary school, and these records were consistent with the adult's current underachieving problems. Shaw and McCuen cited that underachievement in gifted children is, in fact, a chronic problem.[29] This problem, they believed, would remain consistent throughout life without long and arduous early intervention. Girls, interestingly, do not display their underachieving patterns until approximately the ninth grade, and it is believed that this has to do more with sex identification than with academic know-how. Unless a major attempt is made to counteract these patterns at an early age, underachievers run the risk of becoming relatively unproductive members of society, both to their detriment and to ours. There is a continuing problem in these children that stems from their personality and social interactions. Early education, therefore, must include remediation in the realms of both the academic and the emotional. The teacher, in effect, is asked to not only be understanding, but to translate that understanding into a program that can improve both the underachiever's performance and her confidence.

Perkins stated that one of the most prominent features of an underachieving child was the characteristic of withdrawal, especially in the area of mathematics.[30] He explained this phenomenon as directly related to the student's defense mechanisms. If a child is insecure and fearful, he will, in effect, block those feelings in an effort to defend himself against them and their pain. The brain, however, is unable to clearly compartmentalize that blocking, and as a result, the pupil blocks out everything. Math is especially affected because it requires a logical progression of thought, and the high anxiety of the underachiever prohibits that pattern.

Some other trends cited by Perkins include frequent engaging in nonacademic work; more time spent in social non-work-oriented interaction with peers; classroom behavior that was nonadaptive for effective learning; the student's desire to escape from unpleasant experiences kept him from effective confrontation with his environment; the escape patterns and defense reactions were trends that defended the self at all costs; and withdrawal.

Morrow and Wilson found that underachievers were more compulsive, more adventurous, more restless, more dissatisfied with life, had a negative and often hostile peer group, and sought and operated within a nonproductive environment.[31]

French and Carden believed the underachieving gifted child to be vocationally confused. Not only did he feel pressured to conform to school, but also to the academic orientation of school. This child struggles for individuation and is therefore often viewed as a rebel. Many bright dropouts, in fact, are more interested in vocational courses than college preparatory courses. As a result, French and Carden suggest that a more sensible vocational program be created within the public school system, supported by an appropriate guidance system.[32]

To better understand the scope of this problem, one must first realize that underachievement is a total way of life. Therefore, an educational program for underachievers must include a comprehensive base. Baymur and Patterson suggest that such a program include family counseling; a special school environment, which might include homogenous grouping; peers who are better models for imitation; and personal counseling, which would aid in defining both goals and aspirations.

In a study conducted by Baymur and Patterson in which they divided underachievers into four groups and offered each group a different type of counseling, they demonstrated that parent-child group therapy was the most effective.[33] The least effective type of counseling was one in which the pupil was reprimanded for his underachievement and given a pep talk to remediate it. This is the type of approach that parents and teachers use most often. One of the reasons given for the success of the parent-child group therapy remediation was that by placing the child on an equal footing with his parents, he felt more self-respect and more self-esteem. Therefore, the underachiever is given a sense of independence as well as adult acceptance. Ultimately, a result of this type of therapy led the student to recognize the abstract concept that if others could accept him, he might be able to accept himself. Of course, this kind of therapy, though most effective, is quite time-consuming. The profile of the most successful therapist is, of course, the professional therapist, for he is trained well enough to be able to transfer to the underachiever the recognition that he is okay. One other significant factor of this type of counseling is that the child realizes that he is not alone with his problems or in his world. One effect of breaking down this feeling of isolation is the building up of self-worth. It is at this point that real communication can begin between parent and child, for once his reactions and feelings of resentment and hostility are effectively expressed, he can begin to constructively build appropriate behavioral techniques.

Another facet of this educational program should include classroom modification, which would, in fact, bring a remedial concept into school. A very successful classroom modification was studied by Goldberg, in which all children with IQs over 120 were placed in the same classroom and all classes were self-contained.[34] This allowed the underachiever to be exposed to children with similar intellectual ability and superior academic know-how. The study stated that underachievers grouped in such a way did perform better than they did before. Some reasons for this success:

1. The children were given more interesting and stimulating information.
2. They had better peer-group identification.
3. They had ample opportunity for teacher help with both personal and academic problems.

As a result of these findings, Goldberg concluded that manipulating the educational environment was a very successful tool for helping underachievers.

HOW TO FOSTER YOUR CHILD'S UNIQUE GIFTS

If there is one thing attending TED 2013 proved, it is this: no matter how young or how old we are, we all have unique gifts and talents. When sixteen-year-old Jack Andraka took the stage, I was impressed by this young man's ability to develop an early detector for pancreatic cancer. I wondered: what sort of encouragement must this child have received at home to doggedly pursue lab access from two hundred different professors before finally receiving a positive reply from Dr. Anirban Maitra of Johns Hopkins School of Medicine?

Andraka's mother once told the *Baltimore Sun*, "We're not a super athletic family. We don't go to much football or baseball. Instead we have a million [science] magazines and sit around the table and talk about how people came up with their ideas and what we would do differently."[35]

This sort of encouragement follows the discovery learning model. Discovery learning is a way of exploring concepts in order to develop new ideas, and new models of thinking and behavior. Instead of being given concrete answers, children learn by trying, and discarding, as well as investigating options and discussing possibilities.

For example, when my children were young, my husband would drive a different route to school each day. This simple activity showed my children that there was more than one way to solve a problem. Andraka's family, by providing a print-rich environment with exposure to science books and magazines, created easy access to exploration and experimentation.

While your child may not necessarily develop a medical breakthrough, as Andraka did, encouraging your child with activities that support the discovery learning model can help foster the discovery of her unique gifts and talents.

Here are six simple ways you can incorporate the discovery learning model into your family life today:

1. After school, ask your child to share one thing she enjoyed about her day. What surprised her about that one thing? How did she feel about it?

2. The next time you read a book to your toddler or preschool age child, pause and ask her what she thinks will happen next, or how she thinks a character is feeling or what a character is thinking at that moment.

3. When your child is faced with a problem that has her stumped, do not give her a definite answer, but instead ask questions such as "What would happen if you chose Path A versus Path B? How would that choice make you feel?"

4. If a toy or machine breaks in the house, ask your children to help come up with different solutions to fix it.

5. Have your child cook dinner and allow her to decide what to cook, which ingredients to use, and how the meal should be prepared. When your child asks a question about the proper way to cook something, respond with another question that helps her figure out the answer on her own.

6. Let your child experiment with different creative opportunities without judgment or commitment. For example, if your child is interested in trying a new musical instrument, rent the instrument instead of buying it. Another example is visiting your local interactive museums, such as the Museum of Science in Boston. Childhood is a time for creative play, and children must test their boundaries without formal instruction or constraint.

The discovery learning model is a simple, yet effective way of engaging your child's brain in a thoughtful way. By encouraging your child to seek out answers, tapping into her innate curiosity and removing the roadblocks of what is correct and incorrect, you allow room in your child's brain for the associations that stimulate creativity and innovation. This can lead to amazing discoveries of your child's unique gifts and talents that might otherwise never have come to the forefront.

YOUR 3-TO-5-YEAR-OLD'S NUTRITION

Children today are showing earlier signs of food-related health problems. Paying attention to their diet can be as important as focusing on any other developmental problem. For example, blueberries can actually alleviate stress and increase concentration. So eating blueberries before a test or any other stressful event is using food for its truest values, as it helps your child gain control by deliberately affecting his own behavior. Learning about food and its effect on a growing mind and body can be an important asset in your child's developmental bank. There is a lot of general information out there on nutrition, and contemporaneous studies indicate that because organic foods are free from pesticides, they are healthier. As a result, anything that you can purchase that's organic, such as fruits, vegetables, legumes, and grains, will serve your child better by helping to reduce the potential for allergens and toxins. If your child does not have to fight toxic chemicals and allergens in his body, he will feel and perform at his optimal level.

Sadly, even our oceans have been corrupted by chemicals, and now you have to be aware of the mercury levels in fish such as tuna, swordfish, shark, tilefish, and mackerel. These fishes should be avoided when you are pregnant or breastfeeding, because mercury can be dangerous to a growing fetus and infant. Salmon, on the other hand, is lower in mercury and higher in essential fatty acids. So educate yourself to be a wise shopper, read labels, and keep nutritional information current.

Along with modernity, one of the unintended consequences of an affluent society is its abundant and excessive consumption of culinary delights, especially those prepared with sugar. Exposed to a sweet taste right in the womb, and later in mother's breastmilk, your baby is primed, right from the start, to eat sugar. However, these sugars are simple carbohydrates, basically empty calories that not only absorb rapidly in the blood, but also cause a rise in insulin levels and a spike in blood sugar. All of this converges to accelerate the conversion of calories into fat. Moreover, deviations in blood sugar can cause your child to feel tired on the down sugar load, and hyper when blood sugar zooms up. This scenario is one of the factors contributing to both hyperactivity and the epidemic of childhood obesity.

On the other hand, organic vegetables, legumes, whole grains, fruits, and organic soy products are all rich in fiber and necessary to a balanced, healthy diet. Additionally, fiber has the advantage of filling your child up without burdening her body with a high caloric intake, while slowing down food absorption and stabilizing her blood sugar.

HOW TO HELP YOUR OVERWEIGHT CHILD

First and foremost, it is important to know your child. Know your child's emotional history and pay attention to her eating habits. You have to be able to identify a problem before you can craft a solution. Obesity is complex and individual. Childhood obesity has become a national epidemic with many health risks. Type 1 or juvenile diabetes, for example, is on the rise among children, while emotional problems such as self-esteem, depression, anorexia, and bulimia are right behind it.

Children with obesity problems find themselves out of step with their peers. They look different; they may feel embarrassed and experience self-loathing, and they are often shunned by other students, teachers, and parents. Parents play a crucial role in helping their children regain a positive self-image, as well as self-control. This can only happen if children are taught how to manage their own eating habits and develop coping skills to handle stress. The difficulty here is that unlike other addictive behavior, food cannot be given up—it has to be moderated. Children have to feel that it's hip to be fit, and reeducated to understand the role that food plays in their lives—both emotional and physical. Only then can children be taught stress-reduction techniques, healthy eating habits, and physical exercise.

THE THREE KEYS TO A LIFELONG PATTERN OF HEALTH AND VITALITY
1. PARENTS MUST BE WHAT THEY WANT TO SEE

It is true that the role-modeling that parents do at home in relation to physical exercise, nutrition, and self-esteem is the first social learning that their children encounter. Parents must step into their adult and, in a sense, override their own addictive behavior to organize a kitchen that is weight-healthy. That means a refrigerator filled with fruits, vegetables, and proteins, as well as low-fat dairy, sets the tone for healthy eating. Remember not to throw out the baby with the bathwater and include healthy complex carbohydrates in your family's food repertoire. The pantry should consist of low-fat, low-sugar snacks, and breads should be of the whole wheat, rye, or pumpernickel variety, so that the calories taken in have value.

Shopping can be a family affair and a lot of fun. It can be used as a teaching moment, bringing children along and shopping around the perimeter of the store, where all the healthy items can be found—the fruits, the vegetables, the fish, the meat—all wholesome, and real energy-producing calories. Menus can be planned for the week with the family, keeping in mind that Mother and Father can be teaching all along things like blueberries are rich in Vitamin B, and therefore brain food; fish is high in nucleic acid, and therefore good for your skin; celery is good for your micro biome and is mostly water, and therefore minus calories; and so on. When food is looked at in this way, different foods can be eaten for different outcomes, such as blueberries with cereal in the morning before a test at school. In fact, when low-calorie foods are chosen for meals, children can actually eat more and weigh less.

Cooking is a great adventure and an expressive art in itself. Children love activities where they can interact with their parents, and what better activity than the alchemy of cooking in the kitchen—the heart of the house? It is exciting for children when parents create recipes with them that are both good-tasting and good for you. This can be a fun adventure in good eating, and the beginning of a pattern of creating lifelong healthy eating habits.

Eating should be promoted as something sacred, a ritual. It shouldn't be a mood elevator, a stress reducer, or a reward or consequence. It shouldn't be done in any room in the house other than the dining room or kitchen, and, most important, it should be done at the table, deliberately and consciously, not on the run. Children should be taught about digestion, and that chewing their food for a certain amount of time helps it break down, so that it can be used by the body more efficiently.

Gratitude before meals sets the stage for sanctity, recognizing the importance of food to survive. This helps children make the connection between food and their bodies. With children who have anorexia or bulimia, we see a disconnect between food and body image. All of us remember a favorite relative who filled her food with love . . . and we knew it. That is because food is a source of energy that actually reflects the emotional energy of its maker. Therefore, children can become aware of not only what they eat and put in their bodies, but who prepared it.

Finally, it is also important to remember that fluid has calories: fruit juices, though healthy, may have too many, if overused. Diet drinks and colas are loaded with sodium, empty calories, and sometimes caffeine. One makes you retain fluid, while the other increases your appetite. Be aware of what you prepare for your children. Stay away from fast foods because of their high fat content, as well as sugar and sugar substitutes that may contain a lot of salt. If children like the idea of TV dinners, buy the containers in the grocery store and fill them up together with your own healthy foods. Then, freeze your homemade TV dinners and save them for a special occasion, when you and your child share the joy of having created your own TV dinner together.

2. STAY ACTIVE

A walk after dinner with the whole family can become a family tradition, as well as biking and hiking on the weekends. Exercise doesn't have to be excessive or stressful, but it does have to be consistent, as it has two very important functions—to burn calories and reduce stress, two very significant players in the role of weight reduction. Even gardening with your child as a weekend project will burn calories and has the added advantage of seeing something grow out of a family effort. Every gardener knows what a great reward that is.

3. STRESS REDUCTION, WEIGHT, AND SELF-ESTEEM

By limiting sedentary activities such as watching television, we are also restricting mindless eating, often stimulated by food commercials, which are created to subliminally entice eating. There is a direct link between eating and television-viewing, and parents are called upon to both control and inhibit excessive behavior in both things.

Parents need to monitor media marketing and discuss commercials with their children as a way to dispel misinformation about food. This is a way to return to the basics of family relationships. Balance is the answer to healthy eating, and a healthy lifestyle.

Since children, especially overweight children, often deal with a lot of stress, teaching them stress-reduction strategies can help them manage their own stress. Progressive relaxation, breathing, and meditation techniques can be easily taught and practiced by the whole family every morning for ten minutes before school and work. If done consistently, this can be the most fun period of the day, looked forward to by one and all. When children learn how to reduce their own stress, they become self-actualized. This develops a sense of control and self-value, and as a result positive regard and self-esteem. These skills foster positive behaviors that have collateral rewards for life.

Remember that children take their cue from their parents—don't be too restrictive, critical, or judgmental and approach your child's obesity with positive goals. Change happens one step at a time, and real change can only happen consistently, day by day. If your child missteps, don't manipulate her with guilt or shame, don't pressure her, and don't make her feel that your love is based on approval—but rather that the whole family is involved in making subtle but healthy life changes.

Communication is the most important part of this process, and listening is the way to communicate. Once a week, go back to that kitchen table where parents and children can talk about their feelings in relation to discipline, health, and fitness. Be sensitive to the emotions of each family member; listen attentively and never discount, shame, humiliate, or insult. Talk about empathy so that parents can meet their children where they are without defense or criticism. The role of a parent is to parent—to stay above the fray, and guide their children to learn successful living habits. Invest your children in the conversation and encourage them to offer up problem-solving options, so that together you can find vehicles for stress reduction other than food. Include your child in the conversation. If you invest him in the process, he will try his best to follow the rules with a new sense of responsibility. Also, let your child help plan family vacations that are activity filled, such as campouts, hiking, biking, and spas.

You and your children are on a journey together—weight control doesn't have to be a lifelong battle, but rather a positive process—a fun experience in living.

8

MAKING THE INVISIBLE VISIBLE: MOTHERING FOR THE NEUROLOGICAL HEALTH OF OUR UNBORN CHILDREN

By Melani Walton

A significant amount of scientific research in North America and elsewhere today has been looking at new concepts and therapies that make *visible* what was previously *invisible*, and the field of mitochondrial health as it relates to fetal brain development is becoming ever more relevant in this study. The simple truth is that healthy mitochondria equate to a healthier mom and a healthier baby brain, and when a mother supports her mitochondrial health, she is supporting the brain health of all future generations.

Our mitochondria represent probably the most vital subatomic information we carry, yet we are only just now starting to unveil their importance. We now know mitochondrial dysfunction is responsible for *as much as 85 percent* of the incidence of modern diseases,[1] many of which target the brain[2] and heart, the areas of the body with the highest density of mitochondria.[3] While we may have previously thought we were completely at the mercy of our genetics, we now know that supporting our mitochondrial health can lower the chronic and excessive inflammation that is often at the heart of many diseases.[4] This has the potential to dramatically change the trajectory of our health and well-being.

Although mitochondrial health hasn't received much mainstream attention, these tiny universal "fuel cells" are located in almost every cell of the human body. They are vitally important for life to exist, and they carry a unique type of DNA called mitochondrial DNA (mtDNA). One of the hallmarks of many modern diseases is the fact that our mitochondria cannot produce the energy our body needs to function properly.[5]

It is important to clarify that there is a big difference between mitochondrial *disease* and mitochondrial *dysfunction*. While mitochondrial disease is relatively rare, genetic testing of a woman's mtDNA has not made it into the mainstream of pregnancy care yet, and most people do not know before their first child is born whether or not they are carriers of a mitochondrial disease. The options for women who carry the genetic signature for a mitochondrial disease—and who know they do—are limited, but a fairly radical procedure called a mitochondrial transfer is now available. This involves removing the damaged mtDNA from the mother and replacing it with healthy mtDNA from another woman's mitochondria.[6] If this is something you find especially concerning, there are agencies that will provide genetic testing for mitochondrial disease and provide consultation about the results.

Mitochondrial dysfunction, by contrast, results in health issues that are more common and perhaps less severe than mitochondrial disease but can affect many aspects of the brain. These tend to express symptomatically, depending on where in the brain the cell impairment is located.[7] Our concern here is primarily with mitochondrial dysfunction and what can be done to support your mitochondrial health and that of your developing baby. While further studies are needed and are ongoing, the new science is effectively showing that living healthier lives and reducing exposure to the toxins that are frequently present in our everyday lives are key to this mission. Generally speaking, a woman *can* take steps to optimize her own mitochondria and support the mitochondrial health and brain development of her unborn child.

I invite you to join me now in a sweeping journey through the world of mitochondria and mtDNA. We will look at mitochondria and why they are important, how they affect cellular functioning and overall health, and finally we will examine a roster of actions women can take in order to safeguard the neurological wellness of their unborn children.

WHAT IS MTDNA, AND WHY IS IT SO IMPORTANT?

While scientists have known about mtDNA for decades, the study of genetics has intensified in recent years. The mysteries of mtDNA are being probed with mounting excitement.

Most of us are familiar with the double-stranded deoxyribonucleic acid (DNA), which is resident in the nucleus of every cell in the human body except the red blood cells. This DNA—also called nuclear DNA (nDNA)—carries genetic instructions that determine, among many other characteristics, the color of your hair, your skin, and your eyes, and even your height and your bone structure. Half of these instructions were contributed by your father through his sperm, and half by your mother through the egg, which was fertilized by your father's sperm and eventually developed into you.[8]

A small amount of another type of DNA can also be found in your cell mitochondria. Unlike nDNA, this mtDNA is not located in your chromosomes or even in the nuclei of your cells: it is lodged in the mitochondria located in the cytoplasm of your cells.[9]

The mitochondria themselves are structures within our cells that take the energy from food and transform it into a type of chemical energy our cells need in order to function. This substance is called adenosine triphosphate (ATP). In other words, our mitochondria provide energy to our cells, and some people refer to mitochondria as the "powerhouse of the cell."

While nDNA contains coding for about 20,000 genes, scientists have determined that the DNA found in our mitochondria contains coding for only 37 genes. This means our mtDNA is a kind of "elite squad" crucial to the functioning of our body. While nDNA comes from both parents, a child receives mtDNA almost exclusively from its mother. Men do have mtDNA, and although most researchers believe it is rarely if ever passed on to their offspring,[10] new research seems to indicate this could be more common than previously believed.[11]

Some scientists say our mtDNA has been passed down from mother to child, virtually intact, for as many as 200,000 years; some think the chain reaches back even further. Either way, this is called "maternal inheritance," and it is the reason scientists have been able to trace the origins of humanity back to what many believe is one single woman—"Mitochondrial Eve"—who lived in Africa eons ago. Genetic research has shined a light on this previously "invisible" female and made her "visible" to our understanding today, thus unlocking a piece of human history we had not previously known.

Our mtDNA changes over time as a natural outcome of aging and damage to our cells caused by bad habits or poor sleep routines. Since more than one-third of our mtDNA relates to energy production, mutations over time can have a big impact on our energy production and, therefore, on our health.[12] Simply put, cellular energy production and disease are linked.[13]

As we study this fascinating piece of the human puzzle, we are learning that while mtDNA mutations resulting in mitochondrial diseases will be passed down to our babies in utero as a matter of course, the toxicity in our environment and the habits we form can also result in mitochondria-related dysfunction in our children.[14]

NATURE'S WARNING: ORCA WHALES AND TOXINS

We are wise to be concerned about toxicity, and we are seeing worrying signs in nature that could give us a taste of things to come for the human population of the planet. As a philanthropist working around the world on projects related to environmental sustainability, I have become alert to the damage we are doing to the planet by dumping massive amounts of pollutants and toxins into our global ecosystem.

It appears nature is approaching a tipping point: the death rate of baby orca whales, for example, is now up to 50 percent,[15] particularly off the west coast of North America. Pollution has decimated the populations of salmon on which the orcas feed, putting nutritional stress on pregnant female whales.[16] In one study, two-thirds of orca pregnancies were unsuccessful. At the same time, lack of food forces a mother whale to metabolize her stores of fat, thus releasing into her system the toxins that have accumulated there, further endangering her unborn baby. We are facing the possible extinction of this magnificent mammal.[17]

While the plight of whales may not be something we all focus on in our daily lives, we need to recognize human beings are also ingesting and absorbing the pollutants in our environment.

Has the concept of safeguarding the health of the next generation ever been so poignant?

CHILLING STATISTICS: WHAT IS GOING ON?

In the human world, we are seeing chilling statistics that point to a serious increase in the number of disorders and diseases affecting the brains and nervous systems of our children. For example, the Centers for Disease Control report that the incidence of autism and autism spectrum disorders has risen from 1 in 150 in 2000 to 1 in 59 today.[18] We are also seeing increasing concerns over the prevalence of neuroimmune disease, a dysregulation of the immune and nervous systems that results in a range of debilitating symptoms and conditions.[19]

And what about the incidence of PANDAS—Pediatric Autoimmune Neuropsychiatric Disorders Associated with Streptococcal Infections? This is a relative newcomer to the field of childhood diseases, and its rate of incidence has not even been fully calculated yet. However, it can cause anxiety, depression, irritability and aggression, behavioral regression, and sensory and/or motor abnormalities. Researchers are still investigating the causes of this disease, but it is thought to be the result of an inappropriate immune system response to a streptococcal infection.[20]

The creation of life is a complicated process, and the slightest genetic mutation can have dramatic consequences. Some forms of the neurological disorder dystonia, for example, result from a genetic mutation that affects brain chemistry. Those who receive this mutation end up with seriously compromised muscle motor movement, which at this point can only be treated with the neurotransmitter levodopa.[21]

These are just a handful of neurological disorders that can affect the brains of our children. Armies of highly dedicated and compassionate researchers, scientists, and medical practitioners have to date been unable to stem the tide of disease threatening to engulf the next generation.

Mitochondrial disease and dysfunction represent another piece of the neurological puzzle. Scientists have determined that about 15 percent of mitochondrial diseases—most of which have a neurological link—are due to a defect in the mtDNA itself.[22] Researchers and clinical specialists are familiar with several dozen mitochondrial diseases, including Alper's Disease, Leber's Hereditary Optic Neuropathy (LHON), Leigh's Disease, and MELAS.[23] Today, it is thought that some of these genetic defects are acquired, rather than inherited—often through a mother's exposure to harmful radiation, toxins, stress, and exposure to harmful man-made (non-native) electromagnetic frequencies (nnEMFs). While genetic testing and mitochondrial transfer provide some tools for understanding and dealing with the issue of mitochondrial disease, therapeutic options for treating it are limited.

While mitochondrial disease is one thing, mitochondrial dysfunction is quite another. We now know that many conditions—for example, Lou Gehrig's disease, Alzheimer's, diabetes, muscular dystrophy, and cancer—can cause secondary mitochondrial dysfunction.[24] Mitochondrial dysfunction can also be created by environmental pollutants or lifestyle choices. This is especially challenging in our world today: toxicity is ever-persistent in our environment, and it can damage our mitochondria, causing dysfunction that generates health issues for adults and children and, more seriously, for our unborn children.

Just like mother orca whales, human females today are the unwitting repositories of the toxins in our environment. We absorb them into our system, and these toxins, in turn, get passed on to the next generation. For example, there is evidence that environmental toxins are so concentrated in some mothers' breast milk that if it were a commercial product, it would be illegal to sell.[25] One study discovered 287 toxic industrial chemicals in the umbilical cords of newborns.[26]

What makes the situation especially alarming is that high toxicity exposure can trigger mitochondrial gene mutation in a mother that results in neurological disorders in her children.[27] This does not even take into account the danger nnEMFs pose to our mitochondrial health and our ultimate well-being. Thus, the "invisible" toxins in our environment have a very "visible" impact on our children and our community.

Forewarned is forearmed, however: we do have some control over our toxicity exposure and, therefore, the amount of exposure our unborn children receive through us. But we are bombarded daily by thousands of toxins we cannot even see. Time is of the utmost urgency.

THE NEUROLOGICAL CONNECTION

From the time we are conceived and on into adulthood, we suffer ongoing free-radical damage to our mitochondria. It is no coincidence that people with cancer, diabetes, heart disease, Alzheimer's, Parkinson's, and other degenerative diseases of the brain all test positive for substantial cellular free-radical damage and mitochondrial breakdown.[28] What's more, at least one study has shown that the older the mother, the higher the possibility she will pass damaged mtDNA to her offspring.[29]

This becomes an even more serious concern when we understand that damage to a woman's mitochondria can result in mitochondrial dysfunction in her children. This can cause neurological impairment and disorders that can seriously impair their health.[30] If damaged mitochondria are transmitted to the next generation, they have the potential to create disorders that will continue to be passed down for generations to come. This could explain, in some cases, the increase in incidence of diseases that have not been prevalent before: the toxic load on our bodies has been quietly—invisibly—damaging our mtDNA, and that damage is showing up visibly in the health of our children and our grandchildren.

Mitochondrial dysfunction occurs when mitochondria cannot produce enough energy to allow for proper cell function. The mitochondria become depleted, and cell function becomes impaired to the point where the cell may even die. This is a particular risk when the dying cells are located in organs that require the most energy in our bodies—such as our brain, which alone uses 20 percent of our energy resources.[31]

It is important to note that our mtDNA, at birth, is mostly all the same. Over time, environmental and other factors begin damaging our mtDNA. As we age, and/or if we do not take care of our mitochondrial health, our mtDNA becomes increasingly differentiated. This impairs mitochondrial energy production and changes how our mitochondria handle incoming information, increasing our likelihood of creating disease.[32]

This is a complicated topic and gives rise to the opportunity to address another issue that can cause mitochondrial dysfunction: some people are born with one of a number of mitochondrial single nucleotide polymorphisms (SNPs). Some of these genetic aberrations can make a body less adept at detoxifying itself, which is a particular issue for people of child-bearing age who have been born and raised in a time of major pollution and nnEMF overload. In fact, 40 percent of the population have the DNA SNP known as methylene tetrahydrofolate reductase (MTHFR).[33] This SNP makes it hard for your body to detoxify and also interferes with the control of inflammation and the repair and regeneration of cells,[34] among other issues.

People with MTHFR produce inadequate supplies of glutathione, an important ingredient in the body's ability to detox. This, in turn, means they have a higher toxic load to carry, which ultimately ends up damaging their mitochondria.[35] Glutathione supplements are often recommended in order to assist with detoxification; however, as with anything, this should be discussed with members of your medical team.

Ninety-eight percent of children with autism have a mutation in their MTHFR gene, although people with this SNP do not necessarily have autism.[36] While it may cause no symptoms at all, MTHFR can also manifest through one of a long list of other conditions, including fibromyalgia, schizophrenia, and epilepsy.[37] This is an issue that is currently not being addressed in our modern medical practices, but you can be tested to determine if you have this SNP through one of a number of services offering genetic testing.

If a mother has a SNP, she may pass it along to her children, and they, too, may have health complications, particularly if they inherit the MTHFR SNP, which interferes with their ability to detox. Detoxing is an important tool in the maintenance of good health, and if your body struggles with this issue, there are a number of actions you can take to support it. Noted expert on MTHFR and detoxing Dr. Ben Lynch notes that cleaning up one's gut biome is one of the most important first steps to take in detoxing.[38]

We will talk about the key relationship between gut health and brain health in a moment, but for now it is important to note that toxic overload and high-stress circumstances provide the perfect environment for inflammation in the body. We mentioned earlier that chronic, excessive inflammation is at the root of many modern diseases, and it is important to note that inflammation can also cause, in particular, the demyelination[39] of our myelin sheath. This, also, can lead to health issues.[40] Myelin is a fatty substance insulating our nerves, including the ones in our brain and spinal cord. It allows the fast, efficient transfer of electrical impulses throughout your central nervous system. If it becomes damaged, you may experience a range of neurologically related impairments, including vision loss, speech impediments, and/or physical disability.

About two-thirds of a child's brain is made up of fat,[41] and we know that adequate healthy fat consumption and proper nutrition in both mother and child (both before and after birth) is crucial. It will ensure proper brain development[42] while maintaining the health of the myelin sheath covering your baby's nerve cells[43] and supporting mitochondrial health.[44]

GUT HEALTH: A VITAL ASPECT OF BRAIN HEALTH

We mentioned earlier that a healthy gut biome is important for detoxing, but it also plays a key role in our neurological health—and that of our children—in other ways. Our gut is populated by thriving colonies of bacteria, some of which are beneficial and some of which are not. As long as the beneficial bacteria predominate, our immune system, and therefore our health, can stay strong. But research suggests imbalances in the microbiome of our gut can cause immune system responses and inflammation, which can trigger anxiety, depression, obsessive-compulsive disorder, and even other, more serious, psychological and neurological disorders. Did you know that up to 80 percent of serotonin, the "feel-good" neurotransmitter, is produced in our gut, and that bacteria there can either promote or interfere with its production?[45] Evidence shows these issues and others can often be mitigated by ensuring the "good" bacteria in our gut biome flourish.[46]

Newborn babies have vulnerable intestinal systems, and we know that colostrum, the first milk a mother's body produces after her baby is born, helps support gut health. It provides immunity to help baby fight off harmful pathogens, as it is rich in nutrients, antibodies, and enzymes. Plus, it helps your baby grow while sealing holes in his or her gut that could otherwise allow pathogens and other harmful bacteria[47] and viruses[48] to alter the gut biome and potentially generate neurological imbalances. Colostrum is a strong supporter of brain health.[49] This is why it is so important for a baby to be breastfed, although it can be a tough call for some mothers who are worried the potential for toxins in their breast milk might outweigh the benefits of breastfeeding. To date, medical professionals still feel the benefits outweigh the risks.[50]

Adults can benefit from supplementing their diet with commercially available colostrum, as well. Studies have shown that colostrum, taken as a nutritional supplement, can provide a major boost to an adult's health—it can:

- Increase energy and stamina
- Enhance nutrient absorption

- Reduce inflammation
- Balance blood sugar levels
- Regulate serotonin and dopamine
- Stimulate the production of antibodies, natural killer cells, macrophages, and t-cells to prevent and eliminate infections
- Build lean muscle
- Improve digestion and plug a "leaky gut"

Colostrum, sometimes called "liquid gold," is nontoxic and nonallergenic and has no known negative interactions with any drugs, foods, or other supplements.[51] However, as with all things, make sure you check with your medical team before consuming it.

Some people feel we have barely tapped into the mystery of our gut-brain connection. While scientists believe our mitochondria play into this relationship, the study of exactly how this works is still in its infancy.[52] But there are other factors that can help the mitochondria within us and in our developing babies stay strong and healthy. Would it surprise you to learn that sunlight and water have a big impact on our mitochondrial health?

OPTIMIZING MITOCHONDRIAL HEALTH

The sophisticated relationship between sunlight and water is a critical aspect of maintaining mitochondrial health and, beyond that, the neurological well-being of our unborn children. In fact, researcher Jack Kruse asserts that "The water created by your mitochondria has a mission in your body. It is a mission tied to energy and information transfer of wireless data from the sun and from the magnetic field."[53]

At one time, we were much more connected to nature, generally, than we are now. We lived according to the rising and the setting of the sun, and there were no artificial lights emitting incompatible light waves; nor was there any of the interference we get today from harmful nnEMFs.[54]

It is common knowledge today that we get countless benefits from the vitamin D in sunlight,[55] and sunlight has been shown to elevate mood, make our metabolism run more efficiently, and improve sleep patterns.[56] It is important to note that many of our biological processes are triggered by relevant light frequencies from the sun, as well.[57] Sunlight is key to mitochondrial health and energy production. As Dr. Fritz-Albert Popp said, "We are still on the threshold of fully understanding the complex relationship between light and life, but we can now say emphatically, that the function of our entire metabolism is dependent on light."[58]

The journey begins with oxygen and its essential relationship to our mitochondria in the production of cellular energy. Our blood picks up oxygen from our lungs and transfers it to our cells, where our mitochondria use it to produce energy using a number of elements, including hydrogen and electricity. This produces carbon dioxide and water.[59] The process by which these chemical reactions occur is uncannily similar to photosynthesis, which allows plants to transform sunlight into cellular material. In fact, the structure of hemoglobin in human blood is almost identical to the structure of plant chlorophyll.[60] But while plants create sugar and oxygen from carbon dioxide, our mitochondria create carbon dioxide (and water) from sugars or fat.[61]

The overall message here is that our mitochondria need oxygen in order to produce energy. Over time, aging and mitochondrial damage caused by environmental factors or unhealthy habits cause our stock of healthy mitochondria to dwindle; it becomes significantly harder for them to handle oxygen and generate the energy we need to stay strong and healthy.

Further complicating the issue is the fact that oxygen levels on the planet are declining. Two hundred and fifty million years ago, oxygen levels on Earth held steady at 35 percent. By 1850, they had dropped to 22 percent, and today they are hovering around 19 percent or less at sea level in most westernized cities.[62] Healthy human life and efficient mitochondrial functioning require oxygen levels of 19.5 percent.[63] So, not only are we faced with the challenge of deteriorating mitochondrial function over time, but the availability of oxygen in our environment is dropping, making it even more challenging for our cells to generate the energy we need.

What is fascinating about all this is that sunlight kick-starts the process of energy production in human beings in a fashion similar to how it triggers photosynthesis in plants. Mitochondria decode information from their environment, and one of the factors they consider in their calculations is light. If your mitochondria are impaired in any way, not only will they have difficulty processing oxygen, but they will be unable to effectively process the light your body is taking in. Energy production will break down, which in turn increases the likelihood of disease for you and, by extension, your unborn child.

Even more interesting is the idea that light is a type of "food." We need a well-rounded—full-spectrum, or sunlight-based—"diet" of light in order for our mitochondria to work properly. Full-spectrum sunlight is critical for triggering multiple processes within our body and brain, but light can do harm or good depending on its frequency. Some wavelengths of light are now being used for healing. For example, infrared light can be used for reducing inflammation.[64] Red light has been proven to reduce wrinkles, pain, inflammation, and stretch marks; increase weight loss; and improve athletic performance.[65]

Meanwhile, ionizing radiation waves, such as ultraviolet and X-ray, can damage DNA.[66] Blue and green light are emitted by our computers, telephones, televisions, and other Wi-Fi-compatible and Bluetooth equipment, and many experts feel we are getting an overdose of blue light. Studies show Americans are spending up to 90 percent of our time indoors,[67] often under fluorescent lighting. Even worse, we spend up to 42 percent of our time looking at a screen.[68]

Excessive exposure to blue and green light, or fluorescent light, particularly prior to bedtime, can limit our body's ability to manufacture melatonin, which interferes with our sleep cycle[69] and limits our mitochondria's ability to repair and recharge itself. This creates further stress on our health.[70] Damaged or malfunctioning mitochondria are repaired or replaced when we sleep, so lack of sleep means this important work cannot proceed. Ultimately, it means we end up with greater numbers of ineffective mitochondria, which can lead to any one of a number of diseases[71] for us and our developing baby.

Sleep is highly dependent on our circadian rhythm, a twenty-four-hour internal clock that cycles between sleepiness and alertness at regular intervals. We know that light can support or interfere with our circadian rhythm,[72] and some experts say morning sunlight helps set our circadian rhythm for the day. The type of light we encounter throughout the day can affect the release of the sleep hormone melatonin, which is an important support for good sleep. Too much screen time too late in the day gives us excessive exposure to blue light, which is how our sleep cycle can be disrupted.

As noted earlier, our brain consumes 20 percent of our entire energetic requirement, which means brain function is one of the hardest-hit aspects of our physiology when oxygen, solar light input, and mitochondrial function are impaired or reduced.

It is interesting to note that we strive to possess every modern convenience hitting the market in the belief it will help us live more happily, but in fact these devices actually serve to keep us inside more, exposed to ever higher levels of nnEMFs, and limit our exposure to the full-spectrum light that is so vital to our health and well-being.

Light enters our system through our eyes, of course, but we also have photoreceptors all over our bodies.[73] When light hits our cells, it creates a negatively charged "fourth phase" of water (a phase beyond liquid, vapor, or solid), which biomedical engineer and water researcher Dr. Gerald Pollack calls Exclusion Zone (EZ) water.[74] This type of water holds and transports the energy our mitochondria make, which is so vital to the maintenance of life. In fact, as Dr. Pollack asserts, nonfluoridated, "structured" water is best for our cells,[75] and it is key to cellular health and organ function optimization.[76]

Structured water occurs wherever there is naturally moving water, but it can also be created by stirring water to create a vortex,[77] or by cooling it.[78] Natural spring water is already structured, and there are a number of devices available online that will structure your water for you. Another way to stay effectively hydrated is to pursue a routine of juicing, since the water in plants is EZ water.[79] Unlike regular tap water, EZ water molecules are hexagon-shaped and layered, so they are highly structured and act like liquid crystals.[80]

One issue that plays effectively into a discussion of light frequencies and water molecules is that of Earth's energy. Earth has a natural resonating frequency, known as the Schumann resonance, that is so important, astronauts need to artificially recreate it while in space in order to avoid illness.[81] One study showed that any electromagnetic energy that is in disharmony with Schumann resonance pollutes the natural environment and affects our health.[82] So the more we can connect with Earth's resonance, the better. Another important aspect of this conversation is the practice of grounding (also known as earthing). Grounding is finding increasing favor with people in search of optimal health, especially those who understand the importance of EZ water: grounding allows your body to absorb negatively charged ions from the Earth, enhancing your natural ability to structure the water content of your body.[83]

When we ground ourselves, the negatively charged electrons we absorb act as powerful antioxidants. Because they have a negative charge, and the toxic free radicals in our body are positively charged, any free radicals we may be carrying inside us are electrically neutralized by these negatively charged electrons. We'll be addressing free radicals in a little more detail later in this chapter. For now, suffice to say they have the potential to be highly damaging to our health.

Remember we discussed the importance of sunlight? In a beautiful cycle of compatibility, sunlight makes EZ water expand,[84] facilitating mitochondrial function. The inescapable conclusion is that mitochondria need sufficient quantities of light and adequate EZ water hydration in order to function optimally.[85] This is particularly important for pregnant women and their developing babies.

Our age of technology means we are constantly living within a range of frequencies, some harmful and some beneficial. In fact, everything we see around us is vibrating at one frequency or another, but the frequency we haven't talked about yet is the frequency of emotion. Let's look at that now.

TUNING IN TO YOUR INNER FREQUENCIES

The work of Japanese scientist Dr. Masaru Emoto demonstrated that the structure of water molecules is affected by energetic vibration. He also showed that water can hold data.[86] Dr. Emoto proved that higher energetic vibration directed at water by people in a prayerful or meditative state, for example, creates patterns of harmonious molecular organization; energetic vibrations emitted by people in a state of anger generate asymmetrical molecular arrangements.[87] He also found that writing words such as "thank you" or "gratitude" on a bottle of water can create structured water.[88]

Researchers at the Aerospace Institute of the University of Stuttgart in Germany expanded upon Dr. Emoto's research and confirmed that water retains memory and responds to energetic vibrations.[89] Today, many scientists and health-care practitioners are realizing the quality of our thoughts and emotions affect the health of our bodies (which have a high water content), and it is clear from this research there is a very direct correlation between the two.

Everything in the universe is energy vibrating at different frequencies, and the work of Dr. Emoto and others is showing how emotions affect water. In many ways, we humans are capacitators for experiences, and our brain functions as both a transmitter and a receiver of information. It can drive our behavior—behavior that will either supercharge or toxify our body. Our tendency to do either affects our health outcomes. In point of fact, we are highly advanced biological devices.

Your unborn baby, whose body is made up of a high percentage of water, is swimming in a liquid environment that is encapsulated by your body, which is also made primarily of water. Your baby is a transmitter and receiver of information in a highly vulnerable state, and you and your emotions are creating your baby's environment.

A number of studies have been done on the impact of music on the unborn child, and although the "Mozart Effect" is largely misunderstood and in some quarters discredited, we do know that music and other sounds affect a baby's well-being.[90] A fetus develops the ability to hear twenty weeks after conception, and we've discovered that twelve months after they are born, they can remember, and prefer, music they heard before they were born.[91] Music helps babies relax and stimulates their brain structure, thereby enhancing learning and development.[92]

On another front, we also know that fears and sensitivities may be inherited.[93] Taken together, it appears the maintenance of a vibrationally peaceful state is an important priority for a pregnant woman and her family[94] so she can support the structuring of water within her body and that of her unborn child, stimulate baby's brain development, and enhance mitochondrial function to optimize baby's neurological well-being. Again, this pursuit is largely invisible to the human eye; however, the impact may be very visibly demonstrated in the lives of our children and our families.

SUPPORTING OUR CHILDREN'S HEALTH ON ANOTHER FRONT

Another process that occurs, invisibly to most of us, is the generation of reactive oxygen species (ROS—often also known as "free radicals") as a byproduct of mitochondrial functioning. We mentioned the topic earlier, and the application that is important here surrounds the fact that free radicals cause unavoidable degeneration of our mitochondria. At the same time, we know free-radical damage is linked to many diseases.[95] Although we cannot do anything about the natural production of free radicals in the process of mitochondrial functioning, the maintenance of our health depends on eliminating or neutralizing, as much as possible, the free radicals in our system and boosting our intake of antioxidants. What might be news to many is:

- Nonnative electromagnetic frequencies (nnEMFs) cause an excessive assault on our mitochondria,[96] and therefore our bodies ... and their effects can be mitigated by antioxidants; and
- Research is showing that antioxidants can support our mitochondria and help increase their ability to generate energy.[97]

We live within a sea of invisible electromagnetic waves emitted by cell-phone and hydro towers and equipment, our television and computer equipment, and almost anything electrical. They are affecting us every moment of our lives.[98] American neurosurgeon Dr. Jack Kruse says that when nnEMF exposure is excessive, a person's mitochondria become inefficient in processing electrons across their inner mitochondrial membrane.[99] They become less efficient at burning fat[100] and less oxygenated, as well.[101] Dr. Kruse believes rampant levels of obesity, melanoma, and autoimmune diseases in Australia, for example, are due to high levels of solar EMF, which are changing the chemistry of water in the atmosphere above that country.[102]

Meanwhile, elsewhere on the planet, we are seeing a decline in bee populations and a decrease in wildlife, some of which is being blamed on nnEMFs[103] and some on pesticides.[104] Aside from the threat nnEMFs pose to human beings, we too are threatened by pesticides and other chemical pollutants: as noted earlier, they are showing up in our urine and breast milk,[105] and in the umbilical cord blood of newborn babies.[106]

In the face of all of these challenges, women are making babies.

The most sacred time for a child's development occurs during gestation. What can a pregnant woman do to support her mitochondrial health and enhance the raw energy inherent in the cells of her children, grandchildren, great-grandchildren, and beyond for generations to come? Here is a gathering of suggestions from qualified sources for improving mitochondrial health for brain health. I invite you to run these by your medical team to see if they are suitable for you:

LIGHT

- Seek opportunities to be outside twenty minutes a day with no sunscreen or sunglasses[107] to help regulate your hormones and support mitochondrial health. In fact, think of light as nourishment: your skin is full of photocells, so exposing your skin is like charging your solar cells.[108]
- Find opportunities to expose your skin to infrared light for short periods of time, if your medical team agrees, which can also support mitochondrial function.[109]
- Switch from fluorescent to incandescent light bulbs, which are more "mitochondria-friendly" than fluorescent or LED lights.[110]
- Limit your exposure to blue and green light, especially in the hours before you retire for the night, as they interfere with the production of melatonin.[111] (Computer software and blue blocker glasses are available to help you do this.)

WATER

- Stay well hydrated with plenty of unfluoridated water—structured water is the best way to support mitochondrial function. (See Dr. Pollack's work.)[112]

NNEMFS

- Limit harmful nnEMF exposure by unplugging as much electrical equipment in your house as you can, and do not ever rest your cell phone or tablet on your belly while there is a baby in there. You can purchase EMF shields for your belly and meters to test the EMF levels within your home.[113]

NUTRITION AND NUTRIENTS

- Consume the brain foods and nutrients that are either known to be antioxidant in nature[114] or that are able to repair the brain, regulate cellular energy production, and reverse free-radical and oxidative stress damage. Blueberries, colorful vegetables, proteins, and healthy fats (including avocados,[115] coconut oil, olive oil, and flaxseed oil[116]), magnesium,[117] vitamins B, C, and D,[118] and Coenzyme Q10[119] are some suggestions.

- Avoid processed foods as much as possible.

- Eat hormone-free meat and butter or ghee from grass-fed cattle, and organic free-range eggs; opt for certified organic foods whenever possible.

- Check with your medical team to see if colostrum supplements are a good idea for you.

ENVIRONMENT

- Decrease or eliminate as much as possible any exposure to toxins you might be experiencing in foods, cleaning supplies, and the environment.[120]

- Work in common with the laws of nature and the physics of the universe: find opportunities to walk barefoot in the grass. This will enable you to pick up the negative ions and help you reset your circadian clock for better sleep, leading to mitochondrial repair and rejuvenation.

STRESS REDUCTION

- Investigate whether complementary, energetic, and environmental therapies offered by accredited professionals are appropriate for you. Make sure they have experience treating pregnant women. Some therapies you might consider include matrix energetics,[121] Reiki,[122] cranio-sacral therapy,[123] vibrational, functional, and environmental medicine, plus homeopathy,[124] meditation,[125] and general efforts to reduce stress. The goal is to maintain as peaceful a state as possible: a body in "fight, flight, or freeze" mode may affect an unborn child.

- Honor your circadian rhythm so you can get plenty of sleep.[126]
- Learn as much as possible about mitochondria and the enormous impact mtDNA has on your child's developing neurology. This is an expanding field, and new information is coming to light all the time. Mainstream medicine does not have much information available on the topic yet, so you might want to discuss the mysteries of mitochondria with an accredited and well-recommended functional medicine practitioner.
- If you are concerned about the status of your mtDNA, find and work with an experienced genetics team to determine an effective course of action for your unique genetic makeup.[127]

YOUR PHYSICAL WELL-BEING

- Get as much exercise as is compatible with the conditions of your pregnancy—strength training has been shown to increase ATP production and thus increase the energy available to you and your unborn child.[128] Exercise, in general, is good for your mitochondrial health.
- Short bursts of exposure to cold temperatures, a process known as thermogenesis, have been found to increase mitochondrial health, so check into whether this is an appropriate option for you.[129]
- As much as we are told our genetics determine our medical destiny, it is encouraging to learn how much our choices can actually influence our mitochondrial health and some of our health-related outcomes. The more we learn about this exciting area on the cutting edge of medical science, the more we will

understand how supporting our mitochondrial health can help us reduce the incidence of disease, from the moment of conception to the moment we take our final breath. We do have some control over our mitochondrial health, and this gives us some control over our destiny and that of our children and, ultimately, the generations of people who will follow them. We now know that the health of our outer environment is intrinsically related to the health of our inner environment. This is our future. Better still, it is our sustainability plan.

CONCLUDING THOUGHTS

I believe there are many things we can do to optimize the health of our unborn children, and safeguarding our own mitochondrial health is a key part of that mission. Imagine: we are more aware than ever before of what it takes to do this, and we have choices available to us that previous generations never even knew existed. We have the tools and knowledge to optimize our mitochondrial health and protect the mtDNA we women have been nurturing within us, probably since the beginning of time itself.

It heartens me to know that one of the biological structures that has the most impact on determining the health of our species—the mitochondria—has been passed from mother to child for millennia in a long unbroken string of care, wisdom, and the power to sustain life itself. We know we are living in a more polluted environment than ever before, and we know our mtDNA has possibly been compromised as a result. But it is truly wondrous to see the scope of research being done on how to move us forward; it is inspiring to know there are countless people working diligently to ensure that valid, scientifically sound solutions be available.

Mothers are the keepers of the sacred flame of humanity, the custodians of the future. And in that sacred trust lies a responsibility to reverently foster our collective health, so our lineage may continue unburdened into a future blossoming with hope for our world.

Together we can create whole-system healing for the sustainability of mankind. It is going to take a focus on supporting our inner and outer environments, and a desire to reignite and revere that which is sacred. Humankind is one of countless species on this planet, and at the heart of the survival of all of us is a determination to cocreate a way to keep our planet clean. It is imperative that we limit the proliferation of nnEMFs, clean up pollution, and support Mother Earth, all while building our mitochondrial resources to optimize the health of ourselves and our communities.

The challenge for each of us—whether we are a pregnant woman or a person acting in support of one, in this generation or a future one—is to learn more about this key issue that affects our health so deeply. We should encourage projects that will highlight the importance of mitochondria and bring information about it into our everyday life and into the mainstream of our medical systems. From the invisible division of cells replicating quietly within the bellies of the pregnant women of our world, to the very visible children who run loudly and joyfully through our world teaching us all how to love ever more deeply: the Invisible becomes Visible.

We want the Visible to be as full of health and promise as possible.

This concept involves an evolution and integration of science and nature, which brings into our consciousness an awareness and an understanding of who we are as dynamic human beings—the nuts and bolts of our physical being and the heart and soul of who we are, as well. At some level, we are all here to heal.

The future is beckoning us to educate ourselves, to act with leadership, and to inspire others to call forth the best in themselves in the challenging journey of living a healthy life.

We live in an invisible connected web, and it is up to us to determine how we can best work creatively with Nature herself, rather than in opposition to Her.

In peace and promise,
Melani Walton

ABOUT MELANI WALTON

As the cofounder of the Rob and Melani Walton Foundation, Melani is committed to making philanthropic impact on a local, national, and global scale. Through her studies in art history and background as a K-12 educator, real estate agent, human performance trainer, multisport clinician and coach, and three-time Collegiate All-American in academics, basketball, and track & field, she brings a diverse set of skills to helping people solve problems and improve lives. Melani is passionate about supporting research and innovation in education, arts and humanities, brain health and consciousness studies, human performance and well-being, and conservation and sustainability.

Melani's leadership and commitment to these causes is reflected in her board and committee service with numerous organizations, including the Arizona Science Center, Phoenix Symphony, Society of St. Vincent de Paul, Aspen Brain Institute, the Rob and Melani Walton Sustainability Solutions Service at Arizona State University, Liberty Wildlife, Conservation International, Phoenix Children's Hospital, Arizona Women's Board, The Nature Conservancy, Dickinson State University, National Park Foundation, Theodore Roosevelt Presidential Library Foundation, and others.

Melani was the founding force behind the creation of the Sustainability in Science and Technology Museums program, which now reaches close to 200 museums in over 30 countries. She also launched The W.O.N.D.E.R. Center (Walton Optimal Neurological Discovery Education and Research Center) at Arizona Science Center, an interactive mind and brain experience impacting approximately half a million children and adults annually. She has since spearheaded numerous related W.O.N.D.E.R. Projects designed to bring heart and healing to her community. These include Phoenix Theatre's "Partners that Heal," which uses theater to share joy with people facing serious health challenges; and Phoenix Symphony's "B-Sharp Music Wellness," an outreach program that uses the power of music as a healing force in the lives of Alzheimer's patients and people facing homelessness.

Melani played a pivotal role in establishing the Neuro-Rehabilitation Gym at the Barrow Neurological Institute in Phoenix. She created recreational camps and programming for Native American youth and donated funds raised to benefit children with fetal alcohol syndrome. Melani has worked with children, adults, and elite athletes across the globe to help them optimize performance through speed, agility, and quickness (SAQ) training. Through athletics, she gained an appreciation for the importance of biohacking our mitochondrial cells to enhance performance, and she began to realize the value of this pursuit, not just for athletes' performance, but for the health of humanity.

In recognition of her ongoing commitment to people and communities at home and abroad, Melani was honored in 2019 with the prestigious ATHENA Global Leadership Award.

BIBLIOGRAPHY

Ader, Robert, and Nicholas Cohen. "Behaviorally conditioned immunosuppression." *Psychosomatic Medicine* 37, no. 4 (1975): 333–340.

Ader, Robert, and Nicholas Cohen. "Psychoneuroimmunology: Conditioning and stress." Edited by 44. *Annual Review of Psychology* (1993): 53–85. https://doi .org/10.1146/annurev.ps.44.020193.000413.

Adler, Jerry. "It's a Wise Father Who Knows . . ." *Newsweek*. (1997):73.

Allen, Sarah, and Kerry Daly. "The Effects of Father Involvement: A Summary of the Research Evidence." *Newsletter of the Father Involvement Initiative - Ontario Network* 1 (2002): 1–11.

Anderson, Craig A., Leonard Berkowitz, Edward Donnerstein, L. Rowell Huesmann, James D. Johnson, Daniel Linz, Neil M. Malamuth, and Ellen Wartella. "The Influence of Media Violence on Youth." *Psychological Science in the Public Interest* 4, no. 3 (2003): 81–110. https://doi.org/10.1111%2Fj.1529–1006.2003 .pspi_1433.x.

Arnold, Chandler. "Archived: Read with Me—A Guide for Student Volunteers Starting Early Childhood Literacy Programs; Making Connections: How Children Learn." *National Institute on Early Childhood Development and Education*. Accessed November 5, 2018. https://www2.ed.gov/pubs/ReadWith -Me/makconn.html.

Badre, David, and Anthony D. Wagner. "Semantic retrieval, mnemonic control, and prefrontal cortex." *Behavioral and Cognitive Neuroscience Reviews* 1, no. 3 (2002): 206–2018.

Bandura, Albert. *Social Learning Theory*. Englewood Cliffs, N.J.: Prentice-Hall, 1977.

Bastien, Celyne H., Annie Vallières, and Charles M. Morin. "Precipitating Factors of Insomnia." *Behavioral Sleep Medicine* 2, no. 1 (2004): 50–62.

Bayliss, S. *Study supports case for more parental involvement. London Times* Educational Supplement, 3561, 1984.

Baymur, F., and Patterson, C.H. "Three methods of assisting underachieving high school students." *Journal of Counseling Psychology* 7 (1960): 83–90.

Begley, Sharon. "How to Build a Baby's Brain." *Newsweek* (1997): 28-32.

Benson, H., Wilcher, M., Greenberg, B., Huggins, E., Ennis, M., Friedman, R. (2000). "Academic performance among middle school students after exposure to a relaxation response curriculum." *Journal of Research and Development in Education*, 33(3): 156–165.

Biehler, Robert F., and Jack Snowman. *Psychology applied to teaching.* 5th ed. Boston: Houghton Mifflin, 1986.

Bjorkqvist, Kaj. "Violent Films, Anxiety and Aggression: Experimental Studies of the Effect of Violent Films on the Level of Anxiety and Aggressiveness in Children." *World Cat.* November 11, 2018. Accessed December 29, 2018. https://www.world -cat.org/title/violent-films-anxiety-and-aggression-experimental-studies-of-the -effect-of-violent-films-on-the-level-of-anxiety-and-agressiveness-in-children /oclc/58507862.

Bjorntop, P., Holm, G. and Rosmond, R. "Hypothalamic arousal, insulin resistance and Type 2 diabetes mellitus." *Diabetic Medicine* 16, no. 5 (1999): 373–383.

Bloom et al. *Taxonomy of Educational Objectives"* Handbook 1. London: Longman, 1956.

Bolger, Kerry E., Charlotte J. Patterson, William W. Thompson, and Janis B. Kupersmidt. "Psychosocial Adjustment among Children Experiencing Persistent and Intermittent Family Economic Hardship." *Child Development* 66, no. 4 (1995): 1107–1129.

Brazelton, T.B., and Stanley Greenspan. "Our Window to The Future," *Newsweek* (2000): 34-36.

Brooks-Gunn, Jeanne, and Greg J. Duncan. "The effects of poverty on children." *Children and Poverty* 7, no. 2 (1997): 55–71.

Bush, Nicole R., Jelena Obradovic, Nancy E. Adler, and Thomas W. Boyce. "Kindergarten stressors and cumulative adrenocortical activation: The 'first straws' of allostatic load?" *Development and Psychopathology* 23, no. 4 (2011): 1089–2001.

Calvo, Manuel G., and Michael W. Eysenck. "Phonological working memory and reading in test anxiety." *Memory 4*, no. 3 (1996): 289–305.

Carrel, Alexis. "L'homme Cet Inconnu." Place of Publication Not Identified: Lulu .com, 2018.

Carrington, Damian. "The Guardian." *Orca 'apocalypse': half of killer whales doomed to die from pollution.* September 27, 2018. https://www.theguardian.com

/environment/2018/sep/27/orca-apocalypse-half-of-killer-whales-doomed-to
-die-from-pollution (accessed April 22, 2019).

"Centers for Disease Control and Prevention." *Data & Statistics on Autism Spectrum Disorder.* April 5, 2019. https://www.cdc.gov/ncbddd/autism/data.html (accessed April 22, 2019).

Cheek, James R., Loretta J. Bradley, JoLynne Reynolds, and Doris Coy. "An Intervention for Helping Elementary Students Reduce Test Anxiety." *Professional School Counseling* 6, no. 2 (2002): 162–164.

Chen, Edith, Sheldon Cohen, and Gregory E. Miller. "How Low Socioeconomic Status Affects 2-Year Hormonal Trajectories in Children." *Psychological Science* 21, no. 1 (2010): 31–37.

Clark, Barbara. *Growing up gifted: Developing the potential of children at school and at home.* 8th Edition. Upper Saddle River, NJ: Pearson Education, 2012.

Cole, Beverly. "American Dads: Loving Their Kids To Success." Accessed April 22, 2019. https://englishhound.com/2018/04/15/american-dads-loving-their-kids-to-success/.

Coles, Robert. *The Moral Intelligence of Children.* London: Bloomsbury, 1998.

Congreve, William. *The Mourning Bride.* Place of Publication Not Identified: Nabu Press, 2010.

Cook, Jimmie E. *"Children in Crisis: The Academic Effect."* ED 234306, Philadelphia, PA, 1982.

Cooney, Adam, and Samantha Jones. "The Educational Theory of Maria Montessori." *NewFoundations.* November 19, 2018. http://www.newfoundations.com/GALLERY/Montessori.html (accessed April 22, 2019).

Cowley, Geoffrey. "The Language Explosion." New York: *Newsweek,* 1997.

Csikszentmihalyi, Mihaly. *Finding Flow: The Psychology of Engagement with Everyday Life.* New York: Basic Books, 2008.

Dass, Ram. *Be Here Now, Remember.* New York: Crown Publishing Group, 1978.

DeChillo, Suzanne. "Stretch. Pose. Rest. It's Kindergarten Yoga." *New York Times.* December 14, 2002. Accessed December 10, 2018. https://www.nytimes.com/2002/12/14/nyregion/stretch-pose-rest-it-s-kindergarten-yoga.html.

Diamond M.C., Law, F., Rhodes, H., Lindner, B., Rosenzweig, M.R., Krech, D., Bennett, E.L. "Increases in cortical depth and glia numbers in rats subjected to enriched environment." *The Journal of Comparative Neurology* 128 (1966): 117–126. https://doi.org/10.1002/cne.9012801102.

Diamond, M. C., Krech, D., and Rosenzweig, M. R. "The effects of an enriched environment on the histology of the rat cerebral cortex." *Journal of Comparative Neurology* 123 (1964): 111–119.

Dictionary. "Each and Every One." Accessed April 22, 2019. https://www.dictionary .com/browse/each-and-every-one.

"Difficult Child Behavior: 4 Tools to Help You Stay Calm." Empowering Parents. Accessed October 25, 2018. https://www.empoweringparents.com /article/4-tools-to-help-you-stay-calm-with-your-difficult-child/.

Douglas, R., "Does TV Rot Your Brain?" January 1, 2016 (Accessed April 25, 2019). https://www.scientificamerican.com/article/does-tv-rot-your-brain/.

Dreher, Henry. "The Immune Power Personality." *Noetic Sciences Review* 39 (1996): 12–22.

Dusek, Jeffery A., and Herbert Benson. "Mind-Body Medicine." *A Model of the Comparative Clinical Impact of the Acute Stress and Relaxation Responses* (Minnesota Medicine) 92, no. 5 (2009): 47–50.

Elkind, David. *Miseducation: Preschoolers at Risk*. New York: Knopf, 1988.

Elkind, David. *The Hurried Child: Growing Up Too Fast Too Soon* (rev. ed.). Reading, MA: Addison-Wesley. (Original work published 1981, 1988.)

Elkind, David. *The Hurried Child: Growing Up Too Fast Too Soon*. 3rd ed. Cambridge, MA: Da Capo Press, 2001.

Ely, Bert. "How do researchers trace mitochondrial DNA over centuries?" *Scientific American*. n.d. https://www.scientificamerican.com/article/how-do-researchers -trace/ (accessed April 22, 2019).

Elzinga, Bernet M., and Douglas J. Bremner. "Are the neural substrates of memory the final common pathway in posttraumatic stress disorder (PTSD)?" *Journal of Affective Disorders* 70, no. 1 (2002): 1–17.

Eppley, Kenneth R., Allan I. Abrams, and Jonathan Shear. "The Transcendental Meditation Program." *Journal of Clinical Psychology* 45, (1989): 957–974.

Estrada, P., Arsenio, F., Hess, R.D., and Holloway, D. (1987). "Affective quality of the mother-child relationship: Longitudinal consequences for children's school-relevant cognitive functioning." *Developmental Psychology* 213, no. 2 (1987): 210–215.

"Executive Summary." *PISA 2009 Results: Learning Trends*, 2010, 13–15. Accessed December 29, 2018. https://www.oecd.org/pisa/pisaproducts/46619703.pdf.

Feuerstein, Georg, and Stephan Bodian. *Living Yoga: A Comprehensive Guide for Daily Life*. New York: G.P. Putnams Sons, 1993.

Flanagan, Constance A. "Families and schools in hard times." In *Economic stress: effects on family life and child development*, by Constance A Flanagan, edited by Vonnie, C. and Flanagan, Constance A. In McLoyd, 7–26. San Francisco, CA: Jossey-Bass, 1990.

Flinn, Mark V., Nepomnaschy, P.A., Muehlenbein, M.P., and Ponzi, D. "Evolutionary functions of early social modulation of hypothalamic-pituitary-adrenal axis development in humans." *Neurosci. Biobehav. Rev.* (2011), doi:10.1016/j.neubiorev.2011.01.005

French, J.L., and Carden, B.W. "Characteristics of high mental ability dropouts." *Vocational Guidance Quarterly* 32 (1968): 162–168.

Friesen, Sharon. *Bridges to Learning: A Guide to Parent Involvement.* Distributed by ERIC Clearinghouse, 1986. https://eric.ed.gov/?id=ED272313.

Frucht, Steven J. *Rare Disease Database.* Dystonia, Danbury: National Organization for Rare Disorders (NORD), 2015.

Gardner, Howard. *Intelligence Reframed: Multiple Intelligences for the 21st Century.* New York: Basic Books, 1999.

Gelman, R., and Gallistel, C.C. *The child's understanding of numbers.* Cambridge, MA: Harvard University Press, 1978.

Genomics Education Programme. June 2014. https://www.genomicseducation.hee.nhs.uk/inheritance-of-genetic-material/dna-from-parent-to-child/ (accessed April 22, 2019).

"Georgia Strait Alliance." *Orca Facts—Did you know?* 2019. https://georgiastrait.org/work/species-at-risk/orca-protection/killer-whales-pacific-northwest/orca-facts/ (accessed April 22, 2019).

Gesell, Arnold, Frances Lillian, Louise Bates Ames, and Janet Learned Rodell. *Infant and Child in the Culture of Today: The Guidance of Development in Home and Nursery School.* New York: Harper & Row, 1974.

Gibran, Kahlil. *The Prophet.* New York: Alfred A. Knopf, 1948.

Glover, Emily. "Kids' energy levels surpass endurance athletes', says science." January 24, 2019. (Accessed April 22, 2019). https://www.mother.ly/news/your-kids-are-in-better-shape-than-you-even-if-youre-a-pro-athlete.

Glover, V. "The Effects of Prenatal Stress on Child Behavioural and Cognitive Outcomes Start at the Beginning." In: Tremblay R.E., Boivin, M., Peters. R. DeV, eds. Glover V., topic ed. *Encyclopedia on Early Childhood Development* [online]. http://www.child-encyclopedia.com/stress-and-pregnancy-prenatal-and-perinatal/according-experts/effects-prenatal-stress-child. Updated April 2019. Accessed April 25, 2019.

Goldberg, Miriam. "A three-year program at DeWitt Clinton High School to help bright underachievers." *High Points* 41 (1959): 5–35.

Goldston, D. B. et al. "Reading problems, psychiatric disorders, and functional impairment from mid-to-late adolescence." *Journal of the American Academy of Child and Adolescent Psychiatry* 46, no. 1 (2007): 25–32.

Goleman, Daniel. *Emotional Intelligence.* New York: Bantam Books, 1997.

Goleman, Daniel. *Social intelligence.* New York: Bantam Dell, 2006.

Goodenough, F. (1926). "A new approach to the measurement of intelligence of young children." *Journal of Genetic Psychology,* 33 (1926): 185–211.

Goodenough, Florence, *The Handbook of Child Psychology*. Minneapolis, MN: University of Minnesota, 1933.

Goodenough, Florence, in L. Carmichael (ed.), *Manual of Child Psychology*. New York: Knopf, 1954, pp. 75–76.

Goodyer, I. M. "Stress in childhood and adolescence." In FIsher, S. and Reason, J. (Eds.). *Handbook of life stress, cognition and health*. New York: Wiley, 1988, pp. 23–40.

Gross, Gail M. "Child Brain Development: Age One." March 4, 2015. Accessed December 31, 2018. http://drgailgross.com/child-brain-development-age-one/.

Gross, Gail M. "How to Use the Empathic Process—January 9, 2015." Accessed April 12, 2019. http://drgailgross.com/use-empathic-process/.

Gross, Gail M. "It Takes a Family to Raise a Smarter, Less Stressed Child—Not a Village." December 20, 2013. Accessed December 31, 2018. http://drgailgross.com/takes-family-raise-smarter-less-stressed-child-village/.

Gross, Gail M. "Parental Involvement and the Reading Achievement of Third Grade Students." PhD diss., University of Houston, May 1995. 1–113.

Gross, Gail M. "Parenting and Educating the Gifted Child, Part 2." November 21, 2013. Accessed December 31, 2018. http://drgailgross.com/parenting-educating-gifted-child-part-2/.

Gross, Gail M. "The Effect of Stress on the Reading Achievement of Fourth- and Fifth-Grade Students." PhD diss., San Francisco, 2012, 1–105

Gross, Gail M. "The Importance of Early Parental Involvement." August 2, 2018. Accessed April 12, 2019. https://www.huffpost.com/entry/the-important-role-of-dad_n_5489093.

Gross, Gail M. "The Important Role of Dad." August 12, 2014. Accessed April 12, 2019. https://www.huffpost.com/entry/the-important-role-of-dad_n_5489093.

Gross, Gail M. *The Only Way Out Is Through: A Ten-step Journey from Grief to Wholeness*. Lanham, MD: Rowman & Littlefield, 2018.

Gross, Gail M. "The Psychology of Aggression, Part 1." September 08, 2017. Accessed December 31, 2018. http://drgailgross.com/the-psychology-of-aggression-part-1/.

Halpin, Gerald W., David A. Payne, and Chad D. Ellett. "Biographical correlates of the creative personality: Gifted adolescents." *Exceptional Children* 39 (1973): 652–653.

Hamer, Dean H., and Peter Copeland. *Living with Our Genes: Why They Matter More than You Think*. London: Macmillan, 1999.

Hayden, Thomas. "A Sense of Self." *Newsweek* (2000): 56–62

Healey, Shevy E, Anthony Kales, Lawrance J. Monroe, Edward O. Bixler, Katherine Chamberlin, and Constantin R. Soldatos. "Onset of insomnia: Role of life-stress events." *Psychosomatic Medicine* 43, no. 5 (1981): 439–451.

Heward, William L. *An Introduction to Special Education.* (6th ed.) Upper Saddle River, NJ: Merrill/Prentice Hall, 2000, pp. 158–159.

Hoffman, J., Neff, J. A., Hanson, S., and Pierce, K. "The Effects of 60 Beats Per Minute Music on Test Taking Anxiety Among Nursing Students." *The Journal of Nursing Education* 29, no. 2 (1990): 66–70. https://doi.org/10.3928/0148-4834-19900201-06.

"How Much Sleep Do I Need?" *National Center for Chronic Disease Prevention and Health Promotion, Division of Population Health.* Atlanta, 2 March 2017. https://www.cdc.gov/sleep/about_sleep/how_much_sleep.html.

Howe, Michael J. A. *Genius Explained.* Cambridge: Cambridge University Press, 2001.

Hyde, Andrea M. "Yoga at the Promise Program: A Feminist Qualitative Case Study of School-Based Yoga." 2017. https://dx.doi.org/10.4135/9781526402912.

"Ivy Tech Libraries: Psychology 101—Fort Wayne: Human Development." Ivy Tech Community College. August 2, 2018. Accessed December 21, 2018. https://library.ivytech.edu/c.php?g=478335&p=3270530.

Jacobs, Gregg D. "The Physiology of Mind-Body Interactions: The Stress Response and the Relaxation Response." *The Journal of Alternative and Complementary Medicine* 7, no. 1 (2001): S85-S92.

Jones, Maryann Clementi. "Life Stress and Reading Comprehension Test Scores in the Middle School Student." *The Educational Resources Information Center (ERIC)* (Kean College of New Jersey), 1994: 1–42.

Karnes, Merle B., Zehrbach, R.R., Studley, W.M., and Wright, W.R. *Culturally disadvantaged children of higher potential: Intellectual functioning and educational implications.* Champaign, III.: Champaign Community Unit 4 School, 1965.

Kerr, Catherine E, and Stephanie R. Jones. "Effects of mindfulness meditation training on anticipatory alpha modulation in primary somatosensory cortex." *Brain Research Bulletin* 85, no. 3–4 (2001): 96–103.

Kiecolt-Glaser, Janice K., and Ronald Glaser. "Psychological influences on immunity." *Implications for AIDS* (*American Psychologist*) 43, no. 11 (1988): 892–898.

Kiselica, Mark S., Stanley B. Baker, Ronald N. Thomas, and Susan Reedy. "Effects of stress inoculation training on anxiety, stress, and academic performance among adolescents." *Journal of Counseling Psychology* 41, no. 3 (1994): 335–342.

Klein, R.J. "Relaxation strategies." *Trauma and Loss: Research and Interventions Journal* 3, no. 2 (2003): 1–14.

Krech, Paul Rock. "Envisioning a Healthy Future: A Re-becoming of Native American Men." *Journal of Sociology and Social Welfare* 29, no. 1 (2002): 77–95.

Larson, H., Yoder, A., Johnson, C., Ramahi, M., Sung, J., and Washburn, F. "Test anxiety and relaxation training in third-grade students." *Eastern Education Journal* 39, no. 1 (2010): 13–22.

"Lawrence Kohlberg Moral Development | Counseling | Pinterest | Kohlberg Moral Development, Morals and Human Development." *Pinterest.* Accessed December 21, 2018. https://www.pinterest.com/pin/465418942734511790/.

Lehrer, Paul M., Robert L. Woolfolk, and Wesley E. Sime. *Principles and practice of stress management,* Third edition. New York: Guilford, 2007.

Linden, Wolfgang. "Psychosocial Interventions for Patients with Coronary Artery Disease." *JAMA.* April 08, 1996. Accessed November 17, 2018. https://jama -network.com/journals/jamainternalmedicine/article-abstract/621809.

Liotti, Mario, Helen S. Mayberg, Stephen K. Brannan, Scott McGinnis, Paul Jerabek, and Peter T. Fox. "Differential limbic–cortical correlates of sadness and anxiety in healthy subjects: Implications for affective disorders." *Biological Psychiatry* 48, no. 1 (2000): 30–42.

Lipton, Bruce H. *The Biology of Belief: Unleashing the power of consciousness, matter and miracles.* New York: Hay Houston, Inc., 2005.

Liu, Shung-Yi S. "Familial and psychological effects on students' reading achievements." *Linear structural relations (LISREL) approach.* 1992. http://hdl.handle .net/2142/22152.

Livingston, Gretchen. "Fewer than half of U.S. kids today live in a 'traditional' family." *Pew Research Center.* December 22, 2014. http://pewrsr.ch/1zW782T.

Low orca birth rates linked to lack of Chinook salmon. June 29, 2017. https://www .cbc.ca/news/canada/british-columbia/low-orca-birth-rates-linked-to-lack-of -chinook-salmon-1.4183609 (accessed April 22, 2019).

Lozanov, G. "The Bulgarian experience." *The Journal of Suggestive-Accelerative Learning and Teaching* 2, No. 3 & 4 (1977): 85–95; and Martindale, C. *The Regressive Imagery Dictionary.* 1975.

Lozanov, G. "A general theory of suggestion in the communications process and the activation of the total reserves of the learner's personality." *Suggestopaedia-Canada,* 1 (1977): 1–4.

Lupien, S. J., Fiocco, A., Wan, N., Maheu, F., Lord, C., Scramek, T., and Tu, M. T. "Stress hormones and human memory function across the lifespan" [Abstract]. *Psychoneuroendocrinology,* 30, no. 3 (2005): 225–242.

Lupien, Sonia J., Bruce S. McEwen, Megan R. Gunnar, and Christine Heim. "Effects of stress throughout the lifespan on the brain, behaviour and cognition." *Nature Reviews Neuroscience* 10, no. 6 (2009): 434–445.

MacLean, P. "A mind of three minds: Educating the triune brain." In *Education and the Brain,* 27th Yearbook of the National Society for the Study of Education. Edited by Chall, J., and Mirsky, A. Chicago, IL: University of Chicago Press, 1978.

Maercker, Andreas, Tanja Michael, Lydia Fehm, Eni S. Becker, and Jurgen Margraf. "Age of traumatisation as a predictor of post-traumatic stress disorder or major depression in young women." *British Journal of Psychiatry* 184 (2004): 482–487.

Maltz, Maxwell. *Psycho-cybernetics.* New York: Essandess, 1968.

Mann, Denise. "Babies Listen and Learn While in the Womb," January 3, 2013. https://www.webmd.com/baby/news/20130102/babies-learn-womb#1. Accessed April 25, 2019.

Marion, Sheri. "Mitochondrial Disease in Autism." *Focus for Health.* April 7, 2016. https://www.focusforhealth.org/mitochondrial-disease-in-autism/ (accessed April 22, 2019).

Martindale, C. "What makes creative people different?" *Psychology Today,* 9, no. 2 (1975): 44–50

Massey, Marilyn S. "Promoting Stress Management: The Role of Comprehensive School Health Programs." *ERIC Digest,* August 1998: 1–7. https://files.eric .ed.gov/fulltext/ED421480.pdf.

May, Kate T. "An early detection test for pancreatic cancer: Jack Andraka at TED 2013." February 27, 2013 (Accessed April 25, 2019) https://blog.ted.com /an-early-detection-test-for-pancreatic-cancer-jack-andraka-at-ted2013/.

McCarthy, Laura F. "What Babies Learn In the Womb." *Parenting.* July 8, 2014. Accessed January 16, 2019. https://www.parenting.com/article /what-babies-learn-in-the-womb.

McEwen, Bruce S. "Stress, adaptation, and disease: Allostasis and allostatic load." *Annuals of the New York Academy of Sciences* 840 (1998): 33–44.

McGreevey, Sue. "Meditation may help the brain 'turn down the volume' on distractions." *Enhanced control of alpha rhythms may underlie some effects of mindfulness meditation,* 2011.

McLeod, Saul. "Concrete Operational Stage." *Simply Psychology.* January 1, 1970. Accessed December 21, 2018. https://www.simplypsychology.org/concrete -operational.html.

McLeod, Saul. "The Preoperational Stage of Cognitive Development." *Simply Psychology.* Accessed December 21, 2018. https://www.simplypsychology.org /preoperational.html.

McLoyd, Vonnie C. "Socioeconomic disadvantage and child development." *American Psychologist* 53, no. 2 (1998): 185–204.

Midwest Center for Stress and Anxiety. *Symptoms of stress.* 2009.

Miller, Kevin F., Catherine M. Smith, Jianjun Zhu, and Houcan Zhang. "Preschool Origins of Cross-National Differences in Mathematical Competence: The Role of Number-Naming Systems." *Psychological Science* 6, no. 1 (1995): 56–60.

Miller, S., and McCormick, J. (Eds.). "Teaching children to cope." *Journal of Physical Education, Recreation & Dance,* 62(2) (1991): 53–54.

Miller, Susan, and Larry Reibstein. "Good Kid, Bad Kid." *Newsweek* (1997): 64–65.

Miller, Susan, and Larry Reibstein. "Good Kid, Bad Kid." *Newsweek* (1997): 64–68.

Montessori, Maria. *The Absorbent Mind.* New York: Henry Holt, 1995.

Montessori, Maria. *The Discovery of the Child.* New York: Ballantine, 1972.

Morales, Julie R., and Nancy G. Guerra. "Effects of Multiple Context and Cumulative Stress on Urban Children's Adjustment in Elementary School." *Child Development* 77, no. 4 (2006): 907–923.

Morén, Constanza, Sandra Hernández, Mariona Guitart-Mampel, and Glòria Garrabou. "Mitochondrial Toxicity in Human Pregnancy: An Update on Clinical and Experimental Approaches in the Last 10 Years." *Int J Environ Res Public Health* 11, no. 9 (September 2014): 9897–9918.

Morrow, W. R., and Wilson, R. C. "Family relations of bright high achieving and underachieving high school boys." *Child Development* 32 (1961): 501–510.

Murray, John P. "Thoughtless Vigilantes." The International Encyclopedia of Media Studies, 2012. https://doi.org/10.1002/9781444361506.wbiems115.

Murray, John P. "TV violence and brainmapping in children." *Psychiatric Times,* 2001.

Napoli, Maria, Paul Rock Krech, and Lynn C. Holley. "Mindfulness Training for Elementary School Students: The Attention Academy." *Journal of Applied School Psychology* 21, no. 1 (2005): 99–109.

Nauert, Rick. "Stress Affects Learning and Memory." *Psych Central,* 2008. https://psychcentral.com/news/2008/03/12/stress-affects-learning-and-memory/2031.html

NICHD Early Child Care Research Network. "Factors associated with fathers' caregiving activities and sensitivity with young children." *Journal of Family Psychology* 14, no. 2 (2000): 200–219.

Norr, Serena. "10 Ways Moms Can Balance Work and Family." *Parents.* Accessed December 16, 2018. https://www.parents.com/parenting/work/life-balance/moms-balance-work-family/.

Noteboom, Jon T., Kerry R. Barnholt, and Roger M. Enoka. "Activation of the arousal response and impairment of performance increase with anxiety and stressor intensity." *Journal of Applied Physiology* 91 (2001): 2093–2101.

Ornish, Dean. *Dr. Dean Ornish's Program for Reversing Heart Disease: The Only System Scientifically Proven to Reverse Heart Disease Without Drugs or Surgery.* New York: The Random House Publishing Group, 1996.

Ornish, Dean. *Stress, Diet, and Your Heart.* New York: New American Library, 1982.

Ostrander, Sheila, Lynn Schroeder, and Nancy Ostrander. *Superlearning.* New York: Delacorte, 1979.

Papalia, Diane E., et al. *Human Development*. 8th ed., New York: McGraw-Hill, 2001.

"Parents as First Teachers." NeuroImage. June 27, 2014. Accessed November 5, 2018. https://www.sciencedirect.com/science/article/pii/B9780080918204500106.

Partanen E., Kujala, T., Huotilainen, M., et al. "Learning-induced neural plasticity of speech processing before birth." *PNAS*. 2013.

Parten, M.B. "Social play among preschool children." *Journal of Abnormal and Social Psychology* 27, no. 3 (1932): 243–269

Paul, Gina, Barb Elam, and Steven J. Verhulst. "A Longitudinal Study of Students' Perceptions of Using Deep Breathing Meditation to Reduce Testing Stresses." *Teaching and Learning in Medicine* 19, no. 3 (2007): 287–292.

Perkins, H.V. "Classroom behavior and underachievement." *American Educational Research Journal* 2 (1965):1–12.

Perreira, Krista M., and India J. Ornelas. "The Physical and Psychological Well-Being." *Future of Children* 21, no. 1 (2011): 195–218.

Peyser, Marc, and Anne Underwood. "Shyness, Sadness, Curiosity, Joy. Is It Nature or Nurture?" *Newsweek* (1997): 60-63.

Pierce, J., and Bowman, P. "Motivation Patters of High School Students." In *The Gifted Student*. Cooperative Research Monograph no. 2 (OE-35-16). Washington, D.C.: Office of Education, 1960.

Pierce, J.V. "The educational motivation patterns of superior students who do and do not achieve in high school." (Mimeograph report, University of Chicago, 1959.)

Polkki, Tarja, Anna-Maija Pietila, Katri Vehvilainen-Julkunen, Helena Laukkala, and Kai Kiviluoma. "Imagery-Induced Relaxation in Children's Postoperative Pain Relief: A Randomized Pilot Study." *Journal of Pediatric Nursing* 23, no. 3 (2008): 217–224.

Prichard, Allyn, and Jean Taylor. "A demonstration of the concept "hyper-learning." *Journal of Learning Disabilities* 14 (1981): 19–21.

Prichard, Allyn, and Jean Taylor. *Accelerating Learning: The Use of Suggestion in the Classroom*. Novato, CA: Academic Therapy Publications, 1980.

Radin, N., and Russell, G. "Increased Father Participation and Child Development Outcomes," in *Fatherhood and Family Policy*. Edited by M.E. Lamb and A. Sagi. Hillside, NJ: Lawrence Erlbaum, 1983.

Reiss, Albert J., and Jeffrey A. Roth. *Understanding and preventing violence: Panel on the understanding and control of violent behavior*. Consensus Study Report, Washington, DC: The National Academies Press, 1993, pp. 101–181.

Reiss, David, Jenae M. Neiderhiser, E. Mavis Hetherington, and Robert Plomin. *The Relationship Code: Deciphering Genetic and Social Influences on Adolescent Development*. Cambridge, MA: Harvard University Press, 2000.

Restak, Richard. *The Brain: The Last Frontier.* Garden City, NY: Doubleday, 1979.

Rose, C. *Accelerated learning.* New York: Dell, 1985.

Rose, Charlie. "The Brain Series- Aggression." AREA 17, March 5, 2015. Audio, 52:45. https://charlierose.com/videos/20942.

Roykulcharoen, Varunyupa. "Systematic relaxation to relieve postoperative pain." *Journal of Advanced Nursing* (2004): 140–148.

Sandberg, Jared. "Multimedia Childhood." North Seattle. Accessed May 7, 2018. http://webshare.northseattle.edu/fam180/topics/computers/Multimedia Childhood.htm.

Sapolsky, Robert M., Lewis C, Krey, and Bruce S. McEwen. "The Neuroendocrinology of Stress and Aging: The Glucocorticoid Cascade Hypothesis." *Science of Aging Knowledge. Environment,* no. 38 (2002): 21.

Schuster, Donald. "Suggestive, Accelerative Learning and Teaching: A Manual of Classroom Procedures Based on the Lozanov Method." *Journal of Research in Education.* November 30, 1975. Accessed December 12, 2018. https://eric.ed.gov/?id=ED136566.

Schuster, Donald H., and Charles E. Gritton. *Suggestive-Accelerative Learning Techniques.* New York: Gordon and Breach, 1989.

Science News Staff. "Extra Licking Makes for Relaxed Rats." *Science | AAAS.* September 11, 1997. Accessed December 29, 2018. https://www.sciencemag.org/news/1997/09/extra-licking-makes-relaxed-rats.

Seaward, Brian Luke. *Managing Stress: Principles and Strategies for Health and Wellbeing.* Sudbury, MA: Jones and Bartlett, 2006.

Seligman, Martin E.P. *Helplessness: on depression, development, and death.* New York: W. H. Freeman, 1992.

Selye, Hans. *The stress of life.* New York: McGraw-Hill, 1956.

Shaw, M. C., and McCuen, J. T. "The onset of academic underachievement in bright children." *Journal of Educational Psychology* 51 (1960):103–108.

Shek, Daniel T.L. "Economic Stress, Psychological Well-Being and Problem Behavior in Chinese Adolescents with Economic Disadvantage." *Journal of Youth and Adolescence* 32, no. 4 (2003): 259–266.

Silbereisen, Rainer K., Sabine Walper, and Helfried T. Albrecht. "Family income loss and economic hardship: Antecedents of adolescents' problem behavior." *New Directions for Child and Adolescent Development,* 1990: 27–47.

Silberman, Charles Eliot. *Crisis in the Classroom: The Remaking of American Education.* New York: Random House, 1970.

Skwarecki, Beth. "Babies Learn to Recognize Words in the Womb." Science | AAAS. December 10, 2017. Accessed December 31, 2018. https://www.sciencemag.org/news/2013/08/babies-learn-recognize-words-womb.

Snowman, Jack, and Robert Biehler. *Psychology applied to teaching.* Boston, MA: Houghton Mifflin Company, 1986.

Sophian, C. "Early developments in children's understanding of number: Inferences about numerosity and one-to-one correspondence." *Child Development* 59 (1988): 1397–1414.

Soutar, Richard. *Training Meditational States with Neurofeedback in a Clinical Setting.* n.d. https://newmindcenter.com/About-Neurofeedback /Neurofeedback-and-Meditation.

Spalding, Baird T. *India Tour Lessons on Life and Teaching of the Masters of the Far East.* Los Angeles: DeVorss & Publishers, 1948.

Springen, Karen. "This Is Your Brain on Violence." *Newsweek.* March 13, 2010. Accessed December 30, 2018. https://www.newsweek.com/violent -videogames-change-teen-brains-106937.

Staff, Newsweek. "A Bundle of Emotions." *Newsweek.* March 13, 2010. Accessed October 17, 2018. https://www.newsweek.com/bundle-emotions-174922.

Staff, Newsweek. "Cultivating the Mind." *Newsweek.* March 14, 2010. Accessed December 30, 2018. https://www.newsweek.com/cultivating-mind-174976.

Staff, Newsweek. "Turning On the Motor." *Newsweek.* March 13, 2010. Accessed December 30, 2018. https://www.newsweek.com/turning-motor-174928.

Stillman, Jessica. "Why Success Depends More on Personality Than Intelligence." *The Inc. Life.* January 11, 2017. https://www.inc.com/jessica-stillman/success -depends-more-on-personality-than-intelligence-new-study-shows.html (accessed April 24 2019, 2019).

Strodtbeck, F. L. "Family interaction values, and achievement." In McClelland, D.C. (Ed.), *Talent and society.* Princeton, NJ: Van Nostrand Reinhold, 1958, pp. 135–194.

Stuart, Elieen M., Margaret Caudill, Jane Lesermen, Claudia Dorrington, Richard Freidman, and Herbert Benson. "Nonpharmacologic treatment of hypertension: A multiple-risk-factor approach." *The Journal of Cardiovascular Nursing* 1, no. 4 (1987): 1–14.

Syrjala, Karen L., Gray W. Donaldson, Martha W. Davis, Michael E. Kippes, and John E. Carr. "Relaxation and imagery and cognitive-behavioral training reduce pain during cancer treatment: A controlled clinical trial." *Pain* 63, no. 2 (1995): 189–198.

"Tabula Rasa." Wikipedia. October 24, 2018. Accessed December 10, 2018. https://en.wikipedia.org/wiki/Tabula_rasa.

Talbot, Margaret. "The Placebo Prescription." *New York Times* magazine. January 9, 2000. (Accessed April 25, 2019.) https://www.nytimes.com/2000/01/09 /magazine/the-placebo-prescription.html.

Taylor, Shelley E., and Rena L. Repetti. "HEALTH PSYCHOLOGY: What is an unhealthy environment and how does it get under the skin?" *Annual Review Psychology* 48 (1997): 411–447.

Teale, W.H. "Toward a Theory of How Children Learn to Read and Write Naturally." *Language Arts* 56, no. 6 (1982): 555–570.

Teicher, Martin H., Akemi Tomoda, and Susan L. Andersen. "Neurobiological Consequences of Early Stress and Childhood Maltreatment: Are Results from Human and Animal Studies Comparable?" *Annals of the New York Academy of Sciences* 1071 (2006): 313–323.

Terman, L. M., and Oden, M. H. *The gifted group at mid-life: Thirty-five years' follow-up of the superior child. Genetic studies of genius,* vol. 5. Stanford, CA: Stanford University Press, 1959.

Thompson, R.F., Berger, T.W., and Berry, S.D. "An introduction to the anatomy, physiology and chemistry of the brain." In M.C. Wittrock (Ed.), *The Brain and Psychology.* NY: Academic Press, 1980, pp. 3–32.

Torrance, Ellis Paul. "Creative positives of disadvantaged children and youth." *Gifted Child Quarterly* 13, no. 2 (1969): 71–81. https://doi.org/10.1177 -%2F001698626901300201.

Toynbee, Arnold. "Has America Neglected Her Creative Minority?" *Sooner Magazine* 34, no. 5 (January 1962): 7–9. https://digital.libraries.ou.edu /sooner/articles/p7-9_1962v34n5_OCR.pdf.

Trafton, Anne. "The benefits of meditation." *MIT News Office.* May 5, 2011. http://news.mit.edu/2011/meditation-0505 (accessed May 8, 2019).

Tysinger, Jeffrey A., P. Dawn Tysinger, and Terry Diamanduros. "The Effect of Anxiety on the Measurement of Reading Fluency and Comprehension." *Georgia Educational Researcher Online Edition* 8, no. 1 (2010): 1–8.

Underwood, Anne. "Hey—Look Out, World, Here I Come." *Newsweek.* (1997): 12–15.

Underwood, Anne. "Shyness, Sadness, Curiosity, Joy. Is It Nature or Nurture?" *Newsweek.* February 28, 1997. Accessed November 15, 2018. https://www .newsweek.com/shyness-sadness-curiosity-joy-it-nature-or-nurture-174968.

Anne Underwood, "Hey—Look Out, World, Here I Come," *Newsweek* (1997): 12-15.

Van Boven, Sarah. "Giving Infants a Helping Hand." *Newsweek* (1997).

Vygotsky, L.F. *Vygotsky's psychology: A biography of ideas, Alex Kozulin.* Cambridge, MA: Harvard University Press, 1990.

Wadsworth, Martha E., Tali Raviv, Christine Reinhard, Brian Wolff, Catherine DeCarlo, and Lindsey Einhorn. "An Indirect Effects Model of the Association Between Poverty and Child Functioning: The Role of Children's Poverty-Related Stress." *Journal of Loss and Trauma* 13, no. 2–3 (2008): 156–185.

Walsh, Ann. *Self concepts of bright boys with learning difficulties.* New York: Teachers College, Columbia University, 1956.

White, Burton L. *The New First Three Years of Life.* New York: Fireside, 1996.

Williams, Mike. "Taming the wolf: Domesticating the dog." September 27, 2010. https://www.independent.co.uk/life-style/history/taming-the-wolf-domesticating-the-dog-2090768.html. Accessed April 25, 2019.

Woolfolk, Robert L. *Principles and practice of stress management.* New York: Guilford, 1984.

Zuckerman, Catherine. "A Musical Milestone." *National Geographic*, January 2019, 31.

ACKNOWLEDGMENTS

To the memory of my beloved daughter, Dawn Gross, whose deep wisdom, positive attitude, powerful drive, and loving and gentle feminine energy guided me through, to the end of this project.

To my beloved son and writing partner, Shawn Gross, whose wise counseling, brilliant editing, and great ideas supported this project every step of the way. His tremendous drive and people skills helped me keep my eye on the ball. Thank you for always being there.

To my beloved daughter, Kate Gross, your inner and outer beauty, intelligence, generous spirit, and grace once again fills our lives with happiness and joy . . . every day.

To my beloved grandchildren, Maxwell and Samantha Gross, the sparkling light of intellect, compassion, generosity, and kindness that shines from your eyes is a constant reminder to me of why I am.

To the memory of my beloved mother and father, Ida and Samuel Meyrowitz, you set my feet upon this journey of life and learning as my first friends, my first teachers, and my first supports. Thank you.

To the memory of my beloved mother-in-law and father-in-law, Anna and Edward Gross: you gave me the greatest gift of all, an extraordinary husband.

To my beloved brother, Dr. Michael Meyrowitz, my almost twin, thank you for your unfailing support, great advice, big-brother shoulders, and for saving my life.

To my beloved sister-in-law Michele Meyrowitz, you are the sister I always wanted. Your authentic kindness, compassion, and creative thinking remind me daily of how fortunate I am to have you in my life.

To my beloved nieces, nephews, great nieces and great nephews: Dr. Samuel and Aviva Meyrowitz, Dr. Jeff and Ellie Meyrowitz, Elisa and Tom Boyd, Isaac, Josh, and Noah Boyd, Lila, Sadie and Evan Meyrowitz, and Crosby Meyrowitz, because of you, Mother's legacy of love lives on.

To my sister-in-law Marjory, your kindness and thoughtfulness have filled our lives with happy memories, including my nieces, nephews, and grandnephews: Jeff and Marsha Lipsky, Jeniece Lipsky, Brad, Adam, Jami, Nathan, Daniel, Rachel, and to the memory of Gene Lipsky . . . such wonderful adventures.

To my beloved cousins Laura and Mark Zirulnik and Ginny and Barry Zirulnik: growing up together made us more siblings than cousins. And I'm reminded, every day, of the warm and loving memories of our childhood.

To my beloved cousins Ann and Andrew Tisch, who are always there, with open and loving arms, to support and catch me if I fall.

To the whole Rubinstein clan . . . you're great!

To the memory of Richard Rubinstein, a patriot and brave and noble man—you are loved and missed.

To Sol Lesh, thank you for your constant loyalty, kindness, and support always.

To the awesome Dr. Dean Ornish, MD, my brother from another mother. Thank you for always being there.

To the late Dr. William Brugh Joy, MD, the journey continues.

To my wonderful friend and mentor Alma Gildenhorn, who has lovingly inspired, guided, and mentored me throughout the years.

To my amazing friends—inspirational mentors all, thank for your loyalty, love, support . . . and most of all, for listening: Danny Akaka, Elena and Robert Albritton, Anita and Chris Anderson, Missy and Lyle Anderson, Mahnaz and Dari Ansari, Shahla and Ambassador Hushang Ansary, Beverly and Dan Arnold, The Honorable Nancy Atlas, Barbara and the late Gerson Bakar, Susan and The Honorable James Addison "Jim" Baker III, Joy and Hugh Bancroft, Laurel Barrack, Ambassador Barbara and Clyde Barrett, Carol Bartz, Admiral C.R. (Bob) Bell, Lyndie Bensen, B.A. Bentsen, Gayle and Lloyd Bentsen III, Wilma and Ambassador Stuart Bernstein, Tova Borgnine, Nancy and David Boschwitz, Paul Brenner, Renee and William Brinkerhoff, Cathy and Dr. Gary Brock, Sally Brown, Nichole and Eli Buchis, Marj and Tom Callinan, Diane Cassil, Anne and Albert Chao, Donna and Max Chapman, Pamela and Rick Crandall, Danielle and Meredith Cullen, Lorri and Jack Cuthbert, Rania and Jamal Daniel, Teran Davis, Dr. John and Beverly Dawson, Dr. Derbes and Mrs. Marti DeBenedetti and Dr. Ray Lagger, Liz and Dr. Bill Decker, Rinchen Dharlo, Dr. Colin Dinney, Terry Huffington Dittman and Dr. Ralph Dittman, Joy and Leon Dreimann, Liz Dubin, Jerri Duddlesten Moore, Deborah Duncan, Dr. David Eagleman, Eileen Eastham, Suellen Estrin, Gail and Mark Edwards, Diane Farb, Huda & Samia Farouki,

Mike Feinberg, Suzanne and Elliott Felson, Debi and Gary Fournier, Nancy Furlotti, Helen and Rich Gates, Mun Sok Geiger, Alma and Ambassasor Joseph Gildenhorn, Madeline and Harlan Gittin, Dr. Mireille and SirDr. Dennis Gillings, Christine and Sheldon Gordon, Shep Gordon, Adi and Jerry Greenberg, Glenda and Gerald Greenwald, Rabbi Steven M. Gross, Tara Lynda and Peter Guber, Lodi Gyari, Mariska Hargitay and Peter Hermann, Goldie Hawn and Kurt Russell, Paul and Cassandra Hazen, Grant and Jeannette Heidrich, Miriam and Merle Hinrich, Joanne Herring, Dr. Ron Hickerson, Janet and Paul Hobby, Gigi Huang, Arianna Huffington, Mike Huffington, Stormy and David Hull, Caroline Hunt, Dr. Carlos Isada, Lek and Bill Jahnke, Maggie and Ian Joye, Debi and Rick Justice, Barbara and Robert Kildow, Maureen and Gene Kim, Richard & Lauren King, The late Right Honorable Patricia Knatchbull, Countess Mountbatten of Burma, Lord Norton Louis Philp Knatchbill,

Count Mountbatten of Burma and Lady Penelope Knatchbill, Countess Mountbatten of Burma, Susan and Bert Kobayashi, Sima and Masoud Ladjevardian, Lyn and Norman Lear, Sandy Lee, Sara and Tom Lewis, Faith and Dr. Peter Linden, YinYee and Paul Locklin, Adriana Longoria, Sheryl and Rob Lowe, Sally Lucas, Carolyn and Taf Lufkin, Dawn and Duncan MacNaughton, Ann Marie and Jim Mahoney, Marlene and The Honorable Fred Malek, Alexandra Marshall, JoAnn and John Mason, Ann Mather, Leigh and Bill Matthes, Bonnie and Tom McCloskey, Susan and JB McIntosh, Leslie McMorrow, Andrea and Bobby McTamaney, Pat Mitchell, Janet and Thomas Montag, Dr. Courtenay Moore, Ione and Sidney Moran, Joy and Stewart Morris, Jenie Moses, Rosa Mow, and Dr. Bill Mow, Susan and Edward Mueller, The Right Honourable Brian Mulroney and Mila Mulroney, Scott Murray, Jeanette Lerman - Neubauer and The Honorable Joseph Neubauer, Sandi and Bill Nicholson, Dr. Dean and Anne Ornish, Sandy and the late Paul Ortellni, Jane and Carl Panattoni, Renee and Robert (Bob) Parsons, Rhonda and Tom Peed, Cynthia and Tony Petrello, Mary and Andy Pilara, Lexy and Robert Potamkin, Alma Powell, Carolyn Powers, Elsa and C.N. Reddy, Lynda and Stewart Resnick, Elaine and Hans Riddervold, Sogyal Rinpoche, Michelle Robson, Fred and Marian Rosen, Carol and Jay Rosenbaum, John and Judy Runstead, Susan and Pat Rutherford, Kim and Jim Schneider, Joan Schnitzer-Levy, June and Paul Schorr, Walter Scott, Susan and Fayez Sarofim, Louisa Sarofim, Sandi and Ron Simon, Sue Smith, Jennifer and Tony Smorgon, Susan and Randy Snyder, Lois and George Stark, Agapi Stassinopoulos, Paul & Elle Stephens, Kathleen and Bob Styer, Kitch Taub, Mae Thomas, Nena and Dr. Robert Thurman, Sandy and James Treliving, Doan and Dr. Joe Trigg, Phoebe and Bobby Tudor, Gerda and Jerry Ungerman, Dr. Alberto Villoldo, Prince Sangay Wangchuck and the Queen Mother of Bhutan, Joe and Marjorie Walsh, Melani and Rob Walton, Tom and Hilary Watson, Lynda and Doug Weiser, Marcie Taub-Wessel and Tom Wessel, Karin and Paul Wick, Dr. James Willerson, Margaret Williams, Jeannie and Wallace Wilson, Clark and Sharon Winslow, Shannon and Dennis Wong, Gigi Wong, Julie

Wrigley, Lynn and Oscar Wyatt, Gail and Mike Yanney, Pat and Michael York.

To our outstanding Second Tuesday Group: Cathy and Giorgio Borlenghi, William Burge, Susan and Ronald Blankenship, Polly and Murry Bowden, Mo and Ric Campo, Christy and Louis Cushman, Bonnie and Peter Williams Dienna, Patti and Richard Everett, Wendy and Jeff Hines, Suzie and Larry Johnson, Ann and Frank McGuyer, Leila and Walter Mischer, Eileen and John Moody, Kathleen and William Sharman, Sharon Wilkes and Thomas, Simmons, Marcia and David Solomon, Andrea and Bill White, Mary and David Wolff.

To our very special Houston Mediation Group and Hawaii Meditation Group: thank you.

To Don Fehr, my brilliant agent, who has worked tirelessly on my behalf and helped me in more ways than I can enumerate.

To my senior editor Nicole Frail, thank you for all your sensational ideas and generous guidance that encouraged me all the way to the finish line.

To Marlynn Schotland, thank you for your media magic.

To remarkable Kathleen Cuttrell, who is always there when I need her. She started this project with me and saw it through to the end. She worked tirelessly to make sure that we met every deadline. She is just magnificent.

Renée Richards, Thank you for all your help along the way . . . as always.

To Jill Sorensen, thank you for always doing what's needed.

To my loving friends, Angelica and Albert Garza, David Herrera, Kristin Hunt, and Andy Estrada, who are part of our family and take wonderful care of us. To Hanna and Eduardo, our flower-masters.

To Alex and Diane Hamden and their daughter Sarah Gale, You have all been wonderful to our family, throughout the last thirty years.

To everyone at Kukio, Nanea, and Hualalai, thank you all, for always being there to help us and make our lives a true Nanea: Natasha Curran, Kai Fukuda, Marc Hasegawa, Juliana Kasberg, Walter Nakashima, Jr., Gene Namnama, Lauren Pollard, Jacqueline Roses and Shun Tsukazaki at Kukio Golf and Beach Club.

To Daniel Avendano Silva, George Boeckmann, KC Botelho, Adam Condon, Marcial Correa, George Cost, Terry Costales, Joseph Forester, Jorge Garcia, Ben Halpern, Todd Harrington, John Henry, Mavis Hirata, Kaipo Kaahu-Mahi, Chirs Keiter, Kimberly Kim, Tyler Kirkendoll, Kris Kitt, Lance Lawhead, Stacie Loo, Maila Makaena-Pucong, Christopher Manley, Dustin Marin, Keith McGonagle, Kainapau Meheula, Jarren Menke, Darren Naihe, Ian Noonan, Matt Pinstein, Juan Rodriguez, Michael Romero, Les Tengan, Yuri Stuermer, and Channing Tam at Nanea.

To Barbara Eldridge and all the girls in the office, and Brendan Moynahan and all the golf pros at Hualalai.

And a final thank-you to my wonderful publisher, Skyhorse Publishing, and their new collaborators, Simon & Schuster.

ENDNOTES

INTRODUCTION

1 Montessori, Maria. *The Absorbent Mind.* New York: Henry Holt, 1995, p. 8.
2 Carrel, Alexis. *L'Homme Cet Inconnu* (Place of Publication Not Identified: LULU COM, 2018).
3 Elkind, David. *Miseducation: Preschoolers at Risk.* New York: Knopf, 1987, back cover.

CHAPTER 1

1 Dictionary. "Each and Every One." Accessed April 22, 2019. https://www .dictionary.com/browse/each-and-every-one.
2 Santos E., Noggle, C.A. "Synaptic Pruning." In: Goldstein S., Naglieri J.A. (eds.) *Encyclopedia of Child Behavior and Development.* Boston, MA: Springer, 2011. https://doi.org/10.1007/978-0-387-79061-9_2856.
3 Ornish, Dean. *Stress, Diet, and Your Heart.* New York: New American Library, 1982, p. 71.
4 Goodenough, Florence. In L. Carmichael (ed.), *Manual of Child Psychology.* New York: Knopf, 1954, pp. 75–76.
5 Cooney, Adam, and Samantha Jones. "The Educational Theory of Maria Montessori." *NewFoundations.* November 19, 2018. http://www.newfounda tions.com/GALLERY/Montessori.html (accessed April 22, 2019).
6 Goleman, Daniel. *Emotional Intelligence.* New York: Bantam Books, 2006, pp. 273–274.
7 Goleman, Daniel. *Emotional Intelligence: Why It Can Matter More Than IQ.* New York: Bantam Books, 1995.

8 "Executive Summary," *PISA 2009 Results: Learning Trends*, 2010, accessed December 29, 2018, https://www.oecd.org/pisa/pisaproducts/46619703.pdf.

9 Bayliss, Sarah. *Study supports case for more parental involvement. London Times* Educational Supplement, 3561, 6.

10 White, Burton L. *The New First Three Years of Life.* New York: Fireside, 1996.

11 "Parents as First Teachers," NeuroImage, June 27, 2014, accessed November 5, 2018, https://www.sciencedirect.com/science/article/pii/B9780080918204500106.

12 Elkind, *Miseducation*, 36.

13 Gross, *Parental Involvement*, 59.

14 Begley, Sharon. "How to Build a Baby's Brain." *Newsweek*, 30-31.

15 Cole, Beverly. "American Dads: Loving Their Kids To Success." Accessed April 22, 2019. https://englishhound.com/2018/04/15/american-dads-loving-their-kids-to-success/.

16 Adler, Jerry. "It's a Wise Father Who Knows . . ." *Newsweek* (1997):73.

17 Tavernise, Sabrina. "Married Couples Are No Longer a Majority, Census Finds." *New York Times*, May 26, 2011, http://www.nytimes.com/2011/05/26/us/26marry.html.

18 Thriving Workforce, "2016 Global When Women Thrive Report," https://www.mercer.com/our-thinking/when-women-thrive-2016-report.html.

19 Patton, Angela. "A Father-Daughter-Dance—In Prison?" *TED Radio Hour*, April 25, 2014, https://www.npr.org/2014/04/25/301828303/a-father-daughter-dance-in-prison.

CHAPTER 2

1 Arnold and Chandler, "Archived: Read With Me—A Guide for Student Volunteers Starting Early Childhood Literacy Programs; Making Connections: How Children Learn," Home, accessed November 5, 2018, https://www2.ed.gov/pubs/ReadWithMe/makconn.html.

2 Howe, Michael J.A. *Genius Explained.* Cambridge: Cambridge University Press, 2001.

3 Reiss, David. *The Relationship Code: Deciphering Genetic and Social Influences on Adolescent Development.* Cambridge, MA: Harvard University Press, 2003, p. 426.

4 Bloom et al., *Taxonomy of Educational Objectives, Handbook 1.* London: Longman, 1956.

5 Hamer, Dean H., and Peter Copeland. *Living with Our Genes: Why They Matter More than You Think.* London: Macmillan, 1999, p. 11.

6 Hayden, Thomas. "A Sense of Self." http://webshare.northseattle.edu, accessed November 8, 2018, http://webshare.northseattle.edu/fam180/topics/temperament/asenseofself.htm.

7 Underwood, Anne. "Shyness, Sadness, Curiosity, Joy. Is It Nature Or Nurture?" *Newsweek*, March 14, 2010, accessed December 29, 2018, https://www.newsweek.com/shyness-sadness-curiosity-joy-it-nature-or-nurture-174968.

8 Reiss, *The Relationship Code*, 426.

9 Hayden, Thomas. "A Sense of Self." *Newsweek*, 60.

10 Underwood, "Shyness, Sadness, Curiosity, Joy. Is It Nature Or Nurture?"

11 VoosenDec, Paul, et al., "Extra Licking Makes for Relaxed Rats," Science | AAAS, December 11, 2017, accessed December 29, 2018, https://www.sciencemag.org/news/1997/09/extra-licking-makes-relaxed-rats.

12 Underwood, "Shyness, Sadness, Curiosity, Joy. Is It Nature Or Nurture?"

13 Hayden, Thomas. "A Sense of Self." *Newsweek*, 62.

14 Ibid.

15 Ibid.

16 Ibid.

17 Papalia, Diane E., et al., Human Development, 35.

18 Ibid.

19 Miller, Susan, and Larry Reibstein. "Good Kid, Bad Kid." New York: Newsweek, 1997, 64–65.

20 Hayden, Thomas. "A Sense of Self." *Newsweek*, 56–62.

21 Ibid.

22 Ibid.

23 Ibid.

24 Papalia, Diane E., al., *Human Development*, 298.

25 Hayden, Thomas. "A Sense of Self." *Newsweek*, 2000, 56-62. http://webshare.northseattle.edu/fam180/topics/temperament/asenseofself.htm.

26 Rose, Charlie. "The Brain Series-Aggression." AREA 17, March 5, 2015. Audio, 52:45. https://charlierose.com/videos/20942.

27 Ibid.

28 Ibid.

29 Ibid.

30 Ibid.

31 Ibid.

32 Anderson, Craig A., et al. "The Influence of Media Violence on Youth," *Psychological Science in the Public Interest* 4, no. 3 (2003), doi:10.1111/j.1529–1006.2003.pspi_1433.x.

33 Murray, John P., *Thoughtless Vigilantes: The International Encyclopedia of Media Studies*, 2012, doi:10.1002/9781444361506.wbiems115.

34 Springen, Karen. "This Is Your Brain on Violence," *Newsweek*, March 13, 2010, accessed December 30, 2018, https://www.newsweek.com/violent-videogames-change-teen-brains-106937.

35 Murray, *Thoughtless Vigilantes.*

36 Anderson et al. *The Influence of Media Violence on Youth.*

37 Bjornkvist, Kaj. "Violent Films, Anxiety and Aggression: Experimental Studies of the Effect of Violent Films on the Level of Anxiety and Aggressiveness in Children," World Cat, November 11, 2018, accessed December 29, 2018, https://www.worldcat.org/title/violent-films-anxiety-and-aggression-experimental-studies-of-the-effect-of-violent-films-on-the-level-of-anxiety-and-agressiveness-in-children/oclc/58507862?referer=di&ht=edition.

38 "What Babies Learn In the Womb," *Parenting*, July 08, 2014, accessed January 16, 2019, https://www.parenting.com/article/what-babies-learn-in-the-womb.

39 Glover, V. "The Effects of Prenatal Stress on Child Behavioural and Cognitive Outcomes Start at the Beginning." In: Tremblay R.E., Boivin, M., Peters, R. DeV., eds. Glover V, topic ed. *Encyclopedia on Early Childhood Development* [online]. http://www.child-encyclopedia.com/stress-and-pregnancy-prenatal-and-perinatal/according-experts/effects-prenatal-stress-child. Updated April 2019. Accessed April 25, 2019.

40 Mann, Denise. "Babies Listen and Learn While in the Womb." January 3, 2013 https://www.webmd.com/baby/news/20130102/babies-learn-womb#1. Accessed April 25, 2019.

41 Partanen, E., Kujala, T., Huotilainen, M., et al. "Learning-induced neural plasticity of speech processing before birth." PNAS. 2013.

42 Begley, Sharon. "How to Build a Baby's Brain." *Newsweek*, 28-31.

43 Skwarecki, Beth. "Babies Learn to Recognize Words in the Womb." Science | AAAS. December 10, 2017. Accessed December 31, 2018. https://www.science-mag.org/news/2013/08/babies-learn-recognize-words-womb.

44 Zuckerman, Catherine. "A Musical Milestone." *National Geographic*, January 2019, 31.

CHAPTER 3

1 Underwood, Anne, and Marc Peyser. "Shyness, Sadness, Curiosity, Joy. Is It Nature or Nurture?" *Newsweek*, 1997, 60-63. https://www.newsweek.com/shyness-sadness-curiosity-joy-it-nature-or-nurture-174968.

2 Elkind, David. *Miseducation: Preschoolers at Risk.* New York: Knopf, 1987, p. 55.

3 Ibid., 20.

4 Ibid., 21.

5   Montessori, Maria. *The Discovery of the Child*. New York: Ballantine, 1972, p. 46.

6   Elkind, *Miseducation*, 51.

7   Ibid., 22.

8   Estrada, P., et al. (1987). "Affective quality of the mother-child relationship: Longitudinal consequences for children's school-relevant cognitive functioning," 210–215.

9   Van Boven, Sarah. *Giving Infants a Helping Hand*. New York: Newsweek, 1997, p. 45.

10 Ibid.

11 Ibid.

12 Montessori, Maria, and M. Joseph Costelloe. *The Discovery of the Child*. Vancouver: Access and Diversity, Crane Library, University of British Columbia, 2015.

13 Cowley, Geoffrey. *The Language Explosion*. New York: Newsweek, 1997, pp. 16–20.

14 Gross, *Parental Involvement*, 29.

15 Ibid., 28.

16 Ibid., 27.

17 Ibid., 24.

18 Ibid., 23.

19 Ibid., 25.

20 Ibid., 33.

21 Ibid., 32.

22 Elkind, *Miseducation*, 25.

23 Begley, Sharon. "How to Build a Baby's Brain." *Newsweek*. March 13, 2010. Accessed December 30, 2018. https://www.newsweek.com/how-build-babys -brain-174940.

24 Elkind, David. *Miseducation*, 65.

25 Begley, Sharon. "How to Build a Baby's Brain." *Newsweek*, 31.

26 Gross, *Parental Involvement*, 37.

27 Ibid., 37.

28 Ibid., 33.

29 Ibid., 39–40.

30 Underwood, "Shyness, Sadness, Curiosity, Joy. Is It Nature Or Nurture?"

31 Elkind, *Miseducation*, 56.

32 Ibid., 60.

33 Ibid., 39.

34 Ibid., 52.

35 Montessori, *Absorbent Mind*, 28.

36 Begley, Sharon. "How to Build a Baby's Brain." *Newsweek*, 28–32.

37 Papalia, Diane E., et al., *Human Development*, 33

38 Elkind, *Miseducation*, 60.

CHAPTER 4

1 Williams, Mike. "Taming the wolf: Domesticating the dog." September 27, 2010. https://www.independent.co.uk/life-style/history/taming-the-wolf-domesti cating-the-dog-2090768.html. Accessed April 25, 2019.

2 Elkind, *Miseducation*, 79.

3 Sandberg, Jared. "Multimedia Childhood," North Seattle, accessed May 7, 2018, http://webshare.northseattle.edu/fam180/topics/computers/MultimediaChild hood.htm.

4 Ibid.

5 Silberman, Charles E., *Crisis in the Classroom: The Remaking of American Education.* New York: Random House, 1970.

6 Begley, Sharon. "How to Build a Baby's Brain." *Newsweek*, 30.

7 Goodenough, F. "A new approach to the measurement of intelligence of young children." *Journal of Genetic Psychology* (1926): 185–211.

8 Heward, William L. *An Introduction to Special Education.* (6th ed.) Upper Saddle River, NJ: Merrill/Prentice Hall, 2000, pp.158–159.

9 Gross, Gail M. "The Importance of Early Parental Involvement." August 2, 2018. Accessed April 12, 2019. https://thriveglobal.com/stories/the-importance -of-parental-involvement/.

10 Goleman, *Emotional Intelligence.*

11 Norr, Serena. "10 Ways Moms Can Balance Work and Family." *Parents*, accessed December 16, 2018, https://www.parents.com/parenting/work/life -balance/moms-balance-work-family/.

12 "Difficult Child Behavior: 4 Tools to Help You Stay Calm." *Empowering Parents*, accessed October 25, 2018, https://www.empoweringparents.com /article/4-tools-to-help-you-stay-calm-with-your-difficult-child/.

13 Livingston, Gretchen. "Fewer than half of U.S. kids today live in a 'traditional' family." *Pew Research Center.* December 22, 2014. http://pewrsr.ch/1zW782T.

14 Ibid.

15 "Centers for Disease Control and Prevention." *Data & Statistics on Autism Spectrum Disorder.* April 5, 2019. https://www.cdc.gov/ncbddd/autism/dat .html (accessed April 22, 2019).

CHAPTER 5

1 Newsweek Staff, "Turning on the Motor," *Newsweek*, March 13, 2010, accessed December 30, 2018, https://www.newsweek.com/turning-motor-174928.

2 Papalia, Diane E., *Human Development*, 136.

3 Ibid.

4 Ibid.

5 Ibid.

6 Ibid.

7 Ibid.

8 Newsweek Staff, "Turning on the Motor," *Newsweek*, 1997, 26.

9 Newsweek Staff, "A Bundle of Emotions," *Newsweek*, 1997, 78.

10 Papalia, Diane E., *Human Development*, 8th ed. New York: McGraw Hill, 2001, p. 140.

11 Ibid.

12 Ibid., 141.

13 Ibid., 142.

14 Underwood, Anne. "Hey—Look Out, World, Here I Come," *Newsweek*, March 14, 2010, accessed December 30, 2018, https://www.newsweek.com /hey-look-out-world-here-i-come-174964.

15 Papalia, Diane E., et al., *Human Development*, 144.

16 Underwood, Anne. "Hey—Look Out, World, Here I Come," *Newsweek*, 1997, 12–15.

17 Ibid.

18 Ibid.

19 Ibid.

20 Ibid.

21 Ibid.

22 Hayden, Thomas. "A Sense of Self." *Newsweek*, 2000, 56–62. http://webshare .northseattle.edu/fam180/topics/temperament/asenseofself.htm.

23 Papalia et al., *Human Development*, 242.

24 Ibid.

25 Ibid., 243.

26 Ibid., 33.

27 Brazelton, T.B., and Greenspan, Stanley. "Our Window to The Future," *Newsweek*, 2000, 34.

28 Gardner, Howard. *Intelligence Reframed: Multiple Intelligences for the 21st Century.* New York: Basic Books, 1999.

29 Papalia et al., *Human Development*, 343.

30 Ibid., 33.

31 Goleman, *Emotional Intelligence*.

32 Ibid.

33 Ibid.

34 Gross, *Parental Involvement,* 27–28.

35 Stillman, Jessica. "Why Success Depends More on Personality Than Intelligence." *The Inc. Life.* January 11, 2017. https://www.inc.com/jessica-stillman/success -depends-more-on-personality-than-intelligence-new-study-shows.html (accessed April 24 2019, 2019).

36 Schuster, Donald H., and Charles E. Gritton, *Suggestive Accelerative Learning Techniques.* New York: Gordon and Breach, 1989.

37 Papalia, Diane E., et al., *Human Development,* 33.

38 Ibid., 32.

39 Ibid., 32-33.

40 Ibid., 32.

41 Ibid.

42 Ibid.

43 Ibid., 429-432.

44 Ibid., 429.

45 Ibid., 430.

46 "Lawrence Kohlberg Moral Development | Counseling | Pinterest | Kohlberg Moral Development, Morals and Human Development," Pinterest, accessed December 21, 2018, https://www.pinterest.com/pin/465418942734511790/.

47 Papalia, Diane E., et al., *Human Development,* 430.

48 Ibid.

49 Ibid.

50 Ibid, 431.

51 Ibid, 430.

52 Ibid, 431–432.

53 Ibid, 431.

54 Ibid, 431.

55 Ibid, 431.

56 Ibid, 430-431.

57 Friesen, Sharon. "*Bridges to Learning: A Guide to Parent Involvement.*" Distributed by ERIC Clearinghouse, 1986. https://eric.ed.gov/?id=ED272313, page 11.

58 Teale, W.H. "Toward a Theory of How Children Learn to Read and Write Naturally." *Language Arts* 56, no. 6 (1982): 568.

59 Ibid., 556.

60 Snowman, Jack, and Robert Biehler. *Psychology applied to teaching.* Boston, MA: Houghton Mifflin Company, 1986, pp. 63–64.

61 Papalia, Diane E., et al., *Human Development,* 32.

62 Ibid.

63 Ibid.
64 Ibid.
65 Ibid., 37–39.
66 Ibid.
67 Ibid.
68 Ibid.
69 Ibid., 38.
70 Ibid.
71 Ibid.
72 Ibid., 37–39.
73 Ibid.
74 Ibid., 161.
75 Ibid.
76 Ibid., 162.
77 Ibid.
78 Ibid.
79 Ibid., 162–163.
80 Ibid., 162.
81 Ibid.
82 Ibid., 166.
83 Ibid., 164.
84 Ibid., 165.
85 Ibid.
86 Ibid., 173–174.
87 Ibid., 172–173.
88 Ibid., 166.
89 Ibid., 166.
90 Ibid., 163.
91 Ibid., 168.
92 Ibid., 171.
93 Ibid., 170.
94 Ibid., 250.
95 Ibid., 250–251.
96 Ibid., 250.
97 Ibid., 251.
98 Ibid., 251–252.
99 Ibid.
100 Ibid., 252–253.
101 Ibid., 253.
102 Ibid.

103 Ibid.

104 Ibid., 254.

105 Ibid.

106 Ibid., 254–255.

107 Ibid., 255–256.

108 Ibid., 256.

109 Ibid., 254.

110 Ibid., 256–257.

111 Ibid., 257.

112 Ibid.

113 Ibid.

114 Ibid., 257–258.

115 Ibid., 258.

116 Ibid., 260.

117 Ibid., 250–252.

118 McLeod, Saul. "The Preoperational Stage of Cognitive Development." *Simply Psychology*, accessed December 21, 2018, https://www.simplypsychology.org /preoperational.html.

119 McLeod, Saul. "Concrete Operational Stage." *Simply Psychology*, January 1, 1970, accessed December 21, 2018, https://www.simplypsychology.org /concrete-operational.html.

120 Papalia, Diane E., et al., *Human Development*, 32.

121 Ibid., 425–428.

CHAPTER 6

1 Gross, Gail M., *The Only Way Out Is Through*, 112-119.

2 Trafton, Anne. "The benefits of meditation." *MIT News Office*. May 5, 2011. http://news.mit.edu/2011/meditation-0505 (accessed May 8, 2019).

3 Gross, Gail M., *The Only Way Out Is Through*, 112–119.

4 Ibid., 107–108.

5 Ibid.

6 Ibid., 108.

7 Hyde, Andrea M. "Yoga at the Promise Program: A Feminist Qualitative Case Study of School-Based Yoga," 2017, doi: 10.4135/9781526402912.

8 Ibid.

9 Gross, Gail M., *The Only Way Out Is Through*, 108.

10 Feuerstein, Georg, and Stephan Bodian. *Living Yoga: A Comprehensive Guide for Daily Life*. New York: G.P. Putnams Sons, 1993.

11 Gross, Gail M., *The Only Way Out Is Through*, 112–119.

12 Ibid

13 Ibid, 109–111.

14 Ibid, 111–112.

15 Ibid, 112–119.

16 Ibid, 116–117.

17 Ibid, 116–119.

18 Ibid.

19 Congreve. *The Mourning Bride* (Place of Publication Not Identified: Nabu Press, 2010).

20 Hoffman, J., et al., "The Effects of 60 Beats Per Minute Music on Test Taking Anxiety Among Nursing Students." *Journal of Nursing Education*, February 1990.

21 Diane E. Papalia et al., *Human Development*, 255.

22 Ibid., 296.

CHAPTER 7

1   Diane E. Papalia et al., *Human Development*, 8th ed. (New York: McGraw Hill, 2001, pp. 296.

2   Ibid.

3   Ibid.

4   Glover, Emily. "Kids' energy levels surpass endurance athletes', says science." January 24, 2019. (Accessed April 22, 2019). https://www.mother.ly/news /your-kids-are-in-better-shape-than-you-even-if-youre-a-pro-athlete.

5   Papalia, Diane E., et al., *Human Development*, 250.

6   Douglas, R., "Does TV Rot Your Brain?" January 1, 2016 (Accessed April 25, 2019). https://www.scientificamerican.com/article/does-tv-rot-your-brain/.

7   Papalia, Diane E., et al., *Human Development*, 284.

8   Ibid., 315.

9   Ibid., 276.

10 Ibid., 295–296.

11 Miller, Susan, and Larry Reibstein. "Good Kid, Bad Kid." New York: *Newsweek*, 1997, pp. 64–65.

12 Papalia, Diane E., et al., *Human Development*, 298.

13 Ibid., 216.

14 Ibid., 34–36.

15 Clark, Barbara. *Growing up Gifted.* Upper Saddle River, NJ: Pearson Education, 2012.

16 Thompson, R.F., Berger, T.W., and Berry, S.D. "An introduction to the anatomy, physiology and chemistry of the brain." In: Wittrock, M.C. (Ed.). *The Brain and Psychology.* New York: Academic Press, 1980, pp. 29.

17 Restak, Richard. *The Brain: The Last Frontier. Garden City, NY: Doubleday, 1979;* MacLean, P. A. Mind of three minds: Educating the triune brain." In: Chall, J., and Mirsky, A. (Ed.). *Education and the Brain, 27th Yearbook of the National Society for the Study of Education.* Chicago, IL: University of Chicago Press, 1978.

18 Lozanov, G. "A general theory of suggestion in the communications process and the activation of the total reserves of the learner's personality." *Suggestopaedia-Canada,* 1, (1977): 1–4; Martindale, C. "What makes creative people different?" *Psychology Today,* 9, no. 2 (1975): 44–50.

19 Halpin, Gerald W., David A. Payne, and Chad D. Ellett. "Biographical correlates of the creative personality: Gifted adolescents." *Exceptional Children* 39 (1973): 652–653.

20 Torrance, Ellis Paul. "Creative positives of disadvantaged children and youth." *Gifted Child Quarterly* 13, no. 2 (1969): 71–81. https://doi.org/10.1177%2F001698626901300201.

21 Diamond M.C., Law, F., Rhodes, H., Lindner, B., Rosenzweig, M.R., Krech, D., Bennett, E.L. "Increases in cortical depth and glia numbers in rats subjected to enriched environment." *The Journal of Comparative Neurology* 128 (1966): 117–26. PMID 4165855 DOI: 10.1002/cne.901280110.

22 Torrance, Ellis Paul. "Creative positives of disadvantaged children and youth." *Gifted Child Quarterly* 13, no. 2 (1969): 71–81. https://doi.org/10.1177%2F001698626901300201.

23 Terman, L.M., and Oden, M.H. *The gifted group at mid-life: Thirty-five years' follow-up of the superior child. Genetic studies of genius, vol. 5.* Stanford, CA: Stanford University Press, 1959.

24 Pierce, J., and Bowman, P. "Motivation Patters of High School Students." In: *The Gifted Student.* Cooperative Research Monograph no. 2 (OE-35-16). Washington, D.C.: Office of Education, 1960.

25 Ibid.

26 Karnes, Merle B., Allan M. Shwedel, and Susan A. Linnemeyer. "The Young Gifted/Talented Child: Programs at the University of Illinois." *The Elementary School Journal* 82, no. 3 (1982): 195–213. http://www.jstor.org/stable/1001570.

27 Strodtbeck, F. L. "Family interaction values, and achievement." In: McClelland, D.C. (Ed.). *Talent and society.* Princeton, NJ: Van Nostrand Reinhold, 1958, pp. 135–194.

28 Ibid.

29 Shaw, M. C., and McCuen, J. T. "The onset of academic underachievement in bright children." *Journal of Educational Psychology* 51 (1960):103–108.

30 Perkins, H. V. "Classroom behavior and underachievement." *American Educational Research Journal* 2 (1965):1–12.

31 Morrow, W. R., and Wilson, R. C. "Family relations of bright high achieving and underachieving high school boys." *Child Development* 32 (1961): 501–510.

32 Ibid.

33 Baymur, F., and Patterson, C.H. "Three methods of assisting underachieving high school students." *Journal of Counseling Psychology* 7 (1960): 83–90.

34 Goldberg, Miriam. "A three year program at DeWitt Clinton High School to help bright underachievers." *High Points* 41, (1959): 5–35.

35 May, Kate T. "An early detection test for pancreatic cancer: Jack Andraka at TED2013." February 27, 2013 (Accessed April 25, 2019). https://blog.ted.com/an-early-detection-test-for-pancreatic-cancer-jack-andraka-at-ted2013/.

CHAPTER 8

1 Wolbers, Bart. "Mitochondria: Why Your Cells' Functioning—And Not Genetics—Determine Disease." *Nature Builds Health*, April 1, 2018, waww.naturebuildshealth.com/blog/mitochondria#3.

2 "What is Mitochondrial Disease?" United Mitochondrial Disease Foundation, 2017, www.umdf.org/what-is-mitochondrial-disease/.

3 Wolbers, "Mitochondria."

4 Ibid.

5 Ibid.

6 Weiner, Catherine. "Mitochondrial Transfer: The Making of Three-Parent Babies." Science in the News—Harvard University—The Graduate School of Arts and Sciences, August 22, 2018, http://sitn.hms.harvard.edu/flash/2018/mitochondrial-transfer-making-three-parent-babies/.

7 Marina, Shari. "Mitochondrial Disease in Autism." *Focus for Health,* April 7, 2016, www.focusforhealth.org/mitochondrial-disease-in-autism/.

8 "DNA is Passed from Parent to Child." Genomics Education Program. Health Education England, June, 2014, www.genomicseducation.hee.nhs.uk/inheritance-of-genetic-material/dna-from-parent-to-child/.

9 Ely, Bert. "How do researchers trace mitochondrial DNA over centuries?" *Scientific American*, 2019, www.scientificamerican.com/article/how-do-researchers-trace/.

10 Ibid.

11 "Mitochondrial DNA can sometimes come from fathers, too," ZME Science, November 27, 2018, https://www.zmescience.com/science/mitochondrial-dna-fathers-0432432/.

12 Wolbers,"Mitochondria."

13 Ibid.

14 Morén, Constanza, Sandra Hernández, Mariona Guitart-Mampel, and Glòria Garrabou. "Mitochondrial Toxicity in Human Pregnancy: An Update on Clinical and Experimental Approaches in the Last 10 Years," NCBI US National Library of Medicine, National Institutes of Health, September 22, 2014, www.ncbi.nlm.nih.gov/pmc/articles/PMC4199057/.

15 Merrett, Rachael. "Orca Facts: Did You Know?" Georgia Strait Alliance, Caring for our Coastal Waters, 2019, georgiastrait.org/work/species-at-risk/orca-protection/killer-whales-pacific-northwest/orca-facts/.

16 The Associated Press, "Low orca birth rates linked to lack of Chinook salmon." *CBC News*, June 29, 2017, www.cbc.ca/news/canada/british-columbia/low-orca-birth-rates-linked-to-lack-of-chinook-salmon-1.4183609.

17 Carrington, Damian. "Orca 'apocalypse': half of killer whales doomed to die from pollution." *The Guardian*, September 27, 2018, www.theguardian.com/environment/2018/sep/27/orca-apocalypse-half-of-killer-whales-doomed-to-die-from-pollution.

18 "Data & Statistics on Autism Spectrum Disorder." Centers for Disease Control and Prevention, Updated April 5, 2019, www.cdc.gov/ncbddd/autism/data.html.

19 Yildiran, Alisan, Süleyman Kaplan, and Mehmet Emin Önger. "Neuroimmune diseases are increasing. Is there a possible vaccine link?" IOS Press Content Library, 2013, https://content.iospress.com/articles/journal-of-pediatric-neurology/jpn00623.

20 "PANDAS. A Guide for Parents," Healthline, Accessed April 22, 2019, www.healthline.com/health/pandas-syndrome.

21 "Dystonia." National Organization for Rare Disorders, 2015, https://rarediseases.org/rare-diseases/dystonia/.

22 Contributing Author. "What is Mitochondrial DNA and Mitochondrial Inheritance." *ZME Science*, April 10, 2017, www.zmescience.com/other/science-abc/about-mitochondrial-dna-42423/.

23 "Types of Mitochondrial Disease," United Mitochondrial Disease Foundation, Accessed April 22, 2019, www.umdf.org/types/.

24 "Mitochondrial Diseases," The Cleveland Clinic, 2019, my.clevelandclinic.org/health/diseases/15612-mitochondrial-diseases.

25 Potter, Melanie Milam. "The Living Battle Within Breast Milk: Developmental Direction vs A Toxic Toll," *GreenMedInfo*, March 20, 2017, www.greenmedinfo.com/blog/living-battle-within-breast-milk-developmental-direction-vs-toxic-toll.

26 Israel-Berkeley, Brett. "Mom's Exposure to Toxic Chemicals Shows up in Newborn." *Futurity*, November 3, 2016. https://www.futurity.org/pregnancy-toxins-newborns-1288872/.

27 Mercola, Joseph. "Reducing Chemical Exposure Could Save Americans Hundreds of Billions of Dollars in Healthcare Costs," Mercola. Take Care of Your Health, November 2, 2016, articles.mercola.com/sites/articles/archive /2016/11/02/endocrine-disrupting-chemicals-plastics-exposure.aspx.

28 Srivastava, Sarika. "The Mitochondrial Basis of Aging and Age-Related Disorders." NCBI US National Library of Medicine, National Institutes of Health, December 19, 2017, www.ncbi.nlm.nih.gov/pmc/articles/PMC5748716/.

29 Mumal, Iqra. "Older Moms More Likely to Pass Along Mitochondrial DNA with Mutations, Study Finds," *Mitochondrial Disease News*, June 29, 2018, mitochondrialdiseasenews.com/2018/06/29/older-moms-more-likely-to-pass -mutated-mitochrondrial-dna-to-offspring-study-finds/.

30 Virginia Tech, "How Mitochondrial Disease Is Passed Down From Mother To Child: Predicting Severity," *Science Daily*, January 31, 2008, https://www .sciencedaily.com/releases/2008/01/080127130914.htm.

31 Magistretti, Pierre J., and Igor Allaman. "A Cellular Perspective on Brain Energy Metabolism and Functional Imaging," *Neuron Review*, May 20, 2015, www .cell.com/neuron/pdf/S0896-6273(15)00259-7.pdf.

32 Wolbers, "Mitochondria."

33 Asprey, Dave. "The MTHFR Gene Mutation And How To Rewire Your Genetics" Bulletproof Blog, Accessed April 22, 2019, blog.bulletproof.com /the-mthfr-gene-mutation-and-how-to-rewire-your-genetics/.

34 Ibid.

35 "MTHFR, Folic Acid, and Mitochondrial Disease . . . is there a link?" Baby Food Steps, May 14, 2012, babyfoodsteps.wordpress.com/2012/05/14 /mthfr-mito-link/.

36 Asprey, Dave. "Dr. Ben Lynch: MTHFR Gene, Beating Disease, & Folic Acid," Bulletproof Blog, Accessed April 22, 2019, blog.bulletproof.com/dr-ben -lynch-mthfr-gene-overcoming-disease-the-dangers-of-folic-acid-157/.

37 Lynch, Ben, "MTHFR Mutations and the Conditions They Cause." MTHFR.Net, September 7, 2011, mthfr.net/mthfr-mutations-and-the-conditions-they-cause /2011/09/07/.

38 Asprey, Dave. "The MTHFR Gene Mutation.

39 "Demyelination: What Is It and Why Does It Happen?" *Healthline*, Accessed April 22, 2019, www.healthline.com/health/multiple-sclerosis/demyelination.

40 "Demyelinating diseases," *the Journal of Clinical Pathology* NCBI US National Library of Medicine, National Institutes of Health, November, 2006, www .ncbi.nlm.nih.gov/pmc/articles/PMC1860500/.

41 Ipatenco, Sandra. "What Is the Importance of Fat Intake for Children Under 2 Years Old?" *SF Gate*, December 27, 2018, healthyeating.sfgate.com/impor-tance-fat-intake-children-under-2-years-old-4155.html.

42 Ibid.

43 North, Cat. "Can You Repair Myelin Sheath With Diet?" *Livestrong*, Accessed April 22, 2019, www.livestrong.com/article/228947-how-to-repair-myelin -sheath-with-diet/.

44 Maricich, Maria. "Mito Food Plan." The Institute for Functional Medicine, Drmariamaricich.com, 2015, www.drmariamaricich.com/storage/app/media /Mito_Food_Plan_Comprehensive_Guide1.pdf.

45 "Colostrum and the Gut-Brain Axis," Sovereign Laboratories, Accessed April 22, 2019, www.sovereignlaboratories.com/blog/colostrum-gut-brain-axis/.

46 McQuillan, Susan. "The Gut Brain Connection: How Gut Health Affects Mental Health." *Psycom*, Accessed April 22, 2019, www.psycom.net/the-gut -brain-connection.

47 "Colostrum," *Science Daily*, Accessed April 22, 2019, www.sciencedaily.com /terms/colostrum.htm.

48 "Liquid Gold: the wonders of colostrum," *Babysense*, 2017, www.babysense .com/advice-and-tips/liquid-gold-the-wonders-of-colostrum/.

49 "Colostrum-The Superfood for Your Newborn," American Pregnancy Association, 2019, americanpregnancy.org/breastfeeding/colostrum-the-superfood -for-your-newborn.

50 Mead, Nathaniel. "Contaminants in Human Milk: Weighing the Risks against the Benefits of Breastfeeding." NCBI US National Library of Medicine, National Institutes of Health, October, 2008, www.ncbi.nlm.nih.gov/pmc /articles/PMC2569122/.

51 "Answers to Commonly Asked Questions by Our Customers," Sovereign Laboratories, 2019, www.sovereignlaboratories.com/FAQs.html.

52 Clark, Allison, and Núria Mach. "The Crosstalk between the Gut Microbiota and Mitochondria during Exercise." NCBI US National Library of Medicine, National Institutes of Health, May 19, 2017, www.ncbi.nlm.nih.gov/pmc /articles/PMC5437217/.

53 Kruse, Jack. "Reality #13: Can You See the Real Me? Vermont 2017." Reversing Disease for Optimal Health, Accessed April 22, 2019, https://jack kruse.com /reality-13-can-see-real-vermont-2017/.

54 Veon, Kathy. "Non-Native EMF's: An Overlooked Environmental Toxin." Nutrition and Holistic Medicine, Accessed April 22, 2019, www.cfpreventive medicine.com/nutritionist/non-native-emfs-overlooked-environmental-toxin/.

55 Nair, Rathish, and Arun Maseeh. "Vitamin D: The 'Sunshine' Vitamin," NCBI US National Library of Medicine, National Institutes of Health, April, 2012, www.ncbi.nlm.nih.gov/pmc/articles/PMC3356951/.

56 Kruse, Jack. "Time to Rethink Your Truth About the Sun?" LinkedIn, May 19, 2017, www.linkedin.com/pulse/time-rethink-your-truth-sun-jack-kruse/.

57 Kruse, Jack. Time#11: "Can You Supplement Sunlight?" Reversing Disease for Optimal Health, Accessed April 22, 2019, jackkruse.com/time -10-can-you-supplement-sunlight/.

58 "An Introduction to Biophotons," Infoceuticals.co, Accessed April 22, 2019, www.infoceuticals.co/posts/dr-fritz-albert-popp-biophotons.

59 Wolbers, "Mitochondria."

60 "The amazing similarity between blood and chlorophyll," Science2Be, Accessed April 22, 2019, science2be.wordpress.com/2012/09/03/the-amazing -similarity-between-blood-and-chlorophyll/.

61 Wolbers, "Mitochondria."

62 Kruse, Jack. "Energy and Epigenetics 4: Light, Water, Magnetism." Reversing Disease for Optimal Health, Accessed April 22, 2019, jackkruse.com/energy -and-epigenetics-4-light-water-magnetism/.

63 Ibid.

64 Nelson, Scott. "How Red and Near Infrared Light Stimulates Cellular Respiration and Boosts Energy Production." Joovy Go, Accessed April 22, 2019, joovv.com/blogs/joovv-blog/how-red-near-infrared-light-stimulates-cellular -respiration-boosts-energy-production.

65 "Red Light Therapy Benefits," *Healthline*, Accessed April 22, 2019, www .healthline.com/health/red-light-therapy#summary.

66 The American Cancer Society medical and editorial content team. "What is UV Radiation?" American Cancer Society, August 12, 2015, www.cancer.org /cancer/cancer-causes/radiation-exposure/uv-radiation/uv-radiation-what-is-uv .html.

67 Scribner, Herb. "'Indoor generation': Here's how much time we spend indoors." General Filters Incorporated, May 17, 2018, www.generalfilters.com/blog /Indoor-generation-Heres-how-much-time-we-spend-indoors_AE209.html.

68 Schmall, Tyler. "Americans spend half their lives in front of screens." *New York Post*, August 13, 2018, nypost.com/2018/08/13/americans-spend -half-their-lives-in-front-of-screens/.

69 Kruse, Jack. "Artificial Blue Light Dehydrates Your Cells." LinkedIn, January 18, 2017, www.linkedin.com/pulse/artificial-blue-light-dehydrates-your -cells-jack-kruse/.

70 Wolbers, "Mitochondria."

71 Ibid.

72 "What is Circadian Rhythm?" National Sleep Foundation, 2019, www.sleep -foundation.org/sleep-topics/what-circadian-rhythm.

73 Cronin, Thomas. "Seeing without Eyes." *Scientific American*, August 13, 2017, www.scientificamerican.com/article/seeing-without-eyes1/.

74 Pollack, Gerald. "EZ Water." Pollack Laboratory, Accessed April 22, 2019, www.pollacklab.org/research.

75 Ibid.

76 "The Importance of Structured Water to Health," The Sophia Health Institute, Accessed April 22, 2019, www.sophiahi.com/importance-structured -water-health/

77 Mercola, Joseph. "Water: The Single Most Important Element for Your Health." Mercola, January 29, 2011, articles.mercola.com/sites/articles /archive/2011/01/29/dr-pollack-on-structured-water.aspx.

78 Ibid.

79 The Importance of Structured Water to Health.

80 Kruse, Jack. "Is Water the Key to Morphogenesis?" LinkedIn, October 4, 2017, www.linkedin.com/pulse/water-key-morphogenesis-jack-kruse/.

81 "What is Earth Resonance Therapy?" Technology for Life, 2016, www.technol ogyforlife.org/what-is-earth-resonance-therapy/.

82 Ibid.

83 Mercola, Joseph. "Water Supports Health in Ways You May Never Have Suspected." Mercola, January 28, 2017, articles.mercola.com/sites/articles /archive/2017/01/28/ez-water.aspx.

84 Ibid.

85 Mercola, Joseph. "Hydration Is About More Than Just Drinking Water— How to Hydrate at the Cellular Level to Improve Health and Longevity." Mercola, May 6, 2018, articles.mercola.com/sites/articles/archive/2018/05/06 /how-to-hydrate-at-the-cellular-level.aspx.

86 Nemoto, Yasuyuki. "Science of 'Message from Water.'" Masara Emoto's Hado World, Accessed April 23, 2019, hado.com/ihm/subscription/science -of-message-from-water/.

87 Bhavika. "Dr Masaru Emoto on Human Consciousness and Water." *Fractal Enlightenment*, Accessed April 23, 2019, fractalenlightenment.com/14121 /spirituality/dr-masaru-emoto-on-human-consciousness-and-water.

88 "The Importance of Structured Water to Health."

89 Martino, Joe. "Study Shows Water Has Memory. German Scientists Expand On Dr. Emoto's Work." Collective Evolution, December 29, 2015, www .collective-evolution.com/2015/12/20/study-shows-water-has-memory -german-scientists-expand-on-dr-emotos-work/.

90 Partanen, Eino, Teija Kujala, Mari Tervaniemi, and Minna Huotilainen. "Prenatal Music Exposure Induces Long-Term Neural Effects." NCBI US National Library of Medicine, National Institutes of Health, October 30, 2013, www.ncbi.nlm.nih.gov/pmc/articles/PMC3813619/.

91 Parsons, Cheryl. "Rock-a-bye baby: the benefits of playing music to your unborn child." *The National*, January 26, 2017, www.thenational.ae/lifestyle/wellbeing/rock-a-bye-baby-the-benefits-of-playing-music-to-your-unborn-child-1.40360.

92 Ibid.

93 Hughes, Virginia. "Mice Inherit Specific Memories, Because Epigenetics?" *National Geographic*, December 1, 2013, www.nationalgeographic.com/science/phenomena/2013/12/01/mice-inherit-specific-memories-because-epigenetics/.

94 Robinson, Monique. "Health Check: can stress during pregnancy harm my baby?" *The Conversation*, August 20, 2017, theconversation.com/health-check-can-stress-during-pregnancy-harm-my-baby-81825.

95 Villines, Zawn. "How do free radicals affect the body?" *Medical News Today*, July 29, 2017, www.medicalnewstoday.com/articles/318652.php.

96 "Exhibit G: Mitochondrial Dysfunction and Disruption of Electrophysiology," Europa.eu, Accessed April 23, 2019, ec.europa.eu/health/scientific_committees/emerging/docs/emf_3.pdf.

97 Sheua, Shey-Shing, Dhananjaya Naudurib, and M.W. Andersa. "Targeting antioxidants to mitochondria: A new therapeutic direction." Science Direct, February, 2006, www.sciencedirect.com/science/article/pii/S0925443905001535.

98 Cherry, Neil. "Evidence that Electromagnetic Radiation is Genotoxic: The implications for the epidemiology of cancer and cardiac, neurological and reproductive effects." Whale.to, June 2000, www.whale.to/b/cherry6.html.

99 Kruse, Jack. "Energy and Epigenetics 4: Light, Water, Magnetism." Reversing Disease for Optimal Health, Accessed April 23, 2019, jackkruse.com/energy-and-epigenetics-4-light-water-magnetism/.

100 Ibid.

101 Ibid.

102 Ibid.

103 Shepherd, S., Lima, M.A.P., Oliveira, E.E., Sharkh, S.M., Jackson, C.W., and Newland, P.L. "Extremely Low Frequency Electromagnetic Fields impair the Cognitive and Motor Abilities of Honey Bees." Nature.com, May 21, 2018, www.nature.com/articles/s41598-018-26185-y.

104 Goulson, Dave, Elizabeth Nicholls, Cristina Botías, and Ellen L. Rotheray. "Bee declines driven by combined stress from parasites, pesticides, and lack of flowers." *Science Magazine*, March 27, 2015, science.sciencemag.org/content/347/6229/1255957.

105 Mitro, Susanna D., Tyiesha Johnson, and Ami R. Zota. "Cumulative Chemical Exposures During Pregnancy and Early Development." NCBI US National Library of Medicine, National Institutes of Health, December 1, 2016, www.ncbi.nlm.nih.gov/pmc/articles/PMC4626367/.

106 Indiana University, "Banned chemicals pass through umbilical cord from mother to baby, research finds." *Science Daily*, June 29, 2017, www.science daily.com/releases/2017/06/170629085016.htm.

107 Kruse, Jack. "Functional medicine mistakes, EMF, sunlight and your mito-chondria—Podcast #135." Just In Health Wellness Clinic, May 12th, 2017, justinhealth.com/functional-medicine-mistakes-emf-sunlight-and-your -mitochondria-podcast-135/.

108 Krebs, Roy. "5 Ways To Improve Your Health By Boosting Mitochondria." Natural Stacks, May 3, 2017, www.naturalstacks.com/blogs/news/5-ways-to -improve-your-health-by-boosting-mitochondria.

109 Nelson, Scott. "How Red and Near Infrared Light Stimulates Cellular Respiration and Boosts Energy Production." Joovv, 2019, joovv.com/blogs /joovv-blog/how-red-near-infrared-light-stimulates-cellular-respiration -boosts-energy-production.

110 Asprey, Dave. "Light Hacking for Better Energy, Mood, and Performance." Bulletproof Blog, 2019, blog.bulletproof.com/light-hacking-for-better-energy -mood-and-performance/.

111 Harvard Health Letter, "Blue light has a dark side." Harvard Health Publishing, Harvard Medical School, August 13, 2018, www.health.harvard .edu/staying-healthy/blue-light-has-a-dark-side.

112 Pollack, "EZ Water."

113 Kagelidis, Michael. "How to reduce your everyday exposure to artificial electro magnetic fields." *Home Biology*, Accessed April 23, 2019, www.home-biology .com/emf-protection-tips.

114 Husaini, Zara. "Aging Begins in the Womb, Antioxidants Can Help." *Fit Pregnancy*, 2019, www.fitpregnancy.com/nutrition/prenatal-nutrition/aging -begins-womb-antioxidants-can-help.

115 Sorgen, Carol. "Eat Smart for a Healthier Brain." WebMD, 2019, www .webmd.com/diet/features/eat-smart-healthier-brain#1.

116 Bott, Nick. "Coconut oil, olive oil, grape seed oil: which is best for brain health?" *Neurotrack*, March 14, 2017, blog.neurotrack.com/which-oil-is-best-for-brain-health/.

117 Dr. Jockers. "7 Ways Magnesium Improves Brain Health." Dr.Jockers.com, 2019, drjockers.com/7-ways-magnesium-improves-brain-health/.

118 Alban, Deane. "Brain Vitamins: Essential for a Healthy Brain." *Be Brain Fit*, March 9, 2019, bebrainfit.com/brain-vitamins/.

119 Matthews, Russell T., Lichuan Yang, Susan Browne, Myong Baik, and M. Flint Beal. "Coenzyme Q10 administration increases brain mitochondrial concen-trations and exerts neuroprotective effects." US National Library of Medicine,

National Institutes of Health, July 21, 1998, www.ncbi.nlm.nih.gov/pmc
/articles/PMC21173/.

120 Rowe, Keith. "How to Rid Your Life of Harmful Toxins." *Brain MD*, March
9, 2018, www.brainmdhealth.com/blog/how-to-get-rid-of-harmful-toxins/.

121 "Matrix Energetics—a system of healing, self-care and transformation," *Matrix
Energetics*, 2014, www.matrixenergetics.com/WhatIs.aspx.

122 "16 Reasons why reiki could be the best thing for your pregnancy,"
Mumazine, December 12, 2019, www.mumazine.com/article/2013/05/30
/benefits-reiki-while-pregnant.

123 Ananda, Kara Maria. "Craniosacral Therapy in the Midwifery Model of
Care." *Midwifery Today*, Autumn, 2008, midwiferytoday.com/mt-articles
/craniosacral-therapy/.

124 "Homeopathy in Pregnancy and Birth," *Stockbridge Osteopathic Practice*,
Accessed April 23, 2019, www.stockbridgeosteopathicpractice.com/homeopathy
-in-pregnancy-and-birth.html.

125 "Pregnancy Meditation: The Benefits of Mindfulness," *Healthline*, Accessed
April 23, 2019, www.healthline.com/health/pregnancy/meditation-benefits.

126 Wolbers, "Mitochondria."

127 Nesbitt, Victoria, Charlotte L. Alston, Emma L. Blakely, Carl Fratter,
Catherine L. Feeney, Joanna Poulton, Garry K. Brown, Doug M. Turnbull,
Robert W. Taylor, and Robert McFarland. "A national perspective on pre-
natal testing for mitochondrial disease." US National Library of Medicine,
National Institutes of Health, November 22, 2014, www.ncbi.nlm.nih.gov
/pmc/articles/PMC4200441/.

128 Menshikova, Elizabeth V. Vladimir B. Ritov, Liane Fairfull, Robert E. Ferrell,
David E. Kelley, and Bret H. Goodpaster. "Effects of Exercise on Mitochondrial
Content and Function in Aging Human Skeletal Muscle. US National
Library of Medicine, National Institutes of Health, June 2006, www.ncbi
.nlm.nih.gov/pmc/articles/PMC1540458/.

129 Wolbers, Bart. "Cold Thermogenesis: Cold Showers And Ice Baths For
Incredible Fat-Loss, Energy, Well-Being And (Mental) Performance."
Nature Builds Health, Mar 10, 2018, www.naturebuildshealth.com/blog
/cold-thermogenesis-showers-icebaths.

INDEX

empathic process, 21–22, 24, 36, 126, 131, 139, 142, 149, 155, 176, 196, 215, 219, 305, 308–310, 312, 316, 321, 324

empathy, 21–22, 47, 53, 107, 137, 196, 215, 219, 307–313, 316, 342

employer, 127–128

encoding aggressive scripts, 52

energetic vibration, 358

Energizer Bunny, 296

energy production, 346, 350, 354–355, 362

English language, 298

enriched environment, 77, 328

environment, 4–6, 10, 19–23, 26–27, 29, 32–36, 38, 43–45, 54, 57, 66–71, 75–77, 82, 85–89, 93, 99, 101–102, 119, 134–135, 137, 139, 143, 147, 149, 162, 165–167, 171, 173, 175–176, 180, 184, 186, 189, 197–202, 206, 208–209, 218–219, 224, 227, 240, 275–276, 286, 290, 295, 303, 308–309, 325, 327–331, 333, 335, 346–351, 355, 357–359, 362–365

nonstimulating, 328

nurturing, 135, 329

stimulated, 328

environmental toxins, 349

equilibration, 199, 331

Erik Erikson, 88, 169, 182, 183–185, 187, 189, 300

estimate time, 284

Estrada, 72, 83

Europe, 261

excessive inflammation, 343, 351

Exclusion Zone (EZ) water, 356–357

exercises for intellectual development, 274

exhale, 246

eye relaxation exercise, 264

EZ water, 356–357

F

family
  importance of, 151

family identity, 322

family life, 101

family meeting, 131

family of origin, 63–64, 81–82, 141, 144, 215, 305

family roles, 13

family structure, 13, 14, 83, 101, 113, 131, 149, 150, 151, 320

family time, 125–126

Father
  interactions with, 12

feelings
  cope, 46, 48, 50, 312

Feuerstein, Georg, 241

Field, Tiffany, 72

Fifer, William, 55

fight or flight, 84

fight-or-flight, 7, 46, 47, 55, 120

follow-through, 139–140, 310

formal operations stage, 223

formal operations, 198, 220, 222, 223

French, 333

Freud, 43, 182, 223

friends
  learning to make, 302

fuel cells, 343

functional Magnetic Resonance Imaging, 52

G

game of memory, 275

Gandhi, Mohandas, 229, 230

Gardner, Howard, 122, 173

gender 293–295, 301

music, 227, 258–265, 267, 359
importance of, 258
myelin sheath, 351

N
Nadam, 228, 231
National Institute of Child Health and
Human Development, 14
National Institute of Health's Child
Development and Behavioral
Branch, 16
native language, 11, 58
natural curiosity, 9, 70, 227
natural state, 101, 182, 229, 240, 260
nature and nurture, 3, 24, 47
nature's warning, 346
nDNA, 345
neglectful parent, 64
neuroglial cells, 5, 84
neuroimmune disease, 347
neurological connection, 349
neurological development, 11, 59,
155, 159
neurological disorders, 348, 349, 352
neurological health, 343, 352
neurons, 4, 6, 8, 78, 79, 91, 118, 121,
163, 178, 325, 328
Neuroscience Behaviors, 7
neuroscience, 20, 43, 61, 66, 78, 84,
160, 165, 254, 259, 262, 290
New York Times, 240, 25
Newton, Isaac, 101
Newsweek, 18,
nnEMF, 350, 360, 361
nnEMFs, 349, 353, 356, 360, 361,
365
nontraditional families, 149
North America, 343, 346
novelty preference, 207
nuclear DNA (nDNA), 345

number, 204, 206, 212
nutrition and nutrients, 362
Nutrition, 337, 362

O
obesity, 338, 341, 360
OBGYN, 54
object permanence, 203, 204
obsessive-compulsive disorder, 352
Oden, 330
Olympics, 252
om schooling, 240
optimal state, 260
optimal time, 74
orca, 346–348
organization, 124, 144, 197, 199
origins of humanity, 346
Ornish, Dean, 241
overprotective parent, 64–65
overweight child, 338
overweight children, 341

P
Pacific Lutheran University, 57
Pac-Man, 60, 253
Pachelbel, Johann, 264
PANDAS—Pediatric Autoimmune
Neuropsychiatric Disorders
Associated with Streptococcal
Infections, 347
parallel play, 30, 40–41, 166
parental approval, 300
parental attention, 120
parental guidance, 5, 68
parental intervention, 18
parental involvement, 9, 19, 43, 45,
83, 115, 116, 171,
early childhood, in, 19
parental power, 3, 17, 18, 66
parenting plan, 124, 142

sort, 276–278
sound recognition, 57
spanking, 35, 36, 307
spatial
  concepts, 281–281
  knowledge, 203, 206
  relationship, 211, 218, 220, 280, 287, 291–292, 298, 301
  thinking, 210–211
speech development, 79
Springsteen, Bruce, 81
St. Agnes Hospital, 261
St. Luke's Hospital, 261
statistics, 347
stay active, 341
STEM (Science, Technology, Engineering, Mathematics), 293
STEM programs, 293
stimulating objects, 276
storytime, 286
streptococcal infection, 347
stress hormone, 26, 45, 55, 67
stress hormones, 7, 8, 56, 120, 171, 305
stress management, 66
stress reduction, 67–68, 116, 152, 171, 181, 234–235, 237, 241, 339, 341–342, 362
stress, 7–8, 20, 22, 26–27, 35, 38, 41- 42, 45–48, 51- 52, 55–56, 61, 65–68, 72–73, 77, 83–84, 90, 97–98, 102–103, 105–108, 113–114, 116–117, 119–121, 129–130, 133, 136, 147–149, 152–153, 168–169, 171, 179, 181–182, 223, 234–242, 253–256, 261, 263, 305, 320, 337–342, 346, 348, 351, 355, 362–363
  during pregnancy, 55–56
stress-reduction strategies, 341

stress-reduction techniques, 67–68, 116, 171, 181, 234–235, 339
Strodtbeck, 331
structure, 33–34, 113, 132, 139, 152, 286, 305
Studley, 330
successful environment, 134
sunlight, 353–357
Suomi, Stephen, 25, 27
symbolic function, 210, 218
synapses, 4–5, 69, 76, 78–79, 81, 84, 86, 92, 118, 163, 165, 166, 170, 217, 262
synaptic pruning, 4, 91
synaptic, 4, 69, 118, 162, 166, 223, 325, 328

T

tantrum, 30–34, 40, 42, 46, 93
  preventing, 33
  tips for, 32
tau, 229
TED 2013, 335
Teicher, Claudia, 240
Telemann, 263
television viewing, 299, 341
television, 51–53, 105, 108–110, 125, 140–141, 152, 299–300, 341
Terrible Twos, 29, 42, 186–187
Thompson, Berger, 325
three-mountain task, 214
time in, 48, 137, 239, 243, 266
Time magazine, 240
TLC, 42, 66, 218
Todd Elementary School, 240
Tomatis Method, 261
Torman, 330
Torrance, 327, 329
Touch therapy, 73
touch, 72, 278